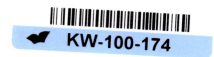

FUTURE OF HEALTH TECHNOLOGY

"Future health technology is perhaps the most exciting field of all in this century. We will see the rise of electronic medicine as a challenger for the chemical near monopoly treatment that we see now. We will also see the human nervous system and brain linked directly with technology, thereby creating a brave new world for us all."

Professor Kevin Warwick

Studies in Health Technology and Informatics

Editors

Jens Pihlkjaer Christensen (EC, Luxembourg); Arie Hasman (The Netherlands);
Larry Hunter (USA); Ilias Iakovidis (EC, Belgium); Zoi Kolitsi (Greece);
Olivier Le Dour (EC, Belgium); Antonio Pedotti (Italy); Otto Rienhoff (Germany);
Francis H. Roger France (Belgium); Niels Rossing (Denmark); Niilo Saranummi (Finland);
Elliot R. Siegel (USA); Petra Wilson (EC, Belgium)

Volume 80

Volume 1 in the subseries
Future of Health Technology Series
Editor: Renata G. Bushko

Earlier published in this series

ISSN: 0926-9630

Future of Health Technology

Edited by

Renata G. Bushko

Future of Health Technology Institute, Hopkinton, MA, USA

IOS
Press

Ohmsha

Amsterdam • Berlin • Oxford • Tokyo • Washington, DC

ISBN 1 58603 091 4 (IOS Press)
ISBN 4 274 90493 8 C3047 (Ohmsha)
Library of Congress Control Number: 2001099063

Publisher
IOS Press
Nieuwe Hemweg 6B
1013 BG Amsterdam
The Netherlands
fax: +31 20 620 3419
e-mail: order@iospress.nl

Distributor in the UK and Ireland
IOS Press/Lavis Marketing
73 Lime Walk
Headington
Oxford OX3 7AD
England
fax: +44 1865 75 0079

Distributor in the USA and Canada
IOS Press, Inc.
5795-G Burke Centre Parkway
Burke, VA 22015
USA
fax: +1 703 323 3668
e-mail: iosbooks@iospress.com

Distributor in Germany, Austria and Switzerland
IOS Press/LSL.de
Gerichtsweg 28
D-04103 Leipzig
Germany
fax: +49 341 995 4255

Distributor in Japan
Ohmsha, Ltd.
3-1 Kanda Nishiki-cho
Chiyoda-ku, Tokyo 101
Japan
fax: +81 3 3233 2426

Cover illustration © 2002, Future of Health Technology Institute (FHTI); designed by Angela Fiori.

Preface

"What Renata Bushko has done over last five years leading the effort to define the future of health technology resulted in many exquisite chapters in this book. "Future of Health Technology" will lend itself to those who want to know now what the future looks like. Understanding that vision of the future is a necessary step in applying health technology to improving healthcare quality in the future. This book sets the direction for the next century."

Michael Fitzmaurice, Ph.D., *Senior Science Advisor for Information Technology Immediate Office of the Director, Agency for Healthcare Research and Quality, US Department of Health and Human Services*

Health technology becomes the center of healthcare systems' strategic planning process. Developing a clear vision of the future of health technology and smart investment in technology are the critical success factors. Healthcare leaders need to develop a vision of future health technology to lead effectively in the new century. The social and economic issues surrounding health care will be inextricably linked to the technological aspects of medicine in the next century. Given rapid progress in nanomedicine, the pressure towards detailed outcomes analysis, growing use of Internet, robotic surgery, genetic therapy, telemedicine, on-line consumer education, and bioinformatics health technology becomes the key to intelligent health care. To embrace technology is the only way health systems can assimilate with the technologically advanced society. On-going massive medical data collection, instantaneous analysis, affective computing with emotional intelligence, and nanosurgery will be possible soon. We are entering the biomechatronics and nano-biomechatronics era.

Last century took us from the first electric switch back in 1880s to the first nanomotor's switch in the year 2000; from 30 ton computer to polymer transistors on a plastic that one can print at home; from electric light to electronic paper, windows, mirrors and wallpaper. In the next century most current diseases will be history and medicine will be focused on maximizing joy and pleasures of long lives of humans augmented with biomechatronics. Most healthcare cost will be shifted from end-of-life to prenatal care. Since everybody will be augmented with biomechatronics, the word "disabled" will not exist anymore – we will all have the same chance to be truly human.

The "Future of Health Technology" book provides a comprehensive vision of the future of health technology by looking at the ways to advance (1) medical technologies, (2) health information infrastructure, and (3) intellectual leadership. It also explores new technology creation and adoption processes including the impact of rapidly evolving technologies. People discover and respond to the future as much as they plan it. Health systems and societies with the clear vision of future health technology will have a better chance of reducing human suffering. This book will make you look technology straight into its glittering eyes and you will see how many tears it can eliminate from the Earth if we all join in the quest for a better tomorrow for us, our children and the generations to follow.

Renata G. Bushko,
Editor, Future of Health Technology book
Founder, Future of Health Technology Institute
Hopkinton, MA, US

Acknowledgements

You will be able to look technology straight into its glittering eyes thanks to the creative spirit of all superb chapter authors of the Future of Health Technology book. They were brave to stretch their imagination and develop topics that I selected for them. Thank you all (please refer to the list of names below) for your dedication to building a better future.

Many thanks to Professor Marvin Minsky, one of the greatest thinkers of our times, who back in 1990 encouraged me to build Dr. Zuzu – an intelligent agent that could reason by analogy using common sense provided by CYC's multi-million-facts knowledge base and the Society of Mind theory.

In 1991 Professor Minsky asked how we could tell if Dr. Zuzu was really adaptive and could do novel things. That made me think of the first order theory of knowledge-rich systems performance as a part of my thesis.

In 1995 he asked: *"How to design an agency that looks at big issues in the future of health technology"* and inspired me to found the Future of Health Technology Institute, focusing on defining the health technology agenda for the new century.

In 2000 Professor Minsky noticed that *"it is annoying to live only 100 years because that's not long enough to get to understand anything"*. That inspired me to work on this book in order to encourage pursuit of better health and longer lives.

We would also like to thank those who will take the time to read this book and engage in creating the vision of the future. As the editor, I invite you to send your ideas to the Future of Health Technology Institute via email at Bushko@fhti.org or by telephone at (508) 497-2577.

Editor
Renata G. Bushko, M.S.
Future of Health Technology Institute
4 Lamplighter Lane, Hopkinton, MA 01748, US

Marina U. Bers, Ph.D.
Maria I. Busquets, M.A.
Mary Jo Deering, Ph.D.
David R. DeMaso, M.D.
Ed Deppert
Robert A. Freitas Jr.
Barbara B.Friedman, M.A., MPA.
    FAHRMM
Jean Garnier, Ph.D.
G. Scott Gazelle, M.D., Ph.D.
Joseph Gonzalez-Heydrich, M.D.
Robert A. Greenes, M.D., Ph.D.
Penny Havlicek, Ph.D.
James J. Kaput, Ph.D..
Colleen M. Kigin, M.S., M.P.A., P.T.
Gary L. Kreps, Ph.D.
Jo Lernout, M.S.

Henry Lieberman, Ph.D.
Cindy Mason, Ph.D.
Blackford Middleton, M.D., MSc, M.P.H.
Alex P. Pentland, Ph.D.
Alice P. Pentland, M.D.
Rosalind W. Picard, Ph.D.
Scott C. Ratzan, M.D., MPA., M.A.S.
Barry Robson, Ph.D., D.Sc.
David Williamson Shaffer, Ph.D.
Richard Spivack, Ph.D.
Albert J. Sunseri, Ph.D.
Graziella Tonfoni, Ph.D.
Kevin Warwick, Ph.D.
Gio Wiederhold, Ph.D.
Meg Wilson, M.S.
Jean Wooldridge, M.P.H.

About
the Future of Health Technology Institute
"Common Sense in Health"

The **Future of Health Technology Institute**, 4 Lamplighter Lane, Hopkinton, MA 01748, US, www.fhti.org is the health technology think-tank dedicated to defining the health technology agenda for the 21st century. Renata Bushko (Bushko@fhti.org) founded the Future of Health Technology Institute in 1996 and has since chaired six annual Future of Health Technology Summits. These summits engage creative minds from the technology and healthcare fields in envisioning the future of technology for global healthcare. Under her leadership, the Future of Health Technology Institute has been recognized as one of the most forward thinking health technology research and training organizations.

Specific goals of the Future of Health Technology Institute are:

1. Develop a vision of future health care supported by current and future health technologies.
2. Define distinct promising health technology research areas.
3. Demonstrate that technology driven cost increases in healthcare can be stopped and possibly reversed by a new allocation of research and development resources.
4. Define productive areas for research and development that will have potential impact on healthcare.
5. Identify new technologies that are practical and necessary in health and wellness maintenance.
6. Identify research and development needed to meet future health challenges.
7. Identify current products best for preparing 21st century healthcare.

Affective Intelligent Caring Creature

In 2057 your personal pharmacists/nurse/physician – Dr. Zuzu – will not be a human but an ICC, an distributed affective Intelligent Caring Creature, with the knowledge of 1000 best physicians, pharmacists, and nurses from different specialties, traditional medicine from 50 cultures and an office in the Cyberspace. You will be able to teleport Dr. Zuzu any time you want to wherever you are.

All Dr. Zuzu's patients will be immersed in the intelligent health environment with data glasses, digital windows, and e-wallpaper. In addition, they will have on-body sensors and nanocomputers inside their bodies allowing continuous screening, monitoring and data collection about their physical and emotional state. They will also have bathroom MRI machines, shower skin mole detectors, toothbrush protein analyzers, smart beds monitoring sleep pattern, and sensors equivalent to a hospital pathology lab checking daily basic lab results.

Their on and in-body sensors will be able to report pain or any unusual physical or emotional state directly to Dr. Zuzu. They could also do it via a voice-enabled telehealth tool at any time since Dr. Zuzu understands 105 human languages and 1005 machine languages. Another communication option will be hybrid brain-machine interface allowing a patient to send a request to Dr. Zuzu just by thinking about requesting an extraordinary pleasant virtual experience such as petting a rabbit on the skyglide to ULURU, or getting rid of terrible nightmares about spiders.

Dr. Zuzu will be prepared to respond to many requests related to maximizing joy and pleasures of life not reducing pain because most of the diseases were eliminated and probability of the rest of them was minimized in the neonatal phase through chromosome replacement. Effective preventors (stress reducers and vitality enhancers) also contributed to low-sickness levels.

Dr. Zuzu will always listen to all its patients (no limit on amount) and will process their vital signs and test results, relating all the findings and looking for unusual patterns. Dr. Zuzu will be able to warn patients about incoming health problem (e.g., pain) using its case-based and memory-based predictive engine: for example, it could warn you "Please, call your surgery robots before leaving for work, to remove a splinter that will cause pain in 3 hour and 15 min – just when you have to change planes in Denver, Colorado."

Dr. Zuzu's will have a rich library of health stories extracted from life-long medical data. These stories will be parsed and represented in the knowledge base for further retrieval and then turned into video scripts out of which context-specific educational health movies will be assembled for other patients in need.

To facilitate ease of patient-physician communication, Dr. Zuzu will have multiple personalities, sex, age, voice and cognitive style depending on the situation and the patient. This includes the ability to become a humanoid version of the best friend from high school in order to maximize its convincing power and emotional closeness. This way Dr. Zuzu will be able to relate well to emotional states of its young and elderly patients in a close and friendly manner.

What if Dr. Zuzu gets sick itself? Dr. Zuzu will use self-treatment through knowledge injections. Another option is to call on other Intelligent Caring Creatures and get a byte of support. Most of the time Dr. Zuzu is in perfect shape – never tired like its human predecessors, never competitive or jealous, never anxious or annoyed.

Based on the genetic profile of each patient Dr. Zuzu will develop a long-term educational and care plan based on personalized interactive movies, illustrating major behavioral points that should be reinforced to maximize life's capacity, length, and pleasure. Dr. Zuzu's ability to annotate and retrieve from image and video libraries allows a just-in-time health education or compliance program. You may ask Dr. Zuzu to whisper a suggestion into your ear based on state of the art medical knowledge and your current situation. Dr. Zuzu will also be able to prescribe and then develop (in its virtual R&D lab) personalized drugs just for its patient.

Dr. Zuzu will help its patients not only to maintain good health but also deal with bad health in a compassionate and emotional way. With Dr. Zuzu you will have a happy environment when you are ill. It will have millions of stories of other people going through a given condition including:

- Encoded mental states
- Most common thoughts they thought and
- Activities and words that helped them to make it through the rough experience.

Dr. Zuzu's collective common sense knowledge will allow it to always say the right thing or to produce a right virtual companion, that you can interact with through direct retinal projection, in difficult cases.

Dr. Zuzu will charge its patients per knowledge injection and per successful interaction that will be automatically recorded based on your positive response recorded in your data stream. The payment will be expected also in the form of knowledge – your permission to use your data to further improve Dr. Zuzu's common sense and medical knowledge. This way your personal ICC will revitalize its curing and educational ability.

Renata G. Bushko

Contents

Looking into the Future

Future of Health Technology
R.G. Bushko (Ed.)
IOS Press, 2002

Defining the Future of Health Technology: Biomechatronics

Renata G. Bushko, M.S.

Chair, Future of Health Technology Institute, Hopkinton, MA, US

Abstract

Future progress in healthcare and medicine depends on today's investment in research, development, and education. We cannot leave such urgent issues to determine themselves, but rather must actively collaborate to ensure a stable healthcare system. This chapter describes efforts made by leading experts in industry, government, and academia to better ascertain future healthcare management. Such collaboration has occurred during a series of Future Healthcare Technology Summits [1] helping in planning investments in health technology. Deliberating and reviewing plans before taking action will accelerate progress as it will (1) save costs, (2) encourage compliance, (3) improve clinical outcomes, and (4) ensure greater patient satisfaction [2]. What we must resolve is: How can we invest a couple billion dollars to save hundreds of billions and, most importantly, increase human health in the future. A new branch of science, Biomechatronics, with millions of Intelligent Caring Creatures– is the answer.

1. Introduction

In early 1990's I worked on national healthcare programs organized by Vice President Gore, Dr. C. Everett Koop, and former secretary of Health and Human Services Dr. Louis Sullivan. I advised on health technology investment issues in US, UK, Puerto Rico, Australia, New Zealand, and Poland. Through my experiences with these healthcare programs I realized that we needed to spend more time on long-term planning. We needed an independent agency to discuss and oversee long-term issues of health technology. This agency would prepare for a future society where computers might outsmart people, where we might be able to stop diseases before they begin, where Affective Intelligent Caring Creatures [3] will aid physicians in 90% of their work and individuals can diagnose and cure themselves with self-health tools and designer drugs. Such an agency would prepare the medical community and consumers for inevitable technological changes and advances.

2. Agency to Look at Long-Term Issues of Health Technology

The Future of Health Technology Institute (FHTI) was founded in 1996 to address the long-term issues of health technology [4]. FHTI is a think-tank aimed at defining an agenda for health technology development and determining the most critical focus areas for health technology investment in the new century. Founded on the 40th anniversary of the field of Artificial Intelligence, FHTI found inspiration in the intellectual legacy of Professor Marvin Minsky. He is one of the founders of Artificial Intelligence and one of the most creative minds of our times. I became his student in 1985 when he was working on the Society of Mind theory.

Since its foundation in 1996, FHTI has been doing what Professor Dertouzos describes as: "Put in a salad bowl the wildest, most forward-thinking technological ideas that you can imagine. Then add your best sense of what will be useful to people. Start mixing the salad. Something will pop up that begins to qualify on both counts" [5]. Professor Dertouzos suggests that we should then "Grab it and run with it," which agrees with the paradigm that the best way to define the future is to invent it.

Unfortunately this optimistic model leaves a lot to random chance. The salad-bowl approach is a good start, but each idea should be attributed impact value and compared against alternative ideas. The ideas rely on both technological novelty and human usefulness. The process of comparing various ideas can be an efficient way to save time and money. FHTI proposes to manage the coordination of the most promising ideas in health technology using top-level experts from the industry, government and academia during Future of Health Technology Summits 1996-2001 [1]. The most investment-productive health technology areas are presented in this chapter (Tables 2-9).

3. Background: Thinking Model from the Field of Artificial Intelligence

In 1956 a diverse group of scientists consolidated various studies into a new field of science: Artificial Intelligence. They aimed to discover the unknown and mysterious machinery of the mind. Future of Health Technology Institute considers their efforts a model of leadership and innovation, representing skills essential in facing the problems of the 21st century.

How can we use this successful example to address emerging complexities that lie ahead? The world has changed in forty years since Marvin Minsky, John McCarthy, Allen Newell, Herbert Simon and other inquisitive minds met to design the field of Artificial Intelligence. In the same forty years the world of biology and medicine faced equally radical changes. FHTI summits address achievements of the last forty years in both medicine and medicine, trying to map out how those fields might come closer and merge in the future.

With the development of new technological innovations, people naturally fear that increased costs are inevitable. FHTI, however, believes that increased expenses can be stopped or even reversed. For example, while computer technology continues to expand, computer costs have decreased exponentially. Why should technological improvements in healthcare not follow the same progression? How can we take advantage of new technologies to improve the quality of life and simultaneously reduce procedure and treatment costs? Perhaps it is a matter of vision and leadership.

Specific goals of the Future of Health Technology Institute are:

1. Develop a vision of future health care supported by current and future health technologies.
2. Define distinct promising health technology research areas.
3. Demonstrate that technology driven cost increases in healthcare can be stopped and possibly reversed by a new allocation of research and development resources.
4. Define productive areas for research and development that will have potential impact on healthcare.
5. Identify new technologies that are practical and necessary in health and wellness maintenance.
6. Identify research and development needed to meet future health challenges.
7. Identify current products best for preparing 21st century healthcare.

4. Health Challenges – Need for Common Sense

4.1 Dare to Guess – Dealing with Hard Problems

Defining the future of health technology is difficult and requires both common sense and intuition. "Common sense is an immense society of hard earned practical ideas – of multitudes of life-learned rules and exceptions, dispositions and tendencies, balances and checks."[6] These balances and checks are especially useful when performing estimation tasks, where we deal with incomplete information. "For a hard problem, it may be almost as difficult to recognize progress as to solve the problem itself". [6] "A problem is hard if it requires common sense knowledge in addition to specialized knowledge and a set of non-obvious to the non-expert heuristics in order to be solved effectively and accurately. A body of knowledge required to solve a hard problem is not algorithmical but it is not totally intuitional either" [7]. A difficult (hard) problem manifests itself by the following facts:

(1) There exist experts that can solve that problem better (significantly faster, with better accuracy) than an average human

(2) Providing solution involves some symbolic reasoning and some common sense reasoning that is perceived as intuition

(3) Training humans to solve this kind of problem is a long-lasting, difficult, and not always successful process

(4) Even single experts accuracy leaves some space for improvement

Hard problems require making educated guesses and then verifying that hypothesis. We do not know the algorithm generating the solution but we can verify the positive solution once a guess is provided [7]. The best way to make some progress in defining the future of health technology is to work with a group of experts in related fields and also reach out to other industries to transfer relevant knowledge and know-how (e.g. hotel industry's customer satisfaction model at FHT99) [7, 8].

4.2 Define Health Challenges

The first step is to define challenges ahead of us. A group of experts was asked to define health challenges of the 21st Century using survey method. The results are listed in Table 1. Experts were energized and inspired to action by the approaching Future of Health Technology Summit.

Table 1. Health challenges of the new century. Order does not reflect importance.

1	Poverty
2	Hunger
3	Escalating costs of drugs
4	Escalating costs of technology
5	Engaging people to be responsible for their health and their family's health
6	Empowering consumers with better information and self help tools
7	Expanding & improving access to quality services including advanced diagnostic/therapeutic technologies while maintaining or reducing costs
8	Improving medical informatics literacy among medical staff
9	Reengineering the medical visit
10	Establishing Internet electronic medical record
11	Better monitoring and treatment of chronically ill patients away from the hospital
12	Finding cure for cancer and heart disease
13	Finding cure for paralysis
14	Coordination of services, transfer of information between providers and provider /patients
15	Effective Knowledge management
16	Providing relevant health information to the people who most need it
17	Creating happy environment for being sick
18	Emotional aspects of getting over healthcare problem and death
19	Assuring medical data integration
20	Improving healthcare workflow
21	Patient-omic data management and analysis (patient genomic, proteomics, physiomics) and patient cross-comparisons &
22	Expanding use of body-pervasive monitoring devices
23	Personalized drug design
24	Improved gene repair
25	Providing high quality health care services to all people, regardless of where they reside, what their socioeconomic status is, or what their cultural characteristics is
26	Reducing healthcare disparity
27	Maintaining high levels of health services (with tight budgets)
28	Inter-disciplinary issues related to the human element, not technology
29	Aging population explosion
30	Healthcare access, especially preventive care, for the large number of the uninsured
31	Shortage of nurses
32	Appropriate selection and use of healthcare resources by clients, self-care, and healthy habits through the dissemination of quality health information
33	Establishing cost-conscious evidence-based practice
34	Stop rising cost of healthcare
35	Increasing expenses and demand for services with decreasing reimbursement
36	Eliminating medical errors (estimated 40,000-98,000 inpatient deaths annually in US[1])
37	Extending human lifespan

---

[1] Institute of Medicine report released on November 29, 1999

4.3 Most Promising Health Technologies – Brainstorming Method

In order to approximate seven most promising health technology areas, the list of most promising health technologies generated by the before-summit survey, was presented to experts for prioritization. Then, seven most promising areas were selected during the brainstorming session. Results are presented in Table 2.

Table 2. Seven most promising health technology areas. Brainstorming method.
Summarized by Dr. Gary Kreps [9].

1	Instant Medical Data Collection and Knowledge Dissemination Technologies and Standards
2	Decision Making and Support Technology (personal and point of care)
3	Individualized Diagnosis and Treatment (e.g. real time protein synthesis, real time genetic testing)
4	Health Systems Methodologies
5	High Tech Intervention (e.g. Robotic Surgery, Sensors, Teleconsultations)
6	Information Access and Feedback Technologies
7	New Technologies Evaluation Methodologies

4.4 Most Promising Health Technologies – Survey Method

Seven technology areas listed in Table 3 were selected as most promising using the survey method. None of these lists or any other lists should be taken as the only lead to follow. They are only useful to attune our common sense and to turn into the right direction in the specific technology investment process.

Table 3. Seven most promising health technology areas selected by experts. Survey method.

1	(A) Tissue Bioengineering & (B) Nanotherapeutic Technologies
2	Knowledge Management Technologies (including decision support and data mining)
3	Electronic Health Record in a Standard Format with Unique Patient Identifier
4	(A) Powerful yet easy to use Self-diagnostic Technologies & (B) Vaccine Biology
5	Affordable information system access with decision support for healthcare professional
6	Internet-driven Technologies
7	Voice Recognition, (B) Psychological Aids & (C) Artificial Intelligence & (D) Controlled Medical Vocabularies

4.5 Seven Health Technology Areas with Highest ROI

As the last step, experts were asked to prioritize technologies given that "most promising" meant technology producing the highest impact with the lowest investment (technologies with highest return on investment - ROI). ROI was evaluated intuitively based on the diverse knowledge of the experts involved. FHTI's graphical Common Sense Squares Method was used in the ranking process.

Table 4. Seven health technology areas with the highest return on investment.
Survey method and FHTI's "Common Sense Squares Method" method.

1	Internet-driven Technologies
2	Electronic Health Record in a Standard Format with Unique Patient Identifier
3	Psychological Aids
4	Vaccine Biology
5	Powerful yet easy to use Self-diagnostic Technologies
6	Intelligent Agents (Intelligent Caring Creatures)
7	Affordable information system access with decision support for healthcare professional & patient

4.6 Most Promising Health Technology Research Areas – Insight

To balance group thinking (Table 3 and 4) FHTI asked one of the leading thinkers, Professor Alice Pentland, to propose a separate list of seven most promising health technology research areas [10]. This list was generated independently from the lists obtained from survey and brainstorming method but all experts involved in prioritization heard a detailed explanation of Professor Pentland's selection just before their brainstorming session.

Table 5. Seven most promising health technology research areas as defined by Professor Alice Pentland.

1	Memory Assistance Aids
2	Tissue Bioengineering and Gene Therapy
3	Perceptual Prostheses
4	Vaccine Biology
5	Rapid Diagnosis
6	3D Mapping
7	Psychological Aids

5. Rapid and Cost-effective Technology Impact Assessment

Technology impact study is an important next step after selection of most promising health technologies. An example of a cost-effective impact study is presented in the chapter "Impact of Voice and Knowledge-enabled Clinical Reporting – US Example" in this book. It uses Unified Quality Framework [2, 11, 12] that helps to examine technology impact on quality of healthcare using four qualitative and quantitative dimensions:

1) Process Quality as measured by cost

2) Organizational Quality as measured by compliance

3) Clinical Quality as measured by clinical outcomes

4) Service Quality as measured by patient and staff satisfaction

It is important that we try to maximize the use of Unified Quality Framework and FHTI's common sense methodology to evaluate quality impact of various technologies. The goal is to generate studies that are not expensive and comparable with each other. We could learn a lot faster if health technology assessment studies, performed by 160 different nations were easily comparable. We would be much closer to the goal of making the process of investment in new technologies less of a random chance. Then one might say – let's leave it all to the market forces. May be it would be a good idea? But then, let's ask ourselves what would have happen if we invested in nanotechnology 20 years ago when Dr. Eric Drexler and others uncovered its potential. How many lives and how much human suffering could we spear? Maybe cancer would be a history by now.

National Quality Cube

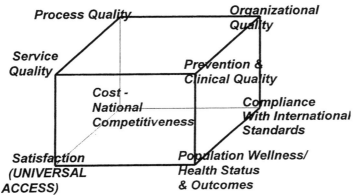

Figure 1. National quality cube in the Unified Quality Framework. Example of a component of the Unified Quality Framework. Top corners illustrate types of quality and bottom corners show the measure of quality.

6. Important Challenges and Technologies in Genetics and Bioengineering

Because of the importance of genetic engineering, a survey regarding most important health challenges and technologies was conducted on a focused group of experts with genetics background. The results are listed in Table 6 and Table 7. Table 8 shows a list of most promising bioengineering areas as defined by the American Medical Association for comparison [13].

Table 6. Health challenges in the beginning of the new millennium. Survey method used on experts with background in genetics.

1	Understanding the genetics of complex traits
2	Curing and preventing disease onset
3	Preventing healthcare and insurance discrimination
4	Delivering mental health focused care (major consumer of healthcare in 2010)
5	Shifting paradigm from reactive to proactive
6	Constraining technology lacking sufficient positive predictive value for treatment/diagnosis
7	Food delivery
8	Preventing cost increase in national healthcare systems
9	Working out disease pathways
10	Development of disease phenotype
11	Establishing interaction of environment and genetics as causes of cancer, diabetes and heart diseases
12	Individualized medicine
13	Lifestyle awareness
14	Wider variety and less expensive drugs

15	Understanding complex molecular networks involved in human diseases
16	Extending medical advances to developing countries
17	Global minimum standards for health
18	Conquering bacterial resistance towards antibiotics
19	Developing cost-effective cures for TB, Malaria, AIDS
20	Deconvolution of clinical disease in terms of genes and function
21	Developing of therapeutics through knowledge of genes and proteins involved
22	Personalized genetic diagnosis and treatment
23	Predictive diagnostic technologies
24	Predictive therapeutic technologies
25	True connectivity for medical professionals and consumers
26	Antibiotic-resistant microorganisms
27	Auto-immune diseases
28	Allergic variations in CYT-P4O (different individuals respond differently to the same drug)
29	Protein folding – function

Table 7. Technologies that can meet health challenges listed in Table 6. Order does not reflect importance

1	Genetic mapping: Genome-wide SNP association studies
2	Diagnostic SNP chips
3	Gene Therapy
4	New antigen delivery systems (molecular biology of peptide expression on cell surfaces)
5	Genome analysis/Genomics
6	Structural genomics
7	Cost-effectiveness analysis technology
8	Bioinformatics
9	Structural biology and drug design
10	Pharmacogenomics
11	Gene/Protein chips
12	Genomic profiling
13	Accurate annotation of genes and prediction of functions

It is also important to keep track of advances in biomedical engineering, especially in the seven areas listed in Table 8.

Table 8. Important areas of biomedical engineering; Order does not reflect importance

1	Molecular Engineering
2	Cell Engineering
3	Tissue Engineering
4	BioMEMS and Microfluidics
5	Virtual Surgery and Nanoinstrumentation
6	Imaging
7	Bioinformatics

7. Technology Areas Important for All Sectors of Economy Including Healthcare

We should never treat healthcare as a separate island, isolated from other parts of the economy. Thus, it is important to keep track of technologies that will change entire economy. Emerging Technology Areas that will soon have a profound impact on the entire economy including healthcare sector are listed in Table 9.

Table 9. Emerging technology areas that will soon have a profound impact on the entire economy including healthcare sector. Order does not reflect importance.

I	**Human-Machine Interaction - Requesting Things from Machines**
	Hybrid Brain-Machine Interfaces (HBMI) – Thought to Computer Communication
	Natural Language Processing
	Automatic Voice Recognition
	Mobile, wireless, wearable, and textile computing
	Computer Implants (connected to tagged smart environment)
	Haptics
II	**Machine Intelligence**
	Processing Requests
	Data Mining
	Common Sense Reasoning
	Reasoning by Analogy
	Flexible Transistors (e.g. on plastic)
	Responding to Requests
	Organic Light Emitting Displays (data glasses, e-paper, smart windows)
	Speech Generation
	Affective Computing (emotional communication)
	Visualization of Data
	Automatic Summarization /Abstracting
	Triggering Action
	Decision Triggers
	Biomechatronic Interfaces (to cells and biomechanical devices)
	Electronic Skin (e.g. triggering payment transaction on the way out of supermarket with no cashiers)
III	**Preservation of Individuality and Security**
	Digital Rights Management
	Biometrics (Face, Voice, DNA, finger print, behavioral pattern recognition)
	Biometronics Ethics and Law
IV	**Human-Machine Global Network**
	Microphotonics (all optical Internet with super high bandwidth)
	High-temperature Superconductivity (inexpensive power quality devices SMES[2])
	Infinite High-density Data Storage
	Restructuring Code (Software Engineering)
V	**Intelligent Creatures**
	Mobile Mechanical Machines
	Nanorobots (Microfluidics)
	Humanoids (Cyborgs)
	Machine Vision
	Machine Learning
	Robot Design
VI	**Sources of Energy**
	Body-heat Batteries
	Chemical Molecular Energy (e.g. ATP)
	Earth tides (Geothermal Energy)
	Solar Energy
	Superconductive Generators

---

[2] Superconducting Magnetic Energy Storage

8. Defining the Future by Vision Statements, Insights and Scenarios

Another way to uncover the future is to envision it and create scenarios. Most of chapter authors whom I invited to focus on specific issues in this book did just that brilliantly. The most convincing vision will have an impact on decision makers and thus on resource allocation decisions today. Selection of topics covered in the book is a result of five years of research by the Future of Health Technology Institute to define health technology agenda for the new century.

8.1 Integrative Vision from Future of Health Technology Summits

8.1.1 Weight-Power Perspective - From 1946 to 2050

In 1946 – ENIAK – the first electronic computer weighted 30 tons and had less computing power than a digital watch; In 2010 one computer could have the same power as all computers on earth in 1999 and it will be printed on plastic with flexible organic light emitting display so we can roll it like a piece of old-fashioned paper. It will be small enough to work inside our bodies powered by molecular chemical reactions (E.g., ATP) or on our bodies as sensors powered by our body-heat. In 2020 computers will be smarter than people and we'll have a choice to augment ourselves to extend our cognition or not. By 2050 most of us will become cyborgs with implanted computers that extend our cognitive powers and give us extra senses (e.g., ultrasonic sense).

8.1.2 Light-Flexibility Perspective – From 1880 to 2006

Electric light, one of the most visible inventions of the 20th Century, was first featured on a steam ship Columbia that traveled from port to port, making headlines by showing the light of 150 light bulbs produced by four generators. The new Millennium has started with a similar story: In May 2000, Quinn Mary in Long Beach California became the showing place for what will become one of the most visible technologies of the 21st Century – technology that will allow flexible, paper-thin, bendable computer and video displays. Future of Health Technology Institute's Cruise to the Future™ planned for the year 2006 will continue Columbia's and Quinn Mary's tradition with specific focus on health technologies.

   Organic light emitting diodes combined with polymer transistors will evolve into electronic paper, personalized hardware that one can print at home, personalized disposable computers woven into textiles, wallpaper that is also a control center of a hospital or electronic skin that is able to respond mechanically to changing conditions. This means that making healthcare paperless does not make sense anymore and that there is hope for rapid computerization of medicine because the biggest obstacle to computerization – computer itself (the way it looks in early 2001) – will change dramatically.

8.1.3 From Electronic Care to Smart Care

We should reformulate "electronic health record" goal in order to make faster progress in technology introduction to healthcare. Framing this problem as "electronic patient record" suggests that the only thing that we are striving for is moving information about patient and care from paper to electronic format. This is not our primary goal. We do not want electronic care – we want smarter and more sensitive care (high tech combined with high touch).

8.1.4 From Electronic Health Record to Intelligent Health Environment

We should use a term:"Intelligent Health Environment" instead of "Electronic Health Record" to embrace the generative aspect of modern computer technology. Health record in an Intelligent Health Environment will also include not only a mere record of human interactions and health metrics but also machine-generated knowledge (facts and relationships). Machines involved will be both software agents (ICCs) and robots. Intelligent Health Environment will utilize biosensors and machine learning techniques. With time it will lead to the Affective Intelligent Caring System embracing other aspects of our lives like childcare, homes, relationships, finance, shopping, work and pleasure activities.

8.1.5 From Knowledge Management to Self-Health Tools

Intelligent Health Environment will involve wearable, wireless and implantable self-health tools based on personal genomic information and linked to tags and geographic positioning system for ongoing monitoring of people's vital signs and location. Fast progress in microphotonics leading to all optical Internet with huge bandwidth will allow real time video links to every home, school and workplace making telemedicine and telepresence a common place.

8.1.6 From Doctor, Nurse and Pharmacists to Affective Intelligent Caring Creature

In an Intelligent Health Environment each person will have a personal distributed Affective Intelligent Caring Creature (ICC) – a hybrid physician/nurse/pharmacist that processes all the data from biosensors, genomic data sources, medical science and other ICCs. Affective Intelligent Caring Creature has many helpers embedded in our homes and also in our bodies, showers, cars, beds, toothbrushes, and kitchen counters. ICCs use Inter-ICC language that allows them to communicate effectively, interlink facts and predict emergency situations that will reduce to the minimum need to have emergency rooms as they are today.

Some helpers are embedded in robots equipped with computer vision and natural language understanding for remote presence. For example, your ICC embedded in a robot may go through the house of your elderly mother to check on her when you are away. Since you can navigate the robot through the Internet you will be able to see her and talk to her.

Yet, another ICC may specialize in monitoring products on international markets that may have impact on your health and well-being. This ICC – health purchasing agent – may suggest that you buy a car that uses video cameras to eliminate the blind spot and that automatically adjusts car seat for your 5-year old child, when the car turns into an airplane. It may then call your financial ICC to prepare savings strategy to buy that "healthy car" resulting in the cancellation of your virtual trip to Mars in 2058.

8.1.7 From Robotic Surgery to Nanosurgery

We will also have private tele-surgery bubble as a mobile attachment to our homes and cars. Intelligent Caring Creature will schedule surgery for us with the surgeon or a surgical robot most experienced with our particular condition. Telesurgeon will see the operating field through virtual retinal display goggles. With rapid progress in hybrid-brain-machine interfaces (HBMI) in the year 2070 we will have direct brain-surgical-tools interface where surgeon operates using her/his thoughts not hands. Thought operated surgical equipment will be as common as thought operated cars for disabled (eventually we will all want to use them).

We will not use surgery bubble a lot though because nanorobots will do most of the surgical jobs for us – starting before our birth. Chromosome replacement and nanocytosurgery will save us from surgeries that are currently necessary. Nanorobots will voyage through our bodies to repair damage, treat tumors, attack viruses, repair cell walls, deliver drugs, and remove blockages. The first nanotweezers and rotating, chemically powered nanomotors were successfully built in 1999. The year 2000 brought the first molecular switches – a great step towards nanocomputers.

8.1.8 From Pharmaceutical Lab to Cellular Drug Invention and Distribution

By 2020 personalized drug design and production in Intelligent Caring Centers will be a common place. Mergers between pharmaceutical companies, health information systems vendors, and providers will be long forgotten by then.

By 2050 we will have nanopharmacies – tiny cellular pharmacies that produce a drug, store it, and release it when needed inside our bodies. They will replace drug prescriptions, lengthy lab design, clinical trials and eventually mixing procedures. Drugs produced by nanopharmacies and designed by Intelligent Caring Creatures will be personalized to a single individual avoiding any adverse reactions and delivered directly to locations in our bodies that need them. As a new form of entertainment we'll watch on VRDs how cancer cells are eliminated because nonorobots will have tiny video transmitters.

8.2 Closer Look at the Doctor of the Future – Affective Intelligent Caring Creature

In 2057 your personal pharmacists/nurse/physician - Dr. Zuzu - will not be a human but an ICC, a distributed Intelligent Caring Creature, with the knowledge of 1000 best physicians, pharmacists, and nurses from different specialties, traditional medicine from 50 cultures and an office in the Cyberspace.

All Dr. Zuzu's patients will be equipped with computers in their homes and cars in the form of data glasses, windows, mirrors and e-wallpaper. In addition, they will have on-body sensors and nanocomputers inside their bodies allowing continuous screening, monitoring and data collection about their physical and emotional state (e.g. EKG, GSR). They will also have bathroom MRI machines, shower skin mole detectors, toothbrush protein analyzers, smart beds monitoring sleep pattern, and sensors equivalent to a hospital pathology lab, checking daily basic lab results.

Their on and in-body sensors will be able to report pain or any unusual physical or emotional state directly to Dr. Zuzu. They could also do it via a voice-enabled telehealth tool at any time since Dr. Zuzu understands 105 human languages and 1005 machine languages. Another communication option will be hybrid brain-machine interface allowing a patient to send a request to Dr. Zuzu just by thinking about requesting an extraordinary pleasant virtual experience such as petting a rabbit on the skyglide to ULURU, or getting rid of terrible nightmares about spiders.

It is important to note that Dr. Zuzu will be prepared to respond to many requests related to maximizing joy and pleasures of life not reducing pain because most of the diseases were eliminated and probability of the rest of them was minimized in the neonatal phase through chromosome replacement. Effective preventors (stress reducers) helping ICCs also contributed to low-sickness levels.

Dr. Zuzu will always listen to all its patients (no limit on amount) and will process their vital signs and test results, relating all the findings and looking for unusual patterns. Dr. Zuzu will be able to warn patients about incoming health problem (e.g., pain) using its case-based and memory-based predictive engine: for example, it could warn you "Please, call your surgery robots before leaving for work, to remove a splinter that will cause pain in 3 hour and 15 min – just when you have to change plains in Denver, Colorado."

Dr. Zuzu's will have a rich library of health stories extracted from life-long medical data. These stories will be parsed and represented in the knowledge base for further retrieval and then turned into video scripts out of which context-specific educational health movies will be assembled for other patients in need.

To facilitate ease of patient-physician communication, Dr. Zuzu will have multiple personalities, sex, age, voice and cognitive style depending on the situation and the patient. This includes the ability to become a humanoid version of the best friend from high school in order to maximize its convincing power and emotional closeness. This way Dr. Zuzu will be able to relate well to emotional states of its young and elderly patients in a close and friendly manner.

What if Dr. Zuzu gets sick itself? Dr. Zuzu will use self-treatment through knowledge injections. Another option is to call on other Intelligent Caring Creatures and get a byte of support. Most of the time Dr. Zuzu is in perfect shape – never tired like its human predesesors, never competitive or jealous, never anxious or annoyed.

Based on the genetic profile of each patient Dr. Zuzu will develop a long-term educational and care plan based on personalized interactive movies, illustrating major behavioral points that should be reinforced to maximize life's capacity, length, and pleasure. Dr. Zuzu's ability to annotate and retrieve from image and video libraries allows a just-in-time health education or compliance program. Dr. Zuzu will also be able to prescribe and then develop (in its virtual R&D lab) personalized drugs just for its patient.

Dr. Zuzu will help its patients not only to maintain good health but also deal with bad health in a compassionate and emotional way. With Dr. Zuzu you will have a happy environment when you are ill. It will have millions of stories of other people going through a given condition including:
() Encoded mental states
() Most common thoughts they thought and
() Activities and words that helped them to make it through the rough experience.

Dr. Zuzu's collective common sense knowledge will allow it to always say the right thing or to produce a right virtual companion, that you can interact with through direct retinal projection, in difficult cases.

Dr. Zuzu will charge its patients per knowledge injection and per successful interaction that will be automatically recorded based on your positive response recorded in your data stream. The payment will be expected also in the form of knowledge – your permission to use your data to further improve Dr. Zuzu's common sense and medical knowledge. This way your personal ICC will revitalize its curing and educational ability.

8.3 The Integrating Power of Insight – Biomechatronics

Future of Health Technology Summit thinking sessions generate knowledge waves present long after the event. 6th Summit, FHT2001, confirmed that an unprecedented revolution is taking place: molecular biology, computer and medical science, electrical, mechanical, genetic and biomedical engineering, are merging into one field best described as Biomechatronics.

To make progress we need to have not only manageable models of the future but also of the science and technology behind it. Biomechatronics brings together tissue engineering, robot design, information technologies, knowledge management, pharmacogenomics, biometrics, nanotechnology, and bioinformatics.

One reason that back in 1996 I focused on health technology in the era of booming healthcare informatics was an observation that health-related information comes from and is embedded in biological, electronic and mechanical artifacts – it is an integral part of Biomechatronics not an independent island. On-going symbolic reasoning on health data and tools helping humans or cyborgs to make sense out of the multi-layered biomedical, organizational and mechanical processes is an important goal. Creating meaning out of petabytes of personal information requires the same common sense capabilities as generating smart medical advice.

The first Biomechatronics summit will address these issues. It will take place October 28-29, 2002, **www.fhti.org** as a part of the 7th Future of Health Technology Summit focusing on the crucial issue of adaptability and learning on molecular, personal, and organizational levels.

9. Defining the Future of Health Technology as a Dynamic Learning Process

According to Allan Newell, knowledge can only be created dynamically in time [14]. "It is generated by an observer, relative to his point of view, in the process of making sense (modeling)" [15]. It is the same with knowledge in health technology – it should be an adaptive, dynamic process not a one-time event or publication. Current rate of innovation and product creation makes the process of defining what to invest in similar to seating on a raft on a fast, infinite, mountain river trying to decide where to stop. "Knowledge about [healthcare] cannot be captured in a finite structure" [14] – it has to be an ongoing dialog. Results of that dialog could be used by decision makers in different situations and different places on earth as hints and general direction in their own problem solving processes.

More than forty years of research on learning, problem solving, and intelligence conducted by the field of Artificial Intelligence brings hope of making that process more effective. Realizing that information becomes knowledge when it starts guiding decision making, makes it even more obvious that defining future of health technology involves on-going, adaptive dynamic learning by industry, governments and academia.

Seven Strategies to Leadership [2] based on forty years of knowledge science provide a guiding structure.

1. **Sustained Renewal & Growth**
   Treat Sustained Growth as a final goal;You do not want to be successful only once - you want to be continuously successful
2. **Situated Adaptability**
   Change your organization in a specific situation and problem solving context; 21st Century requires ongoing situated adaptability
3. **Sociotechnological Responsibility**
   Learn and use new technologies and do not delegate it to others - "I am non-technical" syndrome; Think about your goal in a context of sociotechnological process; technology and organizations cannot be separated
4. **Strategic Repositioning**
   Look outside your organization and ahead in time; Use Unified Quality Framework
5. **Simplification**
   Avoid bureaucracy and look for unconventional shortcuts
6. **Self-Reinventing**
   Keep learning and developing leadership and innovation skills
7. **Strength, Savings, Satisfaction**
   Spend time absorbing results of work; Bring back child-like joy and celebration spirit

10. Conclusions

Future progress in healthcare and medicine depends on the investments in research, development and education made today. Defining most promising health technology areas by the group of experts from industry, government and academia may help in planning investments in health technology. The answer to the question of how to invest a couple of billion dollars to save hundreds of billions and increase human health in the future is an ongoing effort to point in the right direction. According to opinions gathered at Future of Health Technology Summits (1) Instant Medical Data Collection and Knowledge Dissemination Technologies, (2) Tissue Bioengineering & Nanotherapeutic Technologies, (3) Internet-driven Technologies and (4) Brain-Machine Interfaces are the key investment areas for the next 10 –20 years. Unprecedented technological revolution manifests itself in convergence of molecular biology, computer and medical science, electrical, mechanical, genetic and biomedical engineering (including cell, molecular and tissue engineering) into biomechatronics. It will play an integrative role in the future of health technology accelerating the speed of discoveries leading to dramatic cost reduction. It is necessary to maintain an ongoing watch of new technologies and revisit the issue of resource allocation periodically with different groups of experts. We have a unique chance to define the future not to observe it; to say what should happen instead of saying what will happen if we do not change anything.

References

[1] Future of Health Technology Summits 1996-2000, www.fhti.org
[2] R.G. Bushko, Leadership Challenges in the 21st Century: 7 Strategies to Leadership, Workshop P-6, Healthcare Executive's Challenges in the 21st Century: Leadership, Quality, Technology, and Innovation-driven Process Management, IMIA'95, Vancouver Canada, 1995.

[3] R. G. Bushko, Doctor's Office of the Future, presentation at the Future of Health Technology Summit 1998, Cambridge, MA.

[4] R. G. Bushko, From Artificial Intelligence to Intelligent Healthcare; Position paper for the initiation of the Future of Health Technology Summit series, Future of Health Technology Institute, internal document, 1996.

[5] M. Dretouzos, Kurzweil vs. Dretouzos, Technology Review Vol. 104/NO. 1 (2001) 81-84.

[6] M. L. Minsky, The Society of Mind, Simon and Schuster Inc., New York, NY, 1986.

[7] R. G. Bushko, "Knowledge-Rich Analogy: Adaptive Estimation with Common Sense", thesis, Massachusetts Institute of Technology, Cambridge, MA USA, 1991

[8] R. G. Bushko, Wake-Up USA: Accelerated Cross-Domain Knowledge Transfer to Healthcare, Research proposal; 8/1994, Updated 1996, 7SL International and Future of Health Technology Institute, Hopkinton, MA

[9] G. L. Kreps, B. Glassman, FHT99 Synthesis, in R. G. Bushko (Ed.), Future of Health Technology Summit 1999 CD-ROM, Future of Health Technology Institute, Hopkinton, MA, 1999.

[10] A. P. Pentland, Seven Most Promising Health Technology Research Areas in R. G. Bushko (Ed.), Future of Health Technology Summit 1999 CD-ROM, Future of Health Technology Institute, Hopkinton, MA, 1999, www.fhti.org

[11] G. Edwards, R. Bushko; Business Modeling Tools for Decision Support Systems (Quality Impact on Hospitals), Proceedings of the 8th International Medical Informatics Congress, in Robert Greenes (Ed.); 7/1995, Vancouver, Canada.

[12] R. G. Bushko, Poland: Socio-technological Transformation – its Impact on Organizational, Process, Clinical and Service Quality of Health Care. In: W. Wieners (Ed.), Global Healthcare Markets. Jossey-Bass Publishers, John Wiley & Sons, Inc. 2000, pp. 194-201.

[13] L. G. Griffith, A.J. Grodzinsky, Advances in Biomedical Engineering, JAMA, Vol. 285 No. 5, 2001, p 556-561

[14] A. Newell, The Knowledge Level, Artificial Intelligence 18, 87-127, 182.

[15] W. Clancey, The Knowledge Level Reinterpreted: Modeling How Systems Interact, Machine Learning, 4, 285-291, 1989.

[16] M. Minsky, The Future of Artificial Intelligence Technology, Forum, Risk Management Foundation of the Harvard Medical Institutions, Volume 17, Number 1, April 1996.

[17] M. L. Minsky, Framework for Representing Knowledge, MIT AI Memo No. 306, 1974.

[18] M. L. Minsky, The Future of Artificial Intelligence Technology, Is there a Virtual Doctor in the House? Forum, Volume 17, Number 1, April 1996.

[19] R. G. Bushko, Situated, Strategic, and AI-Enhanced Technology Introduction to Healthcare; Proceedings of the Workshop on the Medical Knowledge Representation, International Joint Conference of Artificial Intelligence, 8/1991, Sydney, Australia.

Future of Health Technology
R.G. Bushko (Ed.)
IOS Press, 2002

Inventing the Future –

Tools for Self Health

Alice P. Pentland M.D.

*Co-Director, Center for Future Health and Professor and Chair, Department of
Dermatology, School of Medicine and Dentistry, University of Rochester, NY, US*
and

Alex P. Pentland Ph.D.

Academic Head, MIT Media Laboratory, Cambridge, MA, US

Throughout the history of medicine, technology has produced radical changes in our understanding of human disease, the therapies that we use to treat it, and how we provide care. A useful example of the potential for technology to transform our approach to health and disease is the invention of the microscope. Prior to its invention, we had little understanding of the existence of microorganisms or the cellular structure of the human body. However, once this tool became available, the groundwork was laid so that it was possible to propose the germ theory of disease. We could also understand the cellular structure underlying human anatomy, and so begin to understand the fine processes of organ function. Medicine was revolutionized as a result.

Currently, we are in the midst of a new technology revolution, illustrated by the many chapters included in this book. The effects produced by this newest wave of technology have already begun to change medicine, and are likely to alter our health care system in the next century as much as it was transformed during the last one. The impact is likely to reshape the processes and tools through which we interact with health professionals, and ultimately how we think about caring for ourselves.

It is very important to visualize how future health technology can affect us, as the editor, Renata Bushko, and contributors to this book have done. For the full potential of new health technologies to be realized, we must collectively try to rationalize and discuss the best ways to capture the opportunities technology provides to serve our needs in health, in disease, as individuals and as a community. This task may prove difficult since our individual needs can be in conflict with those of our communities, necessitating careful implementation of public policy to balance them. Because of the complexity of the issues influencing these decisions, the positive as well as negative effects of technical advances on the state of medicine over the last century are therefore worth examining. We must also consider and test different technology evaluation methodologies, as well as methodologies estimating technology impact as discussed in chapters by Gary Kreps and Renata Bushko. These may help us to understand what goals we may want to set and how we may achieve them in the next hundred years.

Since 1900, the introduction of new technology has had a profound impact on the field of medicine. An example of this is the creation of the Pediatric Intensive Care Unit. Who would believe at the turn of the last century, that a child born at 26 weeks gestation would have a chance at a normal healthy life? We see this with some regularity today. Large machines, ventilators, constant monitoring of heart rate, respiration, pulse, and temperature along with the ability to give tiny increments of fluid in proportion to a tiny infant's size permit us to maintain these fragile beings. Now they can be supported until they are able to prosper in the world outside of the womb and live a long life.

Similarly, we have also seen our understanding of human cellular function permit us to design highly specific new drugs. Our understanding of intracellular mediators and cell receptors have allowed the creation of new "designer" pharmaceuticals. These chemicals can block cellular regulatory pathways, stimulating them to delicately tickle the balance of our blood flow, heart function or kidney excretion and battle such killers as diabetes, and heart disease at their root. The result of all of this success has been a wonderful and dramatic increase in the length of the human life span. People born in the United States can now count on an average life span into the late 70's and the number of centenarians is rising dramatically [1]. This is an increase in average life expectancy of nearly 30 years!

These benefits have come at a cost, however. Many people recall great satisfaction with the human aspects of health care delivery in the middle decades of the century. For the most part, the doctor came to visit the sick at their bedside in their own home. People were born at home and died at home. The cycle of human life was part of the cycle of family life in an integral and community centered way. This integration of health care into the daily activities of the family can have a strengthening effect on families and communities that the modern hospital and clinic-based model does not provide.

However, it has not been possible to provide the advanced medical care that we have invented in a home setting. To treat prematurity, the baby currently must live in an isolette, and perhaps also be on a ventilator for weeks on end. This equipment is very expensive, and its proper use requires a great deal of training. Because of the complex knowledge and expense required to take proper care of such infants, it is currently necessary to centralize where such care is provided. The highly specialized physicians, nurses and other caretakers needed to care for the infant must be available near the equipment that contains their tiny patient. There must also be a library, so that these health professionals can take full advantage of the body of knowledge needed to keep these delicate infants alive. Centralization also allows the equipment to be regularly used, lessening its cost. A medical center environment also supports the large complex of machines needed to perform the array of tests that are necessary in order to monitor changes in the infant's health status. So the technology that created the opportunity to keep the premature infant (or the auto accident victim) alive has enlarged the complexity, expense and centralization of health care. In the process, we find ourselves feeling disconnected from our doctors, and perhaps more importantly, our sick relatives. Health care is too expensive, too tightly focused on care of disease and too separate from our daily lives. Ideally, the changes that are coming should work to reverse this trend without diminishing the benefits to our health we have already achieved through technical innovation.

Until recently, there has been very little success in attempting to extend health care into the home environment, yet there clearly is a huge demand for this. Americans currently spend 27 billion dollars on health care outside of the health care establishment [2] because they find it so difficult to access, expensive, and painful. A clear demand for better integration of the home into the health environment exists. No only that, but a dramatic shift in the composition of our population makes it absolutely necessary to develop such distributed systems.

In the year 1970, there were 25 caregivers for each disabled person [3]. However, the success of our health care system is such that the ratio of caregivers for the at-home disabled is going to be 6:1in the year 2030. How will those six people care for that seventh disabled person? Certainly we cannot have a centralized system of visiting nurses that travel to their homes to take care of them because we will not have enough individuals left working in the economy to support it. Thus, a more highly distributed system is not only something that we desire but it is an absolutely necessary change that must take place. Some efforts to alleviate the problem have been introduced with the advent of telemedicine as discussed in the chapter by Meg Wilson. Visiting nurses have recently begun to make house calls via telemedicine connections. In addition, a small industry is springing up around monitoring of key parameters in those with chronic illnesses such as emphysema, diabetes and congestive heart failure. The Physio Chair by Commwell and Lifeshirt by Vivometrics are examples. These new tools are just beginning to be adopted as reimbursement strategies are created which make them profitable.

In addition to extending the activities of health professionals into the home, optimal health care in the future will require the creation of new tools that extend the capacity of the individual to assess and maintain their own health. The technology required to implement this vision must be user friendly, intuitive, and have the user's trust. The technology will need to help an individual to maintain their normal health profile, allowing detailed information and measurements to be collected so that the earliest signs of disease can be detected. In contrast to the current state of information - measuring one's values against those of entire populations, having knowledge of one's own individual variations should better enable individuals to better determine when they need to seek health care, before they actually feel ill. Armed with his or her own personal information, the individual is also greatly empowered in the doctor's office. The visit can become a discussion between individual and doctor, and more time can be spent discussing the implications of such changes and providing personal support, rather than trying to determine whether or not changes have occurred.

In the current system, a patient visits the doctor at intervals, and health information/data is collected through obtrusive or invasive means. For future health technology to be something that individuals at home will use readily, the ongoing collection of personal information must occur in an unobtrusive and cost-effective manner.

What sorts of devices could be created to help an individual stay well? Collectively, they can be thought of as a "personal medical advisor", which could also be adapted to function in remote areas of the world as a local clinic. Where the health care system is well developed, they can help keep the aging population functional longer, guide parents more successfully through the difficulties of childrearing, and help those with chronic diseases function at their best.

Some of the possibilities fulfilling this vision being explored currently are:

- "Memory Assistance" glasses in which the glass contains an extremely small and lightweight computer monitor readable by the wearer, and cameras which can interact with a tiny wearable computer to help an elderly person maintain their independence and social circle. As an example, this device could identify a person whose name has been forgotten or offer reminders regarding such tasks as taking medication or paying bills.

- Sensate Liner Garments such as shorts or socks for people who have lost sensation in their skin due to diabetes or neurologic injury, to monitor skin integrity and "warn" the wearer that their skin is developing a pressure sore.
- The "Smart Bandage" to measure the bacteria or virus in an injury and let the user know whether antibiotic treatment is needed and which antibiotic to use. Such a device can be easily adapted to monitoring food or water supplies, or identifying allergens in the environment.
- The "Smart Bed" to monitor a person's weight, temperature, electrocardiogram, or even electroencephalogram to identify sleep disorders, early stages of depression, and generally act as a central health data repository in the home.
- "Skin Surface Mapping" imaging devices that collect images of an individual's skin surface, then notes any change over time. This could allow very early detection of skin cancer such as melanoma, greatly increasing survival.

We will see many more such helpful innovations over the next several decades, as we understand better when individuals can effectively act to help themselves, and when assistance from a health professional is needed.

In this volume, there are contributions from an array of experts describing in detail how their particular expertise can reshape aspects of the way we approach health care in the future. To make effective changes, these technical advances must be integrated with new institutional strategies for health care delivery that address the needs of individuals for privacy, but still provide the benefit to communities of shared information resources. Public policy discussions must bring balance to these sometimes contradictory needs and points of view. These discussions are already underway with the new Health Insurance Portability and Accountability Act (HIPAA) legislation [4,5], but more work is needed.

The work presented here is therefore offered in the spirit of advancing this thoughtful debate. We hope that these discussions will not only unlock the tremendous opportunities that new health technology presents for treatment of acute illness and injury, but will also emphasize the potential of the advances being made to remedy the problems caused by the last wave of technical advancement and make preventive health care a reality.

The general areas in which new technology will be integrated to advance health care are information infrastructure, health technology interfaces, advances in the understanding and treatment of disease, and tools for understanding and assisting behavior change. The area of disease understanding and treatment is huge, and the complexity has been greatly expanded by the recent complete sequencing of the human genome [6,7].

One promising aspect of having sequenced the human genome will be the opportunity to understand the impact of one's genetic makeup to prevent episodes of disease. Inexpensive nanoscale sensor technology may allow us to prevent health problems in ways that were previously impossible, as envisioned by Barry Robson. Inexpensive rapid tests that determine an individual's susceptibility to disease or predict the likely side effects of medication may spring from such nanoscale creations. Genetic information combined with inexpensive sensors may allow a person to test themselves at home to ask questions such as "Do I have the susceptibility gene for penicillin allergy?" or "what pollen is triggering my runny nose today?" and help them make decisions about being exposed to drugs before they become allergic, or selectively avoid triggers for allergy in ways that were not possible without these tools. In the case of seasonal allergy, such tools could be used by consumers without the need for a medical consultation – only knowledge and antihistamines (already available over the counter) are needed for the average sufferer.

Much new information about the causes of drug allergy and the markers of it must be collected before such a test is possible, but with microsensor arrays and knowledge of the human genome, the ability is in our hands for the first time.

Similarly, such nanoscale sensors can have a huge impact on traditional hospital-based medicine, where they be used to improve the rapid diagnostic tests available in clinical laboratories to increase speed and sensitivity while reducing cost. Nanorobots as surgical assistants will make possible selective surgery with greatly reduced risk and higher success rates. These new approaches will have the same pervasive impact that microsurgery has had over the past two decades. As nanotechnology is advanced, we can take the opportunity to change the large machines we currently employ to make them radically smaller. Devices such as those envisioned by Robert Freitas utilizing nanofabrication and constructed on a molecular scale, can potentially be made cheaply enough that they can be more widely available. Ideally, such sensors could be cheap enough to be placed in the home, for self-assessment and health maintenance purposes. This change will make it so the afflicted would only need to travel to hospitals and clinics when catastrophic illness strikes, or the desire for the support and sympathy that can be provided by interaction with a health professional is needed. Such nanoscale technology could also be used for creation of implantable devices to supplement inadequate organ function – for instance, it could be utilized to assist in the creation of an artificial pancreas for those with diabetes. We have already seen the earliest form of such a device with the creation of the personal insulin pump[8]. As the scale of the technology needed to support the acutely ill becomes smaller, perhaps the hospital will seem a less threatening place in which to be ill.

The information delivery requirements of the existing centralized architecture will need to change radically as we are better able to move and store information, as discussed by Blackford Middleton, Richard Spivack and others included here. Implementing and making interactive the currently available tools is already a formidable task, and one that is consuming large amounts of effort in health care systems and numerous corporations. Clear advantages in the quality of health care and cost of providing care are evident when the new infrastructure is successfully implemented as shown in the chapter by Mary Jo Deering.

Because of the complexity of health information, and the many needs that health information serves, organizing the architecture to serve the needs of all likely users is an active and fruitful area of research as discussed in the chapter by Gio Wiederhold. Communications between physicians, their patients and their insurers will all be subject to systemization over the next few years. We must be strong advocates for patient ease of use, access and privacy protection as these technologies unfold.

The ideal system will provide access to doctors and medical personnel when appropriate, and will also serve public health and research needs while privacy protection is adequately maintained. While systems providing health care are strongly motivated to reduce costs by moving information freely, this may not be in the best interest of the patient. HIPAA rules now under discussion address this set of issues, but clearly cannot deal with all eventualities. Giving patients better access to their own record may help apply pressure to health systems to create systems that serve patients well. Some health systems are already exploring the role of the patient's personal medical record, and assessing how it should be integrated with the records kept by hospital systems. Soon we will be able to use internet applications for routine interactions with the doctor, nurse or pharmacist

Intelligent agent software and decision support tools will be crucial to this process, as discussed here for use in health care by Henry Lieberman and Robert Greenes. In a distributed system that is personalized, updates of new knowledge to individual users will be crucial to keeping care optimal, and new strategies are likely to be needed regularly as the complexity of the information we require to keep us healthy increases. Information will be pushed to us (hopefully with our permission) about therapies that may be helpful to us. More important will be the direct delivery of warnings as side effects become known – such as the cardiac risk of taking Fen-Phen[9], or notification that flu has broken out in your neighborhood. Intelligent agents will also be available to help us as we ask questions about our health, identifying information sources that are most useful to our health.

Intelligent agents will also be helpful in guiding individuals choices about their medical care. People will be able to look to see whether or not the health care system they are working with provides quality services. Hospitals and physicians will have a report card given regularly - whether they cooperate with the process by which such report cards are generated or not! People will be able to know more about the quality of care that is being provided in their doctor's offices and in their communities. This will actually push doctors to provide better care and improve everyone's health.

Better organization of the information infrastructure in medicine, and use of intelligent agents gives us the opportunity to consider a more distributed health care system without losing the quality we currently have. Those tasks that are less complicated and which people might perform better if they felt they had ownership of them should be put into the home. The new technologies in testing and decision support will permit a redistribution of the kinds of care that occur in a clinic and in a doctor's office. The doctor's office will acquire more of the functions of a laboratory space where tests can be done quickly without having to send the patient off to a central facility at a hospital for testing. Hospitalizations will really be reserved for those times when a person needs to have an intervention such as a surgery and the big tools are absolutely required for health maintenance. Transfer between hospitals will be guided by the type and availability of services needed by the individual, rather than standard policy, maximizing the ability for patients to be treated nearer their homes when they are hospitalized.

The LINCOS project (little intelligent communities) is an experiment in how this kind of redistribution of care using low-cost high, tech interfaces impacts the health of rural communities in the third world. These "digital town centers" built in recycled shipping containers and powered by generator with a satellite uplink if needed, contain the basic equipment for business access to the web, education and telemedicine. By bundling the health care needs of a community with its education and business needs, LINCOS allows the creation of a relatively inexpensive high tech "town center" which can be placed in very remote settings to give individuals and communities who have been cut off from the mainstream the access they need to take action to improve their quality of life and health. Several containers have been placed in Costa Rica and in the Dominican Republic, and 60 more are planned. New strategies for assessing community needs prior to placement of the containers and new technologies for placement in these stand-alone city centers are underway [10]. The information gained can provide a roadmap for how decision support, sensors, telemedicine and health information architecture need to be constructed to optimize a distributed model of health care.

Despite advances in the medical infrastructure, sensors, disease understanding and treatments, a crucial aspect for success of health technology in the future will be the interface between the technology and the person using it, as explored in the chapters by Graziella Tonfoni and Jo Lernout.. Failed implementations of technology are frequent, and are often due to problems in understanding the complexity of the problem - or lack of understanding of the users needs. Bulky, slow and non-intuitive interfaces hamper the adoption of technology, both by health care consumers, providers and administrators. The new capabilities of natural language based interfaces will make it far more likely that future systems will be easily used, and may help to address the problem of technical literacy as well. Because health is everyone's problem, solutions for providing care must be readily usable by EVERYONE who needs care. Keyboards, monitors, wires and multistep instructions are an insurmountable barrier to many people – even in the current environment communication problems regularly precipitate emergency room visits.

The authors included here are addressing the problem of the interface with technology in a variety of ways. Natural language recognition, to avoid training needed for current voice recognition applications is a key goal for the future. Integrating this with affective computing as discussed by Rosalind Picard, will make the interaction with new health technology be more intuitive, and thus more useable. In the more distant future, thought to computer communication as discussed by Kevin Warwick, may be the method of choice – particularly for the handicapped, who have difficulty with manipulating any interface. Preliminary work combining implants with brain-wave operated controls has been promising [11].

Clearly the future of health technology is a bright one, with many opportunities to enhance the quality of our lives. By working to personalize, distribute, and cheapen state of the art disease care – perhaps we may even succeed at emphasizing prevention and health! Shouldn't health care focus on health, after all?

References

[1] Older Americans 2000: Key Indicators of Well-Being ed. by Federal Interagency Forum On Aging Related Statistics. Report available on US Government Heath and Human Services website http://www.agingstats.gov

[2] Eisenberg, D.M., Davis, R.B., Ettner, S.L., Appel, S., Wilkey, S., Van Rompay. M., and Kessler, R.C., "Trends in alternative medicine use in the United States, 1990-1997: Results of a follow-up national survey ", Journal of the American Medical Association 280:1569-1575, 1998.

[3] Chronic Care In America: A 21st Century Challenge ed Ellen Freudenheim Robert Wood Johnson Foundation, 1996. http://www.rwjf.org

[4] Christiansen JR. Miller, Nash, Wiener, Hager & Carlsen, LLP, Health information technology and privacy: the legal perspective. MD Computing. 16(4):15-6, 1999

[5] Haugh R. Confronting HIPAA. Hospitals & Health Networks. 74(3):58-62, 64, 2000

[6] International Human Genome Consortium. The human genome. Nature. 409:860- 958,2001

[7] Venter, C. et al., The sequence of the human genome. Science. 291:1304-1351,2001

[8] Savinetti-Rose B. Bolmer L. Understanding continuous subcutaneous insulin infusion therapy. American Journal of Nursing. 97(3):42-8, 1997

[9] Teramae CY. Connolly HM. Grogan M. Miller FA Jr. Diet drug-related cardiac valve disease: the Mayo Clinic echocardiographic laboratory experience. Mayo Clinic Proceedings. 75(5):456-61, 2000

[10] Manderson, L., and Aaby, P., "An epidemic in the field? Rapid assessment procedures and health research" Social Science & Medicine 35:839-850,1992

[11] Barreto AB. Scargle SD. Adjouadi M. A practical EMG-based human-computer interface for users with motor disabilities. Journal of Rehabilitation Research & Development. 37:53-63, 2000

Advancing Medical Technologies

Future of Health Technology
R.G. Bushko (Ed.)
IOS Press, 2002

Future of Medical Knowledge Management and Decision Support

Robert A. Greenes, M.D., Ph.D.

Professor of Radiology and of Health Science & Technology, Harvard Medical School,
Professor of Health Policy & Management, Harvard School of Public Health &
Director, Decision Systems Group, Brigham and Women's Hospital, Boston, MA, US

Abstract and the hazards of prognostication

Attempts to predict the future are typically off the mark. Beyond the challenges of forecasting the stock market or the weather, dramatic instances of notoriously inaccurate prognostications have been those by the US patent office in the late 1800s about the future of inventions, by Thomas Watson in the 1930s about the market for large computers, and by Bill Gates in the early 1990s about the significance of the Internet. When one seeks to make predictions about health care, one finds that, beyond the usual uncertainties regarding the future, additional impediments to forecasting are the discontinuities introduced by advances in biomedical science and technology, the impact of information technology, and the reorganizations and realignments attending various approaches to health care delivery and finance. Changes in all three contributing areas themselves can be measured in "PSPYs", or paradigm shifts per year.

Despite these risks in forecasting, I believe that certain trends are sufficiently clear that I am willing to venture a few predictions. Further, the predictions I wish to make suggest a goal for the future that can be achieved, if we can align the prevailing political, financial, biomedical, and technical forces toward that end. Thus, in a sense this is a call to action, to shape the future rather than just let it happen. This chapter seeks to lay out the direction we are heading in knowledge management and decision support, and to delineate an information technology framework that appears desirable. I believe the framework to be discussed is of importance to the health care-related knowledge management and decision making activities of the consumer and patient, the health care provider, and health care delivery organizations and insurers. The approach is also relevant to the other dimensions of academic health care institution activities, notably the conduct of research and the processes of education and learning.

1. Information glut is not a good thing

We are not information-starved at present, but it may seem that way. Information comes in many forms, ranging from raw data to summaries of results, from narrative documents such as textbooks and journal article, to formal representations of knowledge, rules and guidelines encapsulating best practices, or automated decision support tools. The information focus may pertain to the domains of basic science, clinical practice, preventive medicine, public health, health services research, or a variety of specialized arenas.

The information sources are widely distributed, ranging from local repositories and programs on one's own desktop, to those within the local enterprise (hospital, university, practice networks), to national or international sites accessible via the Internet. Not only is this panoply of sources distributed, but it is heterogeneous in format, software platform, mode of access, and manner of representation or encoding of information. Even within local enterprise networks, multi-vendor platforms and incompatible protocols often complicate access.

Knowledge may be defined as that which results from the organization, analysis, or extrapolation of data to derive a higher level conceptualization of phenomena or processes. "Knowledge differs from data or information in that new knowledge may be created from existing knowledge using logical inference. If information is data plus meaning then knowledge is information plus processing" [1]. Knowledge can be either in human-readable form only, as are textbook and journal content, or capable of being executed in some fashion, as are the rules in knowledge bases of decision support tools.

With respect to knowledge resources, as with information more generally, we are inundated with so many alternatives that it is difficult to sift out those particular items that are most pertinent and of highest quality. Chaos reigns in the generation of health care-relevant knowledge – many producers, many variations in method, review, sponsorship, dissemination approach, and business models. The traditional publishing industry is in disarray [2], libraries are groping with new roles and missions [3], and Internet-based health knowledge providers are struggling to determine how to sustain and grow their activities [4]. The knowledge dissemination industries in the form of educational institutions are also facing upheavals, as virtual classrooms, distance learning, and other models of education are refined [5].

2. The problem-oriented paradigm as a coping strategy

Although potential users of information are faced with many modes of information access, providers, and types of information, they are typically driven by a single problem or task. They seek high quality information, but restricted to those items relevant for that problem or task. Where the information comes from is less important than its value for the task at hand. The information, in addition, is most useful if it can be made available immediately ("just-in-time"), in the context of the application that is being used for solving the problem or carrying out the task. Ideally, the information resources can be selected automatically based on specific data already known. Furthermore, among those resources selected, decision support tools can be primed with pre-existing data, can be used to update or collect additional targeted data, can implement recommendations, and can facilitate workflow.

My thesis is that problem-based information organization is a particularly useful coping strategy, when it is necessary to select pertinent items from a vast array of possibilities, especially when it is necessary to assemble different kinds of information at the same time.

Yet we note a marked contrast between the production and the use of information – its production is primarily *source-oriented*, whereas the use of it is primarily *problem-oriented* (Fig. 1). The production process can be considered to be the province of a set of vertical silos, those entities and services responsible for the creation and distribution of the information. Settings in which use occurs can be viewed as a horizontal set of cross-cutting planes corresponding to problems or tasks, which ideally intersect the silos at the precise points where information pertinent to the problems reside.

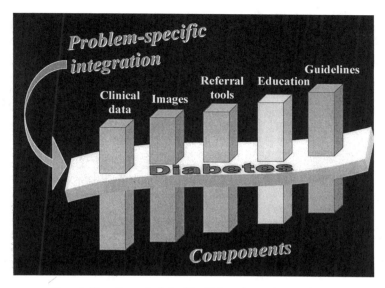

Figure 1. The orthogonal relationship of information producers and users.

In this chapter, we shall discuss a variety of settings in which problem-based organization of information is useful. We then focus on methodologies for providing the necessary infrastructure to support problem-based access and use.

3. Centrality of information needs in the academic health sciences university

The modern academic health sciences center has a combined mission of education, research, and service, where the latter includes both clinical and non-clinical activities. The academic health sciences are now experiencing the birth of many new fields, and the integration of previously separate disciplines, the growth of "big science" initiatives, and the establishment of physical and virtual collaborations spanning multiple disciplines, institutions, and geographic boundaries. As a result, both the opportunity and the necessity exist to rethink traditional approaches to development of an information infrastructure to support the activities of the academic health center.

Integration is the new byword, with most activities increasingly dependent on the information infrastructure. Among the new interdisciplinary and cross-cutting activities with such dependency are, for example: molecular imaging, telesurgery, robotics, nanotechnology, functional genomics, proteomics, drug development, health care or biomedical data warehousing, integrated delivery networks, consumer health, distance education, digital libraries, and networked clinical trials.

4. Health and health care information

4.1 The problem-oriented medical record

The problem-oriented medical record was introduced by Weed in the 1960s [6,7] as a strategy for clinical record keeping, which has at its core the notion that clinical observations (Subjective and Objective), Assessments, and Plans (together referred to as the SOAP note) should be organized by the problems to which they relate. This was proposed both as a means for focusing a clinician's thinking, when writing a progress note, making it easier to review a patient's progress by problem subsequently, and as a means to tie observations to assessments, and assessments to plans, thus enhancing the accountability of the record. Weed and his colleagues developed a computer-based multiple-choice problem-oriented data entry interface for generating the SOAP note for many of the problems in internal medicine, in the 1970s, although no published citations are available describing this ambitious work; the limited success of this project can be attributed in part to the primitiveness, by today's standards, of the user interface technology available at the time, rather than to a fundamental flaw in the concept. While the problem-oriented mode of record keeping has not been popular without use of a computer, many aficionados still do maintain their clinical records that way even manually [8]. With the ability to present the same data in multiple views, either by source (e.g., progress notes vs. labs vs. xrays vs. orders), by chronology, by specialist domain, or by problem, computer systems could today support problem-oriented record keeping more effectively.

Another advantage of a problem-oriented view of a patient's problems is that it allows one to focus on the other associated information resources that could be useful. This might include directories of specialists that might be appropriate for referral for that problem, bibliographic references or textbook materials, guidelines, appropriateness criteria, or other decision support resources for the physician, as well as educational materials or instructions for the patient. Thus delineation of a problem provides a framework for organizing a wide variety of information resources. We shall return to this notion later.

4.2 The Integrated Delivery Network (IDN)

The evolution of the health care environment has been a striking example of the need for integration of information from diverse sources, and focusing them on specific problems or tasks. We have seen a spate of mergers and affiliations in the mid-to-late 1990s, resulting in the formation of integrated delivery networks (IDNs) [9], motivated by the need for increased efficiency and decreased cost. Related goals have been the need to reduce redundancy yet attract referring physicians and patients with a full range of services, improvement in economies of scale by growth of market share and retention of patients and providers in the network, and increased clout for negotiation with payers.

Yet IDNs introduced a new level of complexity in health care, necessitating assimilation of multiple formerly independent hospitals, clinics, practices, and specialty services, each with their own cultures, modes of operation, and information systems. With respect to the latter, disparate electronic medical record systems might often be operating in the entities to be assimilated, along with incompatible information systems and different patient identification schemes. Clinical data and images must be communicated across these multiple systems.

Furthermore, because of the culture of fiscal restraint and cost-effectiveness, practices have been subjected to increasing scrutiny with respect to cost, quality, risk, appropriateness of services or referrals, and adherence to clinical practice guidelines and constraints. Thus, education and decision support must be provided across the IDN to reduce errors and increase safety, and to promote adherence to "best practices". Purely logistical functions become more complicated in an IDN, and help is needed for such tasks as getting oriented and navigating among resources, scheduling of services, finding and initiating consultations, requesting referrals, and learning about and obtaining transportation and parking. Communication support is needed across the network for email, teleconferencing, accessing support groups, obtaining consults, etc. Patient instructions need to be provided and home care services offered and coordinated.

Partners HealthCare System, Inc., the IDN formed in 1993 with the merger of the Brigham and Women's Hospital and Massachusetts General Hospital, plus affiliations and mergers of a number of smaller hospitals and practices in Eastern Massachusetts, provides an example. While parts of the information environment were quite sophisticated, such as the Brigham Integrated Computing System (BICS) [10] at the Brigham, there was no consistent system across the entire IDN.

As efforts were being devoted to beginning the integration of the clinical information systems environment, in 1995, the Decision Systems Group focused on a different problem for Partners HealthCare, that of creating and maintaining a Web site, called PartnerWeb, for the IDN's component health care delivery sites, including Massachusetts General Hospital and Brigham and Women's Hospital. Overall, more than 250 clinical, administrative, and research departments or divisions were producing content. This system, called PartnerWeb [11] was designed to make available information such as descriptions of departments and services, directories of specialists, seminars, educational programs, research activities, training programs, news and announcements, appointment requests, fund raising, and other functions.

Our goal was to have a consistent design for the site, to the extent possible, and to make it easy for these entities to contribute content, and to update their information, without requiring each to have their own Web staff, or to have a huge central Web development organization. The component-based design, one of the first of its kind for Web site management when it was initially developed in 1995, provided interfaces for authors and editors to tools for providing information about administration and organization, profiles of staff, descriptions of services, calendars of events, news items, publications, training programs, and other categories of content. Authors were organized into editing groups, each with an editor responsible, as determined by the department or division, and a hierarchical process was put into place for content development, review, edit and approval, and publication.

Separate form-based tools or components were used for each kind of content (Fig. 2). Components available to editing groups depended on the content domains and foci, and as various departments or divisions identified new requirements that we considered sufficiently generic, we expanded the range of form tools available. This approach provided a number of advantages, including a uniform look and feel, ease of changing the look without redesigning individual pages, the ability to select resources for presentation for specific problems or purposes, and reduction of the need for significant Webmaster services.

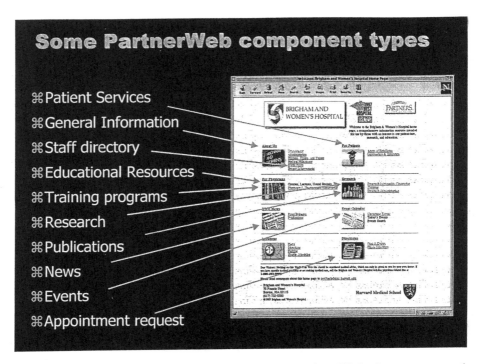

Figure 2. The earliest home page for PartnerWeb shows links to a variety of kinds of content resources, the content for each of which was managed by a different form tool editing component, and the Web display of which was generated dynamically from the component's database.

4.3 Data and knowledge needs of physicians

As noted earlier, a practitioner needs to assemble information that relates to a patient's specific problem, including past medical history, clinical findings, images, diagnoses, and medications, as well as order sets, formularies, lists of relevant specialists, knowledge resources (textbook and journal articles, appropriateness criteria, guidelines, and other decision aids), and instructions and materials to provide to the patient. Health care information systems typically provide each kind of information as a separate resource, or the user must use the Web to go outside of the health care system to find knowledge resources such as articles or decision aids for problems when they need such information. The organization of material is not generally done by problem, and dynamically made available at the point of need, except in some experimental settings.

The issue of sorting quality knowledge content from chaff faces the health professional. Believing that there is a business in providing this knowledge, and developing a relationship with the health professional, multiple entrants have been attracted to this market, with different production approaches and business models. The result is that these resources tend to be in silos reflecting the various producers – resources for journals, textbooks, news, guidelines, clinical trial directories, risk assessment tools, etc. The "dot coms" have epitomized the frenetic exploration of approaches to knowledge generation and delivery to both patients and providers; as the hard times in this sector have shown, identification of viable business models for these entities as alternatives to traditional publishers has still been elusive.

4.4 The health care consumer / patient

Patients or consumers seek information about symptoms, diseases, treatments, or procedures, as well as about healthy lifestyles and disease prevention. This may be in the form of textbook and magazine articles, discussion lists, chat groups or support groups, directories of services or providers, clinical trials databases, logistic information about a health care facility (directions to it, scheduling information, virtual tours, etc.), news items, interactive risk assessments, and other decision aids. Provision of information to this market has also been a broad area of activity in the dot.com sector, with a number of national sites offering content. Other national providers of content include disease-oriented societies (such as the American Diabetes Association or the American Cancer Society), and the government (MedlinePlus from the National Library of Medicine and HealthFinder from the Department of Health and Human Services, coordinated by the Office of Disease Prevention and Health Promotion.

For patients, information relevant to the problem should ideally be organized so as to focus the inquiry, foster easy navigation and pursuit of relevant subtopics, with in-depth exploration where needed, and identification of appropriate related topics. In addition, a feature lacking from most national information sources but being increasingly incorporated into portals associated with health care delivery organizations, is that information about a disease or problem should be coupled, when needed, with resources for follow up – including how to obtain care, from whom, how to schedule it, where to go, and how to get there.

Thus we believe the emphasis should be on "closing the loop", i.e., when a problem is identified, resources for its solution are made available, including the means for obtaining local follow up and care. This was the approach we pursued in a 1997 National Library of Medicine-funded contract to develop and evaluate HealthAware, a prototype resource for consumer health information [12,13]. Distinct from national health information sites, the aim of HealthAware was to provide both generic and locally developed content, through a portal to a health care delivery system, in this case that of Brigham and Women's Hospital, a participant in Partners HealthCare. The HealthAware system was built with the component-based, distributed authoring, dynamic page generation approach used in PartnerWeb, described above. It included in addition to generic content and locally developed materials, a number of tools for interactive risk assessments, finding a doctor for referral, appointment request, ask-a-doctor, chat groups, support groups, search, and problem-specific FAQs (Fig. 3). It was designed to link to resources of the IDN's Web site, such as the doctor directory of PartnerWeb, or its lists of educational seminars, its appointment request function, or "virtual tours" offered by some clinical services. Extensive usability testing and rewriting for appropriateness of literacy level went into the design.

Note that without an approach that links content to local resources, health care information is still readily obtainable, but the user must make all the links. National health information Web sites have largely provided content without local linkages; health care facilities are now seeking to provide health information portals on their Web sites that do a better job of local linkage (to build patient loyalty and to facilitate follow up), and the national sites are changing their business models to offer their content for use in this context through co-branding.

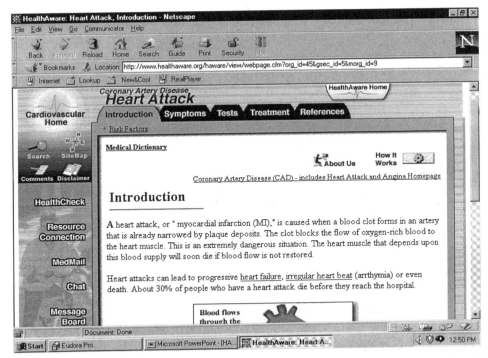

Figure 3. A screenshot from the heart attack topic home page in the cardiovascular disease section of HealthAware. This shows the visual layout into hierarchies of subtopics corresponding to horizontal tabs, plus various interactive tools arrayed along the left margin. In addition, the tools are integrated into the content at appropriate points. The content organization and tool-specific materials were developed through a component-based approach using a distributed authoring environment with editorial responsibility for editing groups.

While HealthAware was only a prototype, and covered only selected medical problem domains, further evolution of the Web strategy at Partners is now incorporating many of the features of the above systems plus others, aimed at providing access to an increased range of resources. Yet the problem still remains how to best organize information in a problem/context-specific way. This involves the development of various user interface paradigms and models of usage. Experimentation is being done for example, in how best to support clinical trial information access, data entry and interface to the EMR of the host environment; integration of clinical practice guidelines into primary care, particularly for chronic disease management.

5. Health Care Education

Problem-based learning has become a popular form of education of medical students, since the introduction of this approach at Harvard Medical School in the mid-1980s [14]. The approach is one in which realistic problem solving scenarios or simulated cases are presented, and the student must determine how to work up, assess, and treat the cases. Case materials are assembled that are relevant to a problem, and supporting references and related materials are provided, or must be found by the student. In so doing, a case becomes a springboard for discussing similar or contrasting conditions or related teaching points. Further, in contrast to the traditional lecture mode, the student learns how to find and assess appropriate information resources, as he or she would often need to do in actual practice, rather than simply memorizing facts, which quickly become outdated. This approach to learning of course also builds on the notion of the problem-based medical record, since the cases are focused on specific problems as instructional paradigms.

In educational contexts in general, not just those involving clinical medicine, it would be useful if study of a topic could be augmented by an information environment that could provide, among other things, such resources as: relevant lecture notes, visual materials, references, access to instructors or experts, access to fellow students, discussion boards, self-test questions, and perhaps databases and software tools for exploration. Ideally, these should be organized and accessible by topic or subtopic primarily, and only secondarily by source. Some Web products are now available that provide collaborative support for discussion groups, and for linking resources such as the above, to foster the establishment of instant communities of individuals pursuing a topic of common interest. A course represents such an instant community. Distance learning environments may find it useful to employ such tools to increase the interactivity and cross-fertilization of learning that is typically lost in non-classroom instruction.

In CME as well, we would like to have a curriculum that organizes resources in a problem-specific fashion. It should reflect one's specialty, the kinds of cases seen, the kinds of problems encountered, updates about recommended approaches, self-assessment questions, and other resources. In the classical study by Covell et al in 1985 [15], it was found that many questions arose in the course of an office clinical session for which answers would have been useful, although not readily available, not only for the immediate care of the patient, but also to enhance the physician's knowledge. What better time to provide such information than when the question is immediate and pertinent? Thus CME should be delivered in the context of care, and when impractical, should be associated with an offline curriculum that reflects the real-time context in which the questions occurred.

6. Multidisciplinary Research

We have discussed the birth of new fields and the development of others at the intersection of existing fields. Biomedical and health care research these days frequently involves many collaborators, multiple disciplines, and often multiple institutions. These areas of research share characteristics with many other fields, and we will not discuss the domains in detail here. The common element, though, appears to be the increase in complexity of many fields, and the need for organizing both access to information and to people.

Collaborative groups must form, often in "virtual space", and must be able to find each other, participate in discussion groups, and provide and access shared data and knowledge of common interest. This is particularly important as a means to break down geographic and disciplinary boundaries. Collaborative tools such as those discussed above for supporting education can also be used to support communities of researchers.

7. Group Collaborative Work

A common theme from the above discussions is that there is a dual requirement for supporting problem solving, whether it is in clinical medicine, education, and research. First, it is necessary to for relevant information resources to be available to the individual participant at the time of need. Secondly, the various human participants must often be able to be brought together around a focus of interest or problem. The problem definition in effect spawns an instant community of interest or affinity group. Early use of the Web was primarily aimed at enabling an individual to have access to multiple information resources. Now the focus is as much on bringing people as well as resources together. This will be important in further evolution of telemedicine for home/office doctor-patient interaction, for medical specialty consultation, for distance-based learning, for collaborative research, and for a large number of other problem solving activities that involve interactions of people as well as access to infromation.

8. Requirements for a Knowledge-Based Infrastructure

The essential challenge of enabling problem-based information access is to have an infrastructure and tools to reconcile the two disparate views of source-oriented producer/distributor and problem-based user of information resources. There are thus dual issues in achieving problem-specific selective access to relevant information resources:

(1) Components: the relevant resources, tools, and services to provide specific kinds of information must be available and identifiable.
(2) Integration methods: the knowledge models, workflow models, and interfaces with user environments must underlie applications, to be able to incorporate information resources at appropriate points.

8.1 Components

There are two primary issues involved in designing and providing component services that function as information sources:

1. *The services must be able to identify and characterize their information content, in terms of descriptive axes and terminologies that are known by and relevant to applications that will be accessing them.*

For the Web to be organized to provide information content as component services, we need to develop standards for encoding the types of information resources that a service contains, and to describe the domain/subdomains to which the information relates. Templates for each of these would need to be defined that provide detailed attributes relating to these, such as form of resource, language, encoding scheme, terminology scheme used, etc. Attributes that enable quality to be assessed should also ideally be standardized, such as sponsoring organization type, source of content, how validated, when updated, etc.

2. *Tools must be able to be located and access information resources.*

A variety of kinds of tools might be used for this purpose. The component services should have APIs that enable them to be queried with respect to their descriptive axes, and searched for particular resources. Further, the component services might be required to register themselves with respect to lookup services, such as provided in distributed object resource environments. The invocation of queries might be via agents, bots, search engines, or other mechanisms.

The coordination of the development of axes and taxonomies for indexing of information resources for specific domains and subdomains needs to be under the aegis of editorial boards, ideally convened by professional specialty organizations focused on those areas of endeavor. Besides their expertise in the areas, such editorial boards are probably in the best position to assess quality indicators.

8.2 Integration methods

Two kinds of capabilities must also exist to enable applications to integrate external information resources into problem-based contexts:

1. *The application must be able to provide a knowledge model that characterize its problem solving approach in terms of the types of information resources that would be useful, ideally identifying specific points in the process where they are most needed.*

For example, in a clinical encounter, the SOAP note in the problem-oriented paradigm has an implied knowledge model, in which identification of a problem determines what data elements (subjective and objective) are relevant. Once data elements have been recorded, their values should determine what assessments are appropriate. Having recorded the assessments, these choices should determine the appropriate plans for further workup or treatment. Thus there is an underlying guideline for management, with a set of rules that go from problem definition to data, from data to assessments, and from assessments to plans.

8.3 A role for guidelines

For clinical practice, we can therefore use clinical guidelines as a basis for creating the underlying knowledge framework. Associated information resources, such as the evidence for a particular decision or action, a dose calculation tool, or instructions for the patient regarding side effects of a medication or preparation for a forthcoming procedure, can be tied to particular steps in a guideline.

We have been carrying out considerable work in development of a sharable representation model for computer-interpretable clinical guidelines, called GLIF (GuideLine Interchange Format) [16,17]. Clinical guidelines are of interest for a number of reasons, primarily to encourage best practices and reduce unjustified practice variation. They can hopefully reduce medical errors [18] and encourage high quality care, and are ideally evidence-based. While guidelines have been produced for decades, and distributed in read-only form, in textbooks, journal and magazine articles, and more recently via CDROM and the Web, they are not typically sufficiently well structured to enable them to be directly executed. Not only are phrases inexact or vague, but logic is not always fully specified, and the medical data elements and actions referred to in decision steps or in recommendations are imprecise.

Computer-based guidelines are potentially useful in a wide variety of applications, including consultation, risk assessment, determination of appropriateness of a procedure or a referral, audit and quality review of care, automated alerts and reminders, the specification of the management protocol of a clinical trial, and in educational simulations.

We are pursuing the goal of trying to standardize the representation of computer-based guidelines, for the variety of applications described above. Because of the enormous effort involved in creating high quality, evidence-based guidelines, and the even greater effort in structuring them sufficiently to enable them to be automated, it would be useful if the representation were sharable. This is because additional adaptation and interfacing is needed to map authoritative guidelines to vendor-specific clinical platforms, to their EMRs, and to local constraints or preferences for medical practice, and to revise these adaptations, when the guideline is updated. GLIF development has been carried out by our group at Harvard, in conjunction with medical informatics groups at Stanford and Columbia, in a collaborative project known as InterMed, funded in part by the National Library of Medicine, the Department of the Army, and the Agency for Healthcare Research and Quality. Recently, the InterMed group initiated cooperation with the HL7 standards development organization, to establish a Clinical Guidelines Special Interest Group within HL7 to further pursue the definition and adoption of a standardized approach to computer-based guidelines (Fig.4).

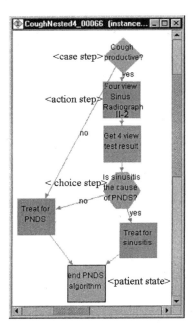

Figure 4. A GLIF-encoded guideline for evaluation of post-nasal drip syndrome (PNDS) as a cause for cough. Underlying the flow chart view for laying out or visualization is a formal representation, based on an object-oriented data model. [Courtesy of M. Peleg, Stanford University]

For the particular purpose described in this paper, that of providing a predictive framework for assembling information resources for a clinical encounter, guidelines appear promising as a basis for representing the knowledge, and our research group is pursuing this. This is particularly feasible for settings in which a patient's problem, and the stage of disease and treatment plan are known from the patient's EMR. Patients with chronic diseases, such as diabetes, hypertension, congestive heart failure, or asthma tend to have multiple clinical encounters over the course of their disease. Not only does the patient have a known problem, but he or she is typically in a particular state of evolution or management of that problem (which we term "clinical management state" or CMS) [19], for example, stable hypertension on beta blocker drug therapy with no comorbidities or complications. Patients tend to stay in a CMS for a period of time, further defining the framework for the clinical encounter, in terms of the data needed, likely assessments and plans, and other information resources that may be useful. Patients may transition to other CMSs, in which case the encounter is based on the new CMS.

The guideline structure for a CMS can be used to predict what data elements need to be retrieved from the EMR, what new data are required, what assessments are likely to be made (and whether they should be automatically triggered or suggested based on the data), the plans that are likely (again, possibly triggered, based on the various possible assessments), other information resources that may be useful, such as instructions or educational materials for the patient, and references, decision aids, and other materials for the provider.

For clinical care, therefore, a knowledge model can be constructed by combining (a) clinical management states identifying classes of patients, and (b) clinical guidelines for the decision making and process flow associated with the states. This framework enables information resources to be associated with classes of patients, and more finely with particular activities represented by guideline steps.

For other arenas of activity, such as education and research, other knowledge models and frameworks would of course be needed. To the extent that activities can be classified by a state model, and the decisions and process flow predicted by a guideline model, the above approach might be useful for them as well.

2. *An interface paradigm must exist for determining how to integrate external information resources into applications, in a form that is helpful to the user, facilitates workflow and task performance, and does not overwhelm.*

Given a knowledge model, we must determine how best to integrate the information access and decision support functions with the workflow and processes of the target application. For example, if the application is one for clinical encounter record keeping, a set of forms can be generated for data entry that are predicted by the guideline. Once data are entered, a set of forms for selecting appropriate assessments can be generated, with highlighted assessments corresponding to those predicted by the guideline based on values of the entered data. Subsequently, forms for entering plans and orders could be generated with highlighted plan/order elements based on the particular assessments that have been chosen. Information buttons can be associated with element for which there are corresponding information resources in the knowledge model (Fig. 5).

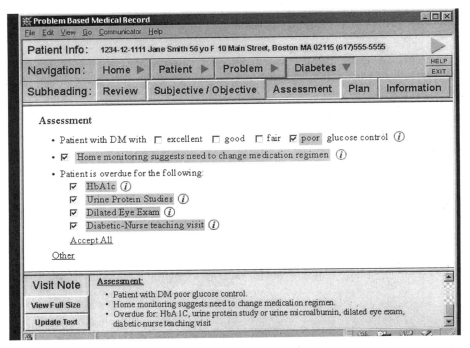

Figure 5. A prototype user interface for entering assessment into a progress note for a clinical encounter in a primary care setting for a patient with moderately well controlled diabetes. An underlying guideline suggests potential assessments by highlighting selections, based on data that have been entered or retrieved from the EMR about the patient's subjective and objective evaluation. The physician may inspect the rationale for highlighted suggestions, and if he or she agrees with them, can accept them with a single mouse click, thus potentially saving time.

A critical pathways/care plan application would use a guideline to extract pertinent data from the record to match against thresholds in the care plan model. An application that used guidelines to determine appropriateness of referrals or procedure orders might be integrated with the order entry or scheduling functions of the information system, such that a form requesting data determined by the guideline to be necessary for assessing appropriateness of the referral or order might be displayed, and explanations and other supporting documentation provided. Other clinical and non-clinical applications might integrate the knowledge in different ways, for which paradigms need to be determined.

9. Other Issues

Many other considerations are important with respect to development of an infrastructure to support knowledge management and decision making. For example, with respect to privacy and confidentiality of data, how should interactive decision support resources access and interact with local data? If the resources are accessed through an API to an external service, how is protection of patient data assured? Or must they be operated only as services internal to a health care institution? More fundamental issues relating to standardized encoding of medical data elements must be solved for generic services to be useful. Further, the data relating to outcomes need to be able to be pooled if we are to be able to do assessments of the decision support tools themselves. For that matter, where should "ownership" of the medical record reside? At present, there is essentially no such thing as a complete patient medical record – portions providing institution- or practice-specific records exist in various places. The whole record would need to somehow be a synthesis of all these disparate sources. This is exactly the reverse of the ideal paradigm, in which the record would exist *in toto* under the aegis of the patient or some trusted authority, and views of it could be obtained, upon authorization, by institutions or practitioners or the patient, based on a need for specific information; they would then in turn update the primary record with new information as it was obtained.

The "holy grail" of clinical knowledge management and decision support is a setting in which all patient data are encoded in structured form using standard terminology, and longitudinal records of all patients are maintained. Cross-sectional research that is appropriately monitored to comply with human research study requirements could be done on this corpus of data. In effect, this would enable every patient to become part of a clinical trial, since it would be possible to retrieve the aggregated experience of patients with similar findings, in order to determine the distribution of diagnoses, responses to therapies, and long term prognoses. Knowledge in this setting would be able to be dynamically derived from such collective experience. We are a long way from achieving this goal, but the essential first steps are to begin to organize problem solving tasks, identify and formalize the data elements required for them, and associate the appropriate decision aids and other knowledge resources with those tasks.

Acknowledgments

This work was supported in part Grant LM06594 with support from the Department of the Army, Agency for Healthcare Research and Quality, and the National Library of Medicine, and by contract N01 LM63539 from the National Library of Medicine.

References

[1] Free Online Dictionary of Computing, http://foldoc.doc.ic.ac.uk.
[2] Markovitz BP. Biomedicine's electronic publishing paradigm shift: copyright policy and PubMed Central. *J Am Med Inform Assoc.* 2000 May-Jun;7(3):222-229.
[3] Tannery NH, Wessel CB. Academic medical center libraries on the Web. *Bull Med Libr Assoc.* 1998 Oct;86(4):541-544.
[4] Rodgers RP. Searching for biomedical information on the World Wide Web. *J Med Pract Manage.* 2000 May-Jun;15(6):306-313.
[5] Curran VR, Hoekman T, Gulliver W, Landells I, Hatcher L. Web-based continuing medical education (I): field test of a hybrid computer-mediated instructional delivery system. *J Contin Educ Health Prof.* 2000 Spring;20(2):97-105.
[6] Weed LL. Medical records that guide and teach. *N Engl J Med.* 1968 Mar 21;278(12):652-657.
[7] Weed LL. The problem oriented record as a basic tool in medical education, patient care and clinical research. *Ann Clin Res.* 1971 Jun;3(3):131-134
[8] Salmon P, Rappaport A, Bainbridge M, Hayes G, Williams J. Taking the problem oriented medical record forward. *Proc AMIA Annu Fall Symp.* 1996;:463-467.
[9] Teich JM. Clinical information systems for integrated healthcare networks. *Proc AMIA Symp.* 1998;:19-28.
[10] Teich JM, Glaser JP, Beckley RF, Aranow M, Bates DW, Kuperman GJ, Ward ME, Spurr CD. The Brigham integrated computing system (BICS): advanced clinical systems in an academic hospital environment. *Int J Med Inf.* 1999 Jun;54(3):197-208.
[11] Karson TH, Perkins C, Dixon C, Ehresman JP, Mammone GL, Sato L, Schaffer JL, Greenes RA. The PartnerWeb Project: A component-based approach to enterprise-wide information integration and

dissemination. *Proc 1997 AMIA Annual Fall Symposium (formerly SCAMC),* Nashville, TN, October, 1997. Philadelphia: Hanley & Belfus. 1997; 359-363

[12] Kogan S, Ohno-Machado L, Boxwala AA et al. HealthAware: A consumer health information destination which links to a health care delivery network. *Proc 1999 AMIA Annual Fall Symposium,* Washington DC, 1999. Philadelphia: Hanley & Belfus. *JAMIA (suppl)* 1999;(1-2):1209.

[13] Greenes RA, Kogan S, Ohno-Machado L, Boxwala A. HealthAware: lessons learned in developing a consumer/patient information portal for a health care system. *Proc Telemedicine and Telecommunications: Options for the New Century.* Bethesda, MD, March, 2001.

[14] Peters AS, Greenberger-Rosovsky R, Crowder C, Block SD, Moore GT. Long-term outcomes of the New Pathway Program at Harvard Medical School: a randomized controlled trial. *Acad Med.* 2000 May;75(5):470-479.

[15] Covell DG, Uman GC, Manning PR. Information needs in office practice: are they being met? *Ann Intern Med.* 1985 Oct;103(4):596-599.

[16] Ohno-Machado L, Gennari JH, Murphy SN, et al. The guideline interchange format: a model for representing guidelines. *J Am Med Inform Assoc.* 1998;5:357-72.

[17] Peleg M, Boxwala AA, Ogunyemi O, Zeng Q, Tu S, Lacson R, Bernstam E, Ash N, Mork P, Ohno-Machado L, Shortliffe EH, Greenes RA. GLIF3: The evolution of a guideline representation format. *Proc AMIA Symp 2000.* Philadelphia: Hanley & Belfus. *JAMIA (suppl)* 2000; 7:645-649.

[18] Kohn LT, Corrigan JM, Donaldson MS. *To err is human: building a safer health system.* Institute of Medicine. National Academy Press, Washington, D.C.; 1999.

[19] Stoufflet PE, Ohno-Machado L, Deibel SRA, Lee D, Greenes RA. GEODE-CM: A state-transition framework for clinical management. *Proc 1996 AMIA Annual Fall Symposium (formerly SCAMC),* Washington, DC. October, 1996. Philadelphia: Hanley & Belfus. 1996; 924.

Future of Health Technology
R.G. Bushko (Ed.)
IOS Press, 2002

The Future of Nanofabrication and Molecular Scale Devices in Nanomedicine

Robert A. Freitas Jr.

Research Scientist, Zyvex Corp.

Abstract

Nanotechnology is engineering and manufacturing at the molecular scale, and the application of nanotechnology to medicine is called nanomedicine. Nanomedicine subsumes three mutually overlapping and progressively more powerful molecular technologies. First, nanoscale-structured materials and devices that can be fabricated today hold great promise for advanced diagnostics and biosensors, targeted drug delivery and smart drugs, and immunoisolation therapies. Second, biotechnology offers the benefits of molecular medicine via genomics, proteomics, and artificial engineered microbes. Third, in the longer term, molecular machine systems and medical nanorobots will allow instant pathogen diagnosis and extermination, chromosome replacement and individual cell surgery in vivo, and the efficient augmentation and improvement of natural physiological function. Current research is exploring the fabrication of designed nanostructures, nanoactuators and nanomotors, microscopic energy sources, and nanocomputers at the molecular scale, along with the means to assemble them into larger systems, economically and in great numbers.

1. Nanotechnology and Nanomedicine

"There is a growing sense in the scientific and technical community that we are about to enter a golden new era," announced Richard E. Smalley, winner of the 1996 Nobel Prize in Chemistry, in recent Congressional testimony [1]. On June 22, 1999, Smalley spoke in support of a new National Nanotechnology Initiative before the Subcommittee on Basic Research of the U.S. House Science Committee in Washington, DC. "We are about to be able to build things that work on the smallest possible length scales, atom by atom," Smalley said. "Over the past century we have learned about the workings of biological nanomachines to an incredible level of detail, and the benefits of this knowledge are beginning to be felt in medicine. In coming decades we will learn to modify and adapt this machinery to extend the quality and length of life." Smalley founded the Center for Nanoscale Science and Technology at Rice University in Texas in 1996. But he became personally interested in the medical applications of nanotechnology in 1999, after he was diagnosed with a type of non-Hodgkin's lymphoma (the same sort that killed King Hussein of Jordan). Smalley then endured an apparently successful course of chemotherapy that caused all the hair on his head to fall out.

"Twenty years ago," Smalley continued, "without even this crude chemotherapy I would already be dead. But twenty years from now, I am confident we will no longer have to use this blunt tool. By then, nanotechnology will have given us specially engineered drugs which are nanoscale cancer-seeking missiles, a molecular technology that specifically targets just the mutant cancer cells in the human body, and leaves everything else blissfully alone. To do this, these drug molecules will have to be big enough -- thousands of atoms -- so that we can code the information into them of where they should go and what they should kill. They will be examples of an exquisite, human-made nanotechnology of the future. I may not live to see it. But, with your help, I am confident it will happen. Cancer -- at least the type that I have -- will be a thing of the past."

The term "nanotechnology" generally refers to engineering and manufacturing at the molecular or nanometer length scale. (A nanometer is one-billionth of a meter, about the width of 6 bonded carbon atoms.) The field is experiencing an explosion of interest. Nanotechnology is so promising that the U.S. President, in his January 2000 State-of-the-Union speech, announced that he would seek $475 million for nanotechnology R&D via the National Nanotechnology Initiative, effectively doubling federal nanotech funding for FY2001. The President never referred to "nanotechnology" by name, but he gushed about its capabilities, marveling at a technology that will someday produce "molecular computers the size of a tear drop with the power of today's fastest supercomputers."

After the President's speech, Walter Finkelstein, president and CEO of NanoFab Inc. in Columbia, MD, agreed that it was conceivable that the technology could be used to develop computers chips so small that they could be injected into the bloodstream -- "Fantastic Voyage-like," he said -- to locate medical problems. In February 2000, John Hopcroft, dean of the College of Engineering at Cornell University, announced plans for a new 150,000-square-foot nanotechnology research center. The facility already has $12 million per year of earmarked funding and is expected to support 90 local jobs and approximately 110 graduate students. "The implications of this research are enormous," Hopcroft asserted, and include "the development of mechanical devices that can fight disease within the human body.

In May 2000, the National Cancer Institute signed an agreement with NASA, the U.S. space agency, to study the medical potential of nanoparticles. Nanoscience has also attracted the attention of the U.S. National Institutes of Health (NIH), which hosted one of the first nanotechnology and biomedicine conferences in June 2000. In July, the National Science Foundation (NSF) announced a Nanoscale Science and Engineering Initiative to provide an estimated $74 million in funding for nanotechnology research. Northwestern University in Evanston, Illinois will spend $30 million on a new nanofabrication facility of its own, joining existing operations such as the Stanford Nanofabrication Facility (started in 1985 with $15 million of backing from 20 industrial sponsors) and the Cornell Nanofabrication Facility, expected to attract 450 researchers in 2000, half of them visiting scientists. Cornell is spending $50 million on a new building for the Facility, and has just won a $20 million, five-year grant from the NSF to operate a new nanobiotechnology center which will make nanoscale tools available to biologists.

Burgeoning interest in the medical applications of nanotechnology has led to the emergence of a new field called nanomedicine [2, 3]. Most broadly, nanomedicine is the process of diagnosing, treating, and preventing disease and traumatic injury, of relieving pain, and of preserving and improving human health, using molecular tools and molecular knowledge of the human body.

It is most useful to regard the emerging field of nanomedicine as a set of three mutually overlapping and progressively more powerful technologies. First, in the relatively near term, nanomedicine can address many important medical problems by using nanoscale-structured materials that can be manufactured today. This includes the interaction of nanostructured materials with biological systems -- in June 2000, the first 12 Ph.D. candidates in "nanobiotechnology" began laboratory work at Cornell University. Second, over the next 5-10 years, biotechnology will make possible even more remarkable advances in molecular medicine and biobotics (microbiological robots), some of which are already on the drawing boards. Third, in the longer term, perhaps 10-20 years from today, the earliest molecular machine systems and nanorobots may join the medical armamentarium, finally giving physicians the most potent tools imaginable to conquer human disease, ill-health, and suffering.

2. Medical Nanomaterials

The initial medical applications of nanotechnology, using nanostructured materials, are already being tested in a wide variety of potential diagnostic and therapeutic areas.

2.1 Tagged Nanoparticles

For example, fluorescent tags are commonplace in medicine and biology, found in everything from HIV tests to experiments that image the inner functions of cells. But different dye molecules must be used for each color, color-matched lasers are needed to get each dye to fluoresce, and dye colors tend to bleed together and fade quickly after one use. "Quantum dot" nanocrystals have none of these shortcomings. These dots are tiny particles measuring only a few nanometers across, about the same size as a protein molecule or a short sequence of DNA. They come in a nearly unlimited palette of sharply-defined colors, can be excited to fluorescence with white light, and can be linked to biomolecules to form long-lived sensitive probes to identify specific compounds. They can track biological events by simultaneously tagging each biological component (e.g., different proteins or DNA sequences) with nanodots of a specific color.

Quantum Dot [4], the manufacturer, believes this kind of flexibility could offer a cheap and easy way to screen a blood sample for the presence of a number of different viruses at the same time. It could also give physicians a fast diagnostic tool to detect, say, the presence of a particular set of proteins that strongly indicates a person is having a heart attack. On the research front, the ability to simultaneously tag multiple biomolecules both on and inside cells could allow scientists to watch the complex cellular changes and events associated with disease, providing valuable clues for the development of future pharmaceuticals and therapeutics. In mid-2000, Genentech began evaluating the dots for commercial utility in a variety of cellular and molecular assays. A related technology called PEBBLES (Probes Encapsulated by Biologically Localized Embedding) [5], pioneered by Raoul Kopelman at the University of Michigan, allows dye-tagged nanoparticles to be inserted into living cells to monitor metabolism or disease conditions.

2.2 Artificial Molecular Receptors

Another early goal of nanomedicine is to study how biological molecular receptors work, and then to build artificial binding sites on a made-to-order basis to achieve specific medical results. Buddy D. Ratner at the University of Washington in Seattle has researched the engineering of polymer surfaces containing arrays of artificial receptors. In a recent series of experiments [6], Ratner and his colleagues used a new radiofrequency-plasma glow-discharge process to imprint a polysaccharide-like film with nanometer-sized pits in the shape of such biologically useful protein molecules as albumin (the most common blood protein), fibrinogen (a clotting protein), lysozyme and ribonuclease (two important enzymes), and immunoglobulin (antibodies). Each protein type sticks only to a pit with the shape of that protein. Ratner's engineered surfaces may be used for quick biochemical separations and assays, and in biosensors and chemosensors, because such surfaces will selectively adsorb from solution only the specific protein whose complementary shape has been imprinted, and only at the specific place on the surface where the shape is imprinted. The RESIST Group at the Welsh School of Pharmacy at Cardiff University [7] and others have looked at how molecularly imprinted polymers could be medically useful in clinical applications such as controlled drug release, drug monitoring devices, and biological and antibody receptor mimics.

2.3 Dendrimers

Dendrimers represent yet another nanostructured material that may soon find its way into medical therapeutics. Starburst dendrimers are tree-shaped synthetic molecules with a regular branching structure emanating outward from a core. Dendrimers form nanometer by nanometer, so the number of synthetic steps or "generations" dictates the exact size of the particles in a batch. Each molecule is typically a few nanometers wide but some have been constructed up to 30 nanometers wide, incorporating more than 100,000 atoms. The peripheral layer of the dendrimer particle can be made to form a dense field of molecular groups that serve as hooks for attaching other useful molecules, such as DNA, which hunker down amongst the outermost branches.

In 1998, James R. Baker Jr. co-founded the Center for Biologic Nanotechnology at the University of Michigan to bring together doctors, medical researchers, chemists and engineers to pursue the use of dendrimers as a safer and more effective genetic therapy agent [8]. For Baker, these nanostructures are attractive because they can sneak DNA into cells while avoiding triggering an immune response, unlike viral vectors commonly employed today for transfection. The dendrimer molecule is decorated with specific snippets of DNA, then injected into biological tissue. Upon encountering a living cell, dendrimers of a certain size trigger a process called endocytosis in which the cell's outermost membrane deforms into a tiny bubble, or vesicle. The vesicle encloses the dendrimer which is then admitted into the cell's interior. Once inside, the DNA is released and migrates to the nucleus where it becomes part of the cell's genome. The technique has been tested on a variety of mammalian cell types [9], and Baker hopes to begin clinical human trials of dendrimer gene therapy in 2001. Donald Tomalia, another co-founder of the Center for Biologic Nanotechnology, recently reported using glycodendrimer "nanodecoys" to trap and deactivate influenza virus particles [10]. The glycodendrimers present a surface that mimics the sialic acid groups normally found in the mammalian cell membrane, causing virus particles to adhere to the outer branches of the decoys instead of the natural cells.

2.4 Smart Drugs

Medical nanomaterials also may include "smart drugs" that become medically active only in specific circumstances. A good example is provided by Yoshihisa Suzuki at Kyoto University, who has designed a novel drug molecule that releases antibiotic only in the presence of an infection [11]. Suzuki started with the common antibiotic molecule gentamicin and bound it to a hydrogel using a newly developed peptide linker. The linker can be cleaved by a proteinase enzyme manufactured by Pseudomonas aeruginosa, a Gram-negative bacillus that causes inflammation and urinary tract infection, folliculitis, and otitis externa in humans. Tests on rats show that when the hydrogel is applied to a wound site, the antibiotic is not released if no P. aeruginosa bacteria are present. But if any bacteria of this type are present, then the proteolytic enzyme that the microbes naturally produce cleaves the linker and the gentamicin is released, killing the bacteria. "If the proteinase specific to each bacterium [species] can be used for the signal," writes Suzuki, "different spectra of antibiotics could be released from the same dressing material, depending on the strain of bacterium." This specificity of action is highly desirable because the indiscriminate prophylactic use of antibiotics is associated with the emergence of strains of drug-resistant bacteria, and most antibiotics apparently have at least some toxicity for human fibroblasts.

Immunotoxins are another class of smart drugs, in this case activating only in the presence of cancer cells. An immunotoxin molecule is an engineered hybrid of functional protein modules fabricated from two different types of proteins: a toxin and an antibody. Toxin proteins are normally produced and released by infectious bacteria. The protein binds to the surface of a host cell, penetrates it, and kills it. Toxin molecules are so potent that just a few of them can kill a cell. Antibodies are proteins produced by the immune system to recognize and bind to specific foreign materials. An immunotoxin molecule is made by fusing a part of the gene encoding a toxin with a part of the gene encoding an antibody that recognizes surface features on cancer cells. This creates a novel gene that can be used to express a new synthetic protein molecule. This new molecule will bind only to a cancer cell (via a module from the antibody protein), then penetrate it and kill it (via modules from the toxin protein). The first experiments with mice showed that these engineered proteins successfully eliminated certain tumors. Then early in 2000, National Cancer Institute researchers confirmed that an immunotoxin made from a truncated form of Pseudomonas exotoxin was cytotoxic to malignant B-cells taken from patients with hairy cell leukemia [12]. A second clinic trial at the Universitaet zu Koeln in Germany also found that a ricin-based immunotoxin had moderate efficacy against Hodgkin's lymphoma in some patients [13].

2.5 Nanopore Immunoisolation Devices

Mauro Ferrari, director of the Biomedical Engineering Center at Ohio State University and chairman of the BioMEMS Consortium on Medical Therapeutics, has created what could be considered one of the earliest therapeutically useful nanomedical devices [14]. Ferrari and his collaborators at the Biomedical Microdevices Center at the University of California at Berkeley employed bulk micromachining to fabricate tiny cell-containing chambers within single crystalline silicon wafers. The chambers interface with the surrounding biological environment through polycrystalline silicon filter membranes which are micromachined to present a high density of uniform nanopores as small as 20 nanometers in diameter. These pores are large enough to allow small molecules such as oxygen, glucose, and insulin to pass, but are small enough to impede the passage of much larger immune system molecules such as immunoglobulins and graft-borne virus particles. Safely ensconced behind this artificial barrier, immunoisolated encapsulated rat pancreatic cells may receive nutrients and remain healthy for weeks, happily secreting insulin back out through the pores, while the immune system remains blissfully unaware of the foreign cells which it would normally attack and reject.

Ferrari believes that microcapsules containing replacement islets of Langerhans cells -- most likely easily-harvested piglet islet cells -- could be implanted beneath the skin of some diabetes patients. This could temporarily restore the body's delicate glucose control feedback loop without the need for powerful immunosuppressants that can leave the patient at serious risk for infection. Supplying encapsulated new cells to the body could also be a valuable way to treat other enzyme or hormone deficiency diseases, including encapsulated neurons which could be implanted in the brain and then be electrically stimulated to release neurotransmitters, possibly as part of a future treatment for Alzheimer's or Parkinson's diseases.

2.6 Nanopore Sensors and DNA Sequencing

The flow of materials through nanopores can also be externally regulated. The first artificial voltage-gated molecular nanosieve was fabricated by Charles R. Martin and colleagues [15] at Colorado State University in 1995. Martin's membrane contains an array of cylindrical gold nanotubules with inside diameters as small as 1.6 nanometers. When the tubules are positively charged, positive ions are excluded and only negative ions are transported through the membrane. When the membrane receives a negative voltage, only positive ions can pass. Future similar nanodevices may combine voltage gating with pore size, shape, and charge constraints to achieve precise control of ion transport with significant molecular specificity. In 1997, an exquisitely sensitive ion channel switch biosensor was built by an Australian research group [16]. The scientists estimated that their sensor could detect a minute change in chemical concentration equivalent to a single sugar cube tossed into Sidney harbor, or roughly one part in a billion billion.

Daniel Branton at Harvard University has conducted an ongoing series of experiments using an electric field to drive a variety of RNA and DNA polymers through the central nanopore of an alpha-hemolysin protein channel mounted in a lipid bilayer similar to the outer membrane of a living cell [17]. As early as 1996, the researchers had determined that the individual nucleotides comprising the polynucleotide strands must be passing single-file through the 2.6 nanometer-wide nanopore, and that changes in ionic current could be used to measure polymer length. By 1998, Branton had shown that the nanopore could be used to rapidly discriminate between pyrimidine and purine segments (the two types of nucleotide bases) along a single RNA molecule. In 2000, the scientists demonstrated the ability to distinguish between DNA chains of similar length and composition that differ only in base pair sequence. A similar research effort at the University of California at Santa Cruz has produced nanopore devices with read rates potentially up to 1000 bases per second [18]. Because nanopores can rapidly discriminate and characterize DNA polymers at low copy number, future refinements of this experimental approach may eventually provide a low-cost high-throughput method for very rapid genome sequencing.

3. Biotechnology Devices

Biotechnology originally contemplated the application of biological systems and organisms to technical and industrial processes, but in recent times the field has expanded to include genetic engineering and the emerging fields of genomics, proteomics, transcriptomics, gene chips, artificial chromosomes, and even biobotics. Biotechnology now takes as its ultimate goal no less than the engineering of all biological systems, even completely designed organic living systems, using biological instrumentalities or "wet" nanotechnology. There are many good summaries of biotechnology elsewhere, so here we focus on efforts to engineer natural nanomachines to create new cellular devices.

During the 1990s, bioengineered viruses of various types and certain other vectors routinely were being used in experimental genetic therapies as "devices" to target and penetrate certain cell populations, with the objective of inserting therapeutic DNA sequences into the nuclei of human target cells in vivo. Retrovirally-altered lymphocytes (T cells) began to be injected into humans for therapeutic purposes. Another example was the use, by Neurotech (Paris), of genetically modified cerebral endothelial cell vectors to attack glioblastoma. This was the first therapeutic use of genetically engineered endothelial cells in humans; Phase I/II clinical studies were underway in 2000.

Engineered bacteria were also being pursued by Vion Pharmaceuticals in collaboration with Yale University. In their "Tumor Amplified Protein Expression

Therapy" program [19], antibiotic-sensitive Salmonella typhimurium (food poisoning) bacteria were attenuated by removing the genes that produce purines vital to bacterial growth. The tamed strain could not survive very long in healthy tissue, but quickly multiplied 1000-fold inside tumors which are rich in purines. The engineered bacteria were available in multiple serotypes to avoid potential immune response in the host, and Phase I human clinical trials were underway in 2000 using clinical dosages. The next step would be to add genes to the bacterium to produce anticancer proteins that can shrink tumors, or to modify the bacteria to deliver various enzymes, genes, or prodrugs for tumor cell growth regulation.

In 1998, Glen Evans, then at the University of Texas Southwestern Medical Center, described the possible construction of synthetic genomes and artificial organisms. His proposed strategy involved determining or designing the DNA sequence for the genome, synthesizing and assembling the genome, then introducing the synthetic DNA into an enucleated pluripotent host cell to create an artificial organism. Genome engineers could modify an existing microbe by adding a biochemical pathway borrowed from other organisms, though this remains a difficult task because tailoring an existing system to match unique requirements demands detailed knowledge about the pathway. But ultimately, says Adam P. Arkin at Lawrence Berkeley National Laboratory, "we want to learn to program cells the same way we program computers." Some genome engineers have started by building the biological equivalent of the most basic switch in a computer -- a digital flip-flop. "Cells switch genes on and off all the time," observes MIT's Thomas F. Knight, Jr., who has pioneered some of this research. A cellular toggle switch, made of DNA and some well-characterized regulatory proteins, might be devised to turn on a specific gene when exposed to a particular chemical. These could be used in gene therapies -- implanted genes might be controlled with single doses of specially selected drugs, one to switch the gene on, another to switch it off.

Arcady Mushegian of Akkadix Corp. [20] has looked at the genes present in the genomes of fully sequenced microbes to see which ones are always conserved in nature. He concludes that as few as 300 genes are all that may be required for life, constituting the minimum possible genome for a functional microbe. An organism containing this minimal gene set would be able to perform the dozen or so functions required for life -- manufacturing cellular biomolecules, generating energy, repairing damage, transporting salts and other molecules, responding to environmental chemical cues, and replicating. The minimal microbe -- a basic cellular chassis -- could be specified by a genome only 150,000 nucleotides bases in length. Glen Evans, now at Egea BioSciences, can already produce made-to-order DNA strands that are 10,000 nucleotide bases in length [21] and is striving to increase this length by at least a factor of ten. The engineered full-genome DNA, once synthesized, would then be placed inside an empty cell membrane -- most likely a living cell from which the nuclear material had been removed. These artificial biobots could be designed to produce useful vitamins, hormones, enzymes or cytokines in which the patient's body was deficient, or to selectively absorb and metabolize into harmless endproducts harmful substances such as poisons, toxins, or indigestible intracellular detritis, or even to perform useful mechanical tasks.

Besides their direct medical applications, biobots might be employed in molecular construction. Gerald J. Sussman at MIT notes that when computer parts are reduced to the size of single molecules, engineered microbes could be directed to lay down complex electronic circuits. "Bacteria are like little workhorses for nanotechnology; they're wonderful at manipulating things in the chemical and ultramicroscopic worlds," he says. "You could train them to become electricians and plumbers, hire them with sugar and harness them to build structures for you."

4. Medical Nanorobotics

The third major branch of nanomedicine -- molecular nanotechnology (MNT) or nanorobotics [2, 22] -- takes as its purview the engineering of all complex mechanical medical systems constructed from the molecular level. Just as biotechnology extends the range and efficacy of treatment options available from nanomaterials, the advent of molecular nanotechnology will again expand enormously the effectiveness, comfort and speed of future medical treatments while at the same time significantly reducing their risk, cost, and invasiveness. MNT will allow doctors to perform direct in vivo surgery on individual human cells.

4.1 Early Thinking

The first and most famous scientist to voice these possibilities was the late Nobel physicist Richard P. Feynman, who worked on the Manhattan Project at Los Alamos during World War II and later taught at CalTech for most of his professorial career. In his remarkably prescient 1959 talk "There's Plenty of Room at the Bottom," Feynman proposed employing machine tools to make smaller machine tools, these to be used in turn to make still smaller machine tools, and so on all the way down to the atomic level [23]. Feynman prophetically concluded that this is "a development which I think cannot be avoided." Such nanomachine tools, nanorobots and nanodevices could ultimately be used to develop a wide range of atomically precise microscopic instrumentation and manufacturing tools -- that is, nanotechnology.

Feynman was clearly aware of the potential medical applications of the new technology he was proposing. After discussing his ideas with a colleague, Feynman offered [23] the first known proposal for a nanomedical procedure to cure heart disease: "A friend of mine (Albert R. Hibbs) suggests a very interesting possibility for relatively small machines. He says that, although it is a very wild idea, it would be interesting in surgery if you could swallow the surgeon. You put the mechanical surgeon inside the blood vessel and it goes into the heart and looks around. (Of course the information has to be fed out.) It finds out which valve is the faulty one and takes a little knife and slices it out. Other small machines might be permanently incorporated in the body to assist some inadequately functioning organ." Later in his historic lecture in 1959, Feynman urged us to consider the possibility, in connection with biological cells, "that we can manufacture an object that maneuvers at that level!"

Extending nanomedicine to molecular machine systems will probably require, among many other things, the ability to build precise structures, actuators and motors that operate at the molecular level, thus enabling manipulation and locomotion. For example, in 1992 K. Eric Drexler of the Institute for Molecular Manufacturing theorized that an efficient nanomechanical bearing could be made by bending two graphite sheets into cylinders of different diameters, then inserting the smaller one into the larger one [22]. By 2000, John Cumings and Alex Zettl at U.C. Berkeley had demonstrated experimentally that nested carbon nanotubes do indeed make exceptionally low-friction nanobearings [24].

4.2 DNA-Based Nanodevices

But early mechanical nanorobots might be made, at least in part, of DNA. The idea of using DNA to build nanoscale objects has been pioneered by Nadrian Seeman at New York University [25]. Two decades ago, Seeman recognized that a strand of DNA has many advantages as a construction material. First, it is a relatively stiff polymer. Its intermolecular interaction with other strands can be readily predicted and programmed due to the base-pair complementarity of nucleotides, the fundamental building blocks of genetic material. DNA also tends to self-assemble. Arbitrary sequences are readily manufactured using conventional biotechnological techniques, and DNA is readily manipulated and modified by a large number of enzymes. During the 1980s, Seeman worked to develop strands of DNA that would zip themselves up into more and more complex shapes -- first tiny squares, then three-dimensional stick-figure cubes comprised of 480 nucleotides each, then a truncated octahedron containing 2550 nucleotides. By the mid-1990s, Seeman could fabricate nanoscale DNA stick figures of almost any regular geometric shape, by the billions per batch.

In 1999, Seeman reported yet another breakthrough -- the construction of a mechanical DNA-based device that might serve as the basis for a nanoscale robotic actuator [26]. The mechanism has two rigid double-stranded DNA arms a few nanometers long that can be made to rotate between fixed positions by introducing a positively charged cobalt compound into the solution surrounding the molecules, causing the bridge region to be converted from the normal B-DNA structure to the unusual Z-DNA structure. The free ends of the arms shift position by 2-6 nanometers during this fully reversible structural conversion, like a hinge opening and closing. "It's a very simple nanomachine," admits Seeman, "but in the scheme of molecular devices it's huge because it generates more than four times the amount of movement produced by typical molecular devices." A large version of the device might function as an elbow, while smaller devices could serve as finger joints.

Bernard Yurke at Bell Laboratories and Andrew Turberfield at the University of Oxford synthesized another DNA actuator using three single strands of artificial DNA which, when placed together, find their complementary partners and self-assemble to form a V-shaped structure [27]. The open mouth of this nanotweezer can be made to close by adding a special "fuel" strand which binds to the single-stranded DNA dangling from the ends of the arms of the tweezers and zips them closed. A special "removal" strand, when added, binds to the fuel strand and pulls it away, opening the nanotweezers again. The cycle may then be repeated.

4.3 Nanotweezers

In 1999, Philip Kim and Charles Lieber at Harvard University created the first general-purpose nanotweezer [28]. Its working end is a pair of electrically controlled carbon nanotubes made from a bundle of multiwalled carbon nanotubes. To operate the tweezers, a voltage is applied across the electrodes, causing one nanotube arm to develop a positive electrostatic charge and the other to develop a negative charge. The attractive force can be increased or decreased by varying the applied voltage -- 8.5 volts completely closes the arms, while lower voltages give different degrees of grip. Using the tool, Kim and Lieber have successfully grasped 500-nanometer clusters of polystyrene spheres, about the same size scale as cellular substructures. They were also able to remove a semiconductor wire 20 nanometers wide from a mass of entangled wires. At present, each of the tweezer's arms is about 50 nanometers wide and 4 microns long. But by growing single-walled nanotubes directly onto the electrodes, the researchers hope to produce nanotweezers small enough to grab individual macromolecules.

4.4 Nanomotors

Other researchers are developing nanomotors for future nanorobots. Most notably, Carlo Montemagno at Cornell University has modified a natural biomotor to incorporate nonbiological parts, creating the first artificial hybrid nanomotor [29]. Montemagno started with natural ATPase, a ubiquitous enzyme found in virtually every living organism and which helps to convert food into usable energy in living cells. The moving part of an ATPase molecule is a central protein shaft (or rotor, in electric-motor terms) that rotates in response to electrochemical reactions with each of the molecule's three proton channels (comparable to the electromagnets in the stator coil of an electric motor). ATP (adenosine triphosphate) is the fuel that powers the molecular motor's motion.

Using the tools of genetic engineering, Montemagno added metal-binding amino acid residues to the ATPase. This allowed each motor molecule to bind tightly to nanoscale nickel pedestals prepared by electron beam lithography. Properly oriented motor molecules 12 nanometers in diameter were then attached to the pedestals with a precision approaching 15 nanometers, and a silicon nitride bar a hundred nanometers long was bound to the rotor subunit of each motor molecule, all by self-assembly. In a microscopic video presentation, dozens of bars could be seen spinning like a field of tiny propellers. The group's first integrated molecular motor ran for 40 minutes at 3-4 revolutions per second. Subsequent motors have been operated for hours continuously by feeding them plenty of ATP. Montemagno has been measuring things like horsepower and motor efficiency, simple tests that would be familiar to any mechanical engineer inspecting a car engine. Montemagno is also trying to build a solar-powered, biomolecular motor-driven autonomous nanodevice, wherein light energy is converted into ATP which then serves as a fuel source for the motor. "We think we'll be able to make autonomous devices that are powered by light on a scale of 1 micron or less, smaller than bacteria," he says.

Montemagno is developing a chemical means of switching his hybrid motors on and off reliably. By engineering a secondary binding site tailored to a cell's signalling cascade, he plans to use the sensory system of the living cell to control nanodevices implanted within the cell. Montemagno envisions tiny chemical factories operating inside living cells. He speculates that these nanofactories could be targeted to specific cells, such as those of tumors, where they would synthesize and deliver chemotherapy agents. Within three years he expects to have a motor assembled within a living cell, with the cell's physiology providing the energy to run it. "My 10-year goal is to make a device that harvests single molecules within a living cell, maybe a cellular pharmacy that produces a drug, stores it within the cell, and then based upon some signal, releases it," Montemagno said in 2000. "For a technology that wasn't expected to produce a useful device before the year 2050, I think we've made a pretty good start. But we have a long way to go before it's safe to turn these little machines loose in the human body."

Nanomotor research is progressing in other laboratories as well. For instance, a 78-atom chemically-powered rotating motor was synthesized in 1999 as a proof of principle by chemist T. Ross Kelly at Boston College [30]. Ben Feringa at the University of Groningen in the Netherlands has built an artificial 58-atom motor molecule that spins when illuminated by solar energy [31]. Another potential nanorobot power source is a modified microbial fuel cell -- laboratory demonstrations of such cells contain captive bacteria or immobilized enzymes [32] which, when fed organic material, convert chemical energy into electricity that could be used to power tiny motors.

4.5 Nanocomputers

Truly effective medical nanorobots may require onboard computers to allow a physician to properly monitor and control their work. Molecular electronics or "moletronics" is a hot research topic in nanotechnology right now. For example, in 2000, a collaborative effort between UCLA and Hewlett Packard produced the first laboratory demonstration of completely reversible room-temperature molecular switches that could be employed in nanoscale memories, using mechanically interlinked ring molecules called catenanes [33].

Two independent companies -- Molecular Electronics Corp. in Texas and California Molecular Electronics Corp. in California -- have sprung up with the explicit goal of building the first commercial molecular electronic devices including memories and other computational components of computers, possibly in the next few years, using techniques of self-assembly.

4.6 Positional Assembly

As machine structures become more complex, getting all the parts to spontaneously self-assemble in the right sequence will be increasingly difficult. To build such complex structures, it makes more sense to design a mechanism that can assemble a molecular structure by what is called positional assembly -- that is, picking and placing molecular parts exactly where you want them. A device capable of positional assembly would work much like the robot arms that manufacture cars on automobile assembly lines in Detroit, or which insert electronic components onto computer circuit boards with blinding speed in Silicon Valley. Using the positional assembly approach, the robot manipulator picks up a part, moves it to the workpiece, installs it, then repeats the procedure over and over with many different parts until the final product is fully assembled.

One of the leading proponents of positional assembly at the molecular scale is Zyvex Corp., a privately-held nanotechnology research and development corporation headquartered in Richardson, Texas [34]. Zyvex is the first engineering company with the explicit goal of creating a molecular assembler that uses positional assembly to manufacture atomically precise structures. As a first step toward this goal, in 1998 Zyvex demonstrated the ability to use three independently-controlled inch-long robotic arms to manipulate tiny carbon nanotubes in three dimensions, under the watchful eye of a scanning electron microscope that can monitor objects and motions as small as 6 nanometers at near-video scan rates. Zyvex still has a very long way to go before it can assemble nanoscale parts into useful machines, but its work is a small step in the right direction and the research continues today. Zyvex engineers are also conceiving and testing various manufacturing architectures that may someday enable massively parallel, or exponential, construction of large batches of identical molecular machines simultaneously. This might allow vast numbers of nanodevices -- ultimately including medical nanorobots -- to be produced relatively inexpensively and to molecular specifications.

4.7 Nanomedical Diagnosis and Treatment

The idea of placing autonomous self-powered nanorobots inside of us might seem a bit odd, but actually the human body already teems with such nanodevices. For instance, more than 40 trillion single-celled microbes swim through our colon, outnumbering our tissue cells almost ten to one. Many bacteria move by whipping around a tiny tail, or flagellum, that is driven by a 30-nanometer biological ionic nanomotor powered by pH differences between the inside and the outside of the bacterial cell. Our bodies also maintain a population of more than a trillion motile biological nanodevices called fibroblasts and white cells such as neutrophils and lymphocytes, each measuring perhaps 10 microns in size. These beneficial natural nanorobots are constantly crawling around inside of us, repairing damaged tissues, attacking invading microbes, and gathering up foreign particles and transporting them to various organs for disposal from the body.

The greatest power of nanomedicine will emerge in a decade or two when we learn to design and construct complete artificial nanorobots using nanometer-scale parts and subsystems including sensors, motors, manipulators, power plants, and molecular computers. If we make the reasonable assumption that we will someday be able to build these complex medical nanorobots, and build them cheaply enough and in sufficiently large numbers to be useful therapeutically, then what are the medical implications? We have space here to describe only a few of the many possibilities [2, 35-38].

One thing that would change dramatically is clinical diagnostics and treatment. Consider a patient who goes to his doctor with a mild fever, nasal congestion, discomfort, and cough. In the nanomedical era, taking and analyzing microbial samples will be as quick and convenient as the electronic measurement of body temperature using a tympanic thermometer in a late 20th-century clinical office or hospital. The physician faces the patient and pulls from her pocket a lightweight handheld device resembling a pocket calculator. She unsnaps a self-sterilizing cordless pencil-sized probe from the side of the device and inserts the business end of the probe into the patient's opened mouth in the manner of a tongue depressor. The ramifying probe tip contains billions of nanoscale molecular assay receptors mounted on hundreds of self-guiding retractile stalks. Each assay receptor is sensitive to the chemical signature of one of thousands of specific bacterial coats or viral capsids.

The patient says "Ahh," [35] and a few seconds later a three-dimensional color-coded map of the throat area appears on a display panel held in the doctor's hand. A bright spot on the screen marks the exact location where the first samples are being taken. Underneath the color map scrolls a continuously updated microflora count, listing in the leftmost column the names of the ten most numerous microbial and viral species that have been detected, key biochemical marker codes in the middle column, and measured population counts in the right column. The number counts flip up and down a bit as the physician directs probe stalks to various locations in the pharynx to obtain a representative sampling, with special attention to sores or exudate. After a few more seconds, the data for two of the bacterial species suddenly highlight in red, indicating the distinctive molecular signatures of specific toxins or pathological variants. One of these two species is a known, and unwelcome, bacterial pathogen. The diagnosis is completed and the infectious microbe is promptly exterminated using a patient-inhaled aerosol of mobile nanorobots which the physician has programmed to seek out and destroy that one microbial strain. After a few minutes the nanorobots have finished their work and are retrieved by the doctor. A resurvey with the diagnostic probe reveals no evidence of the pathogen.

4.8 Improved Human Abilities

Another major change that nanomedicine will bring is the ability to dramatically extend natural human capabilities. As a simple example, a few years ago I designed an artificial mechanical red cell called a "respirocyte" [36]. Still entirely theoretical, the respirocyte measures 1 micron in diameter and just floats along in the bloodstream. It is a spherical nanorobot made of 18 billion atoms precisely arranged in a diamondoid structure to make a tiny pressure tank that can be pumped full of up to 9 billion oxygen (O_2) and carbon dioxide (CO_2) molecules. Later on, these gases can be released from the tank in a controlled manner using tiny molecular pumps. Gases are stored onboard at pressures up to about 1000 atmospheres.

Respirocytes mimic the action of the natural hemoglobin-filled red blood cells. Gas concentration sensors on the outside of each device let the nanorobot know when it is time to load O_2 and unload CO_2 (at the lungs), or vice versa (at the tissues). Each respirocyte can store and transport 236 times as much gas per unit volume as a natural red cell. So the injection of a 5 cc therapeutic dose of 50% respirocyte saline suspension, a total of 5 trillion individual nanorobots, into the human bloodstream can exactly replace the gas carrying capacity of the patient's entire 5.4 liters of blood. But up to 1 liter of respirocyte suspension could safely be added to the bloodstream, which could keep a patient's tissues safely oxygenated for up to 4 hours in the event a heart attack caused the heart to stop beating. Or it would enable a healthy person to sit quietly at the bottom of a swimming pool for four hours, holding his breath, or to sprint at top speed for at least 15 minutes without breathing.

Similarly, an artificial mechanical platelet or "clottocyte" [37] could make possible complete hemostasis in just 1 second, even for moderately large wounds, a response time 100-1000 times faster than the natural system. The basic clottocyte is conceived as a serum oxygen/glucose-powered spherical nanorobot, 2 microns in diameter, that contains a compactly-folded fiber mesh. Upon command from its control computer, the device unfurls its mesh packet in the vicinity of an injured blood vessel -- following, say, a cut through the skin. Soluble thin films coating certain parts of the mesh dissolve upon contact with plasma water, revealing sticky sections (e.g., complementary to blood group antigens unique to red cell surfaces) in desired patterns. Blood cells are immediately trapped in the overlapping artificial nettings released by multiple neighboring activated clottocytes, and bleeding halts at once. While up to 300 natural platelets might be broken and still be insufficient to initiate a self-perpetuating clotting cascade, even a single clottocyte, upon reliably detecting a blood vessel break, can rapidly communicate this fact to its neighboring devices [2], immediately triggering a progressive carefully-controlled mesh-release cascade. Clottocytes may perform a clotting function that is equivalent in its essentials to that performed by biological platelets, but at only 0.01% of the bloodstream concentration of those cells or about 20 nanorobots per cubic millimeter of serum. Hence clottocytes appear to be about 10,000 times more effective as clotting agents than an equal volume of natural platelets.

4.9 Chromosome Replacement Therapy

Medical nanorobots will also be able to intervene at the cellular level, performing in vivo cytosurgery. The most likely site of pathological function in the cell is the nucleus -- more specifically, the chromosomes. In one simple cytosurgical procedure, a nanorobot controlled by a physician would extract existing chromosomes from a diseased cell and insert new ones in their place. This is called chromosome replacement therapy. The replacement chromosomes will be manufactured to order, outside of the patient's body in a laboratory benchtop production device that includes a molecular assembly line, using the patient's individual genome as the blueprint. The replacement chromosomes are appropriately demethylated, thus expressing only the appropriate exons that are active in the cell type to which the nanorobot has been targeted. If the patient chooses, inherited defective genes could be replaced with nondefective base-pair sequences, permanently curing a genetic disease. Given the speed with which nanorobots can be administered and their potential rapidity of action, it is possible that an entire whole-body procedure could be completed in one hour or less. Robert Austin at Princeton University has also begun early thinking along these lines, hoping someday to design a nanoprobe capable of identifying biological markers that are specific for targeted diseases. "Then you just pop open the cells, remove the bad DNA from that cell, and repair it on a single-cell level," he says. "That's a long way down the road, but it will happen."

In the first half of the 21st century, nanomedicine should eliminate virtually all common diseases of the 20th century, and virtually all medical pain [38] and suffering as well. Only conditions that involve a permanent loss of personality and memory information in the brain -- such as an advanced case of Alzheimer's disease or a massive head trauma -- may remain incurable in the nanomedical era. Because aging is believed to be the result of a number of interrelated molecular processes and malfunctions in cells, and because cellular malfunctions will be largely reversible, middle-aged and older people who gain access to an advanced nanomedicine can expect to have most of their youthful health and beauty restored. And they may find few remaining limits to human longevity in this wonderfully vigorous state. It is a bright future that lies ahead for medicine, but we shall all have to work very long and very hard to bring it to fruition.

References

[1] U.S. House Testimony of Richard E. Smalley, 22 June 1999; http://www.house.gov/science/smalley_062299.htm.
[2] Robert A. Freitas Jr., Nanomedicine, Volume I: Basic Capabilities, Landes Bioscience, Georgetown, TX, 1999; http://www.nanomedicine.com.
[3] Robert A. Freitas Jr., "The Nanomedicine Page"; http://www.foresight.org/Nanomedicine/index.html.
[4] Quantum Dot Corporation; http://www.qdots.com/.
[5] H.A. Clark, R. Kopelman, R. Tjalkens, M.A. Philbert, "Optical nanosensors for chemical analysis inside single living cells. 2. Sensors for pH and calcium and the intracellular application of PEBBLE sensors," Anal. Chem. 71(1 November 1999):4837-4843.
[6] H. Shi, B.D. Ratner, "Template recognition of protein-imprinted polymer surfaces," J. Biomed. Mater. Res. 49(January 2000):1-11.
[7] C.J. Allender, C. Richardson, B. Woodhouse, C.M. Heard, K.R. Brain, "Pharmaceutical applications for molecularly imprinted polymers," Int. J. Pharm. 195(15 February 2000):39-43.
[8] J.F. Kukowska-Latallo, A.U. Bielinska, J. Johnson, R. Spindler, D.A. Tomalia, J.R. Baker, Jr., "Efficient transfer of genetic material into mammalian cells using Starburst polyamidoamine dendrimers," Proc. Natl. Acad. Sci. (USA) 93(14 May 1996):4897-4902.
[9] J.F. Kukowska-Latallo, E. Raczka, A. Quintana, C. Chen, M. Rymaszewski, J.R. Baker, Jr., "Intravascular and endobronchial DNA delivery to murine lung tissue using a novel, nonviral vector," Hum. Gene Ther. 11(1 July 2000):1385-1395.
[10] J.D. Reuter, A. Myc, M.M. Hayes, Z. Gan, R. Roy, D. Qin, R. Yin, L.T. Piehler, R. Esfand, D.A. Tomalia, J.R. Baker, Jr., "Inhibition of viral adhesion and infection by sialic-acid-conjugated dendritic polymers," Bioconjug. Chem. 10(March-April 1999):271-278.
[11] Y. Suzuki, M. Tanihara, Y. Nishimura, K. Suzuki, Y. Kakimaru, Y. Shimizu, "A new drug delivery system with controlled release of antibiotic only in the presence of infection," J. Biomed. Mater. Res. 42(October 1998):112-116.
[12] D.H. Robbins, I. Margulies, M. Stetler-Stevenson, R.J. Kreitman, "Hairy cell leukemia, a B-cell neoplasm that is particularly sensitive to the cytotoxic effect of anti-Tac(Fv)-PE38 (LMB-2)," Clin. Cancer Res. 6(February 2000):693-700.
[13] R. Schnell, E. Vitetta, J. Schindler, P. Borchmann, S. Barth, V. Ghetie, K. Hell, S. Drillich, V. Diehl, A. Engert, "Treatment of refractory Hodgkin's lymphoma patients with an anti-CD ricin A-chain immunotoxin," Leukemia 14(January 2000):129-135.
[14] T.A. Desai, W.H. Chu, J.K. Tu, G.M. Beattie, A. Hayek, M. Ferrari, "Microfabricated immunoisolating biocapsules," Biotechnol. Bioeng. 57(5 January 1998):118-120.
[15] Matsuhiko Nishizawa, Vinod P. Menon, Charles R. Martin, "Metal nanotubule membranes with electrochemically switchable ion-transport selectivity," Science 268(5 May 1995):700-702.
[16] B. Cornell, V. Braach-Maksvytis, L. King, P. Osman, B. Raguse, L. Wieczorek, R. Pace, "A biosensor that uses ion-channel switches," Nature 387(5 June 1997):580-583
[17] A. Meller, L. Nivon, E. Brandin, J. Golovchenko, D. Branton, "Rapid nanopore discrimination between single polynucleotide molecules," Proc. Natl. Acad. Sci. (USA) 97(1 February 2000):1079-1084.
[18] D.W. Deamer, M. Akeson, "Nanopores and nucleic acids: prospects for ultrarapid sequencing," Trends Biotechnol. 18(April 2000):147-151.
[19] D. Bermudes, B. Low, J. Pawelek, "Tumor-targeted Salmonella. Highly selective delivery vectors," Adv. Exp. Med. Biol. 465(2000):57-63.
[20] A.R. Mushegian, "The minimal genome concept," Curr. Opin. Genet. Dev. 9(December 1999):709-714.
[21] "Researchers build huge DNA chains," BBC, 27 January 2000; http://www.crystalinks.com/biology5.1.html.
[22] K. Eric Drexler, Nanosystems: Molecular Machinery, Manufacturing, and Computation, John Wiley & Sons, New York, 1992.
[23] R.P. Feynman, "There's Plenty of Room at the Bottom," Engineering and Science (California Institute of Technology), February 1960, pp. 22-36. See at: http://nano.xerox.com/nanotech/feynman.html.
[24] John Cumings, A. Zettl, "Low-Friction Nanoscale Linear Bearing Realized from Multiwall Carbon Nanotubes," Science 289(28 July 2000):602-604.

[25] N.C. Seeman, "DNA engineering and its application to nanotechnology," Trends Biotechnol. 17(November 1999):437-443.

[26] C. Mao, W. Sun, Z. Shen, N.C. Seeman, "A nanomechanical device based on the B-Z transition of DNA," Nature 397(14 January 1999):144-146.

[27] B. Yurke, A.J. Turberfield, A.P. Mills, Jr., F.C. Simmel, J.L. Neumann, "A DNA-fuelled molecular machine made of DNA," Nature 406(10 August 2000):605-608.

[28] P. Kim, C.M. Lieber, "Nanotube Nanotweezers," Science 286(10 December 1999):2148-2150.

[29] C.D. Montemagno, G.D. Bachand, "Constructing nanomechanical devices powered by biomolecular motors," Nanotechnology 10(1999):225-231; G.D. Bachand, C.D. Montemagno, "Constructing organic/inorganic NEMS devices powered by biomolecular motors," Biomedical Microdevices 2(2000):179-184.

[30] T.R. Kelly, H. De Silva, R.A. Silva, "Unidirectional rotary motion in a molecular system," Nature 401(9 September 1999):150-152.

[31] N. Koumura, R.W. Zijlstra, R.A. van Delden, N. Harada, B.L. Feringa, "Light-driven monodirectional molecular rotor," Nature 401(9 September 1999):152-155.

[32] S. Sasaki, I. Karube, "The development of microfabricated biocatalytic fuel cells," Trends Biotechnol. 17(February 1999):50-52.

[33] C.P. Collier, G. Mattersteig, E.W. Wong, Y. Luo, K. Beverly, J. Sampaio, F.M. Raymo, J.F. Stoddart, J.R. Heath, "A [2]Catenane-based solid state electronically reconfigurable switch," Science 289(18 August 2000):1172-1175.

[34] Zyvex Corporation; http://www.zyvex.com.

[35] Robert A. Freitas Jr., "Say Ah!" The Sciences 40(July/August 2000):26-31; http://www.foresight.org/Nanomedicine/SayAh/index.html.

[36] Robert A. Freitas Jr., "Exploratory Design in Medical Nanotechnology: A Mechanical Artificial Red Cell," Artificial Cells, Blood Substitutes, and Immobil. Biotech. 26(1998):411-430; http://www.foresight.org/Nanomedicine/Respirocytes.html.

[37] Robert A. Freitas Jr., "Clottocytes: Artificial Mechanical Platelets," Foresight Update No. 41, 30 June 2000, pp. 9-11; http://www.imm.org/Reports/Rep018.html.

[38] Robert A. Freitas Jr., "Nanodentistry," J. Amer. Dent. Assoc. 131(November 2000):1559-1566.

Future of Health Technology
R.G. Bushko (Ed.)
IOS Press, 2002

Thought to Computer Communication

Kevin Warwick

Professor of Cybernetics, Department of Cybernetics, University of Reading, UK

Abstract

This paper describes some of the implant experimentation presently underway. The basic approach taken is introduced and general techniques are explained. Achievements already attained are summarized and short term plans are expanded. Potential results, as they could impact on healthcare and related issues, are thrown into the arena. The author speculates 'a little' on what might be achieved in the future with implant technology.

1. Introduction

Let's start with a few basics. Humans are, for the most part, successful at being humans. As Homo Sapiens we have though been around for only 100,000 years or so, which is a very brief time span in comparison with many other creatures. Just as Big Macs relate to gourmet food so humans relate to life on earth. But the moving hand of evolution points to the future. Some creatures adapt, surviving or even becoming more successful, those that don't will, almost surely, die out. Even the Big Mac, as we know it now, will not last for ever.

It is possible that humans will slowly change, to utilize more effectively the technical world we are creating. The consequences of not adapting at all are potentially horrific. Could we really end up with machines, far more intelligent than ourselves, becoming the dominant 'life' form on earth? An alternative is for humans to e-volve, to technically upgrade the human form by linking much more closely humans with technology. In science fiction terms this means we will become Cyborgs – part human, part machine.

But what sort of an upgrade are we looking at for humans? It may be that spare arms and legs become the order of the day, but unless we are all going to become Inspector Gadget look alikes, with corkscrew fingers and propeller heads, it is difficult to see where this will get us. No, clearly it is not a physical upgrade where the rewards are greatest, it is a mental one. In fact healthcare problem number one in this new technological world, in that most physical aspects of the human body are rapidly becoming redundant. Some people, as a result, become obese, whilst others take regular, enforced, exercise. What is to be done with physical bodies that are no longer required to perform as they used to, yet are living much longer is indeed a pertinent question. But I will not attempt to answer it here.

Even though humans have been in their way, fairly successful on earth, we are extremely limited in what we can do and how we perform. Clearly we have physical limitations. In the last few centuries in particular we have employed technology to improve our capabilities. So we can lift heavy loads, dig tunnels, accurately and rapidly repeat a mundane task, communicate instantly around the world and fly.

Technology has also been used to improve our senses. Basically we are limited to 5 senses only. However technology gives us indirect information on such as x-rays, infrared or ultrasonic signals; often by converting them to visual images we can understand. Perhaps most important of all, humans have evolved to understand the world around us in terms of only 3 dimensions. (Sometimes even less than that). Whilst computers can understand the world in many (almost infinite) dimensions, it is questionable whether we have yet made much use of this capability at all.

But what are the possibilities for humans to be upgraded to cyborgs to take on board some of these abilities? Could it be possible for ourselves, in cyborg form, to understand the world in many dimensions, by linking our human brain directly with a computer brain? Could we then directly tap into the phenomenal math and memory performance of the computer. What's the use of the human brain remembering things or learning math when the computer brain can do those tasks much better? Whilst human brains will, on their own, evolve relatively slowly, perhaps by gradually expanding over generations; could it be possible for us to bring about a form of designer evolution by connecting computer brains, with near-infinite potential, to our own.

Our senses also might be directly upgraded. Is it possible, for example, for us to take on board x-ray, infrared and ultrasonic signals? Could these be fed directly to our brains? What then would the world feel and look like to a cyborg who senses it also in terms of ultra violet and ultrasonic signals, and comprehends it in 8-dimensions? Surely this would completely change our understanding of the world; what we believe to be possible and what not.

2. Self-Experimentation

In the fall of 1998 I had a silicon chip transponder surgically implanted in my left arm, with this in position the main computer in the Cybernetics building at the University of Reading was able to monitor my movements. Essentially at various doorways large coils of wire within the door frame provided a low power radio frequency signal which energized the small coil within the transponder. This in turn provided an electric current enabling the transponder's silicon chips to transmit a unique signal to the computer, identifying me.

Signals were, in this way, transmitted to/from the computer and inside my body. To demonstrate some of the capabilities, a voice box by the entrance welcomed my arrival each morning with "Hello Professor Warwick", the door to my lab opened as I approached and the computer was aware of what time I entered a room and when I left. It switched on lights for me, automatically, as appropriate. The experiment having been a success, 9 days after its insertion, the implant was removed.

Since that time we have been working on the next step of our research program, a new implant. The operation to put it in position is tentatively scheduled for

September2001, almost exactly 3 years after the previous experiment. Once again the target area is my left arm, just above the elbow. This time however a direct connection will be made with the nerve fibers running up the center of my arm. Electronic signals on the nerve fibers will be picked up and transmitted to a computer, rather like tapping into a telephone conversation. Signals will though also be received from the computer, and played down onto the nervous fibers.

The nerve fibers in the upper arm link the brain to the hand and they carry a variety of signals. In one direction signals from the brain cause movement and dexterity in the hand, whilst in the opposite direction sensory data from touch or pressure is passed. Also apparent are a number of body state signals concerned with temperature, blood flow and the like, along with physical emotional signals such as anger, shock and excitement. Signals relating to pain are also sent via this route. So at any instant in time the nerve fibers carry a very mixed collection. Some people might regard many signals as noise, but this is not really the case at all, as every signal is important. This said, if you are investigating movement then signals relating to anger or pain could be deemed to be noise as they do not directly relate to the study at hand. One thing is apparent however and that is, in the upper arm the nerve fibers are rather like a Freeway in that most of them directly link the brain and hand, with very few turn offs. It is therefore a good place to investigate a nervous system implant if, as a scientist, you are not yet ready to have one positioned in your brain.

Apart from a direct connection onto the nervous fibers, the implant will contain a transmitter, a receiver and some local signal processing and conditioning. The implant will merely be providing an interface between the nervous fibers and the computer, it will not be carrying out any signal understanding itself.

We wish to look at a range of signals. Firstly a series of movement experiments will be conducted. The signals which cause particular fingers to move will be recorded in the computer and then played back again in an attempt to recreate the movement as closely as possible. Secondly signals from an ultrasonic sensor will be directly played down onto the fibers and I will visually learn when objects are close by and when not, thereby relating visually to the signals on my nervous system. We will see if I can directly sense objects close by. Hopefully the movement experiments will contribute to research in that area whilst extrasensory signals could be immediately useful as an alternative sense for people who are blind.

Then come experiments more into the unknown. Pain, anger and shock signals will all be stimulated as much as possible and recorded on the computer, even excitement. The relevant signals will then be played back down again onto the nervous fibers. Will my brain indicate any of the original feelings? This is what we wish to find out. Could it be possible to initiate the feeling of pain electronically? If so perhaps we can send in equalizing signals instead, to counteract the effects of pain in an individual. Can we electronically cause excitement, happiness and so on? If so we are looking at the potential world of e-medicine.

3. Communication

As long as the experiments go well with my implant in place, my wife Irena will join me by having her own implant. What we wish to look at then is communication from one person's nervous system to the other. Potentially across the internet. So the signals from my own nervous system will be played down onto Irena's nervous system and nice versa. Both implants will be positioned at roughly the same point in our upper left arms.

Obviously movement signals will be of interest. When I move my left index finger and the electronic signals that achieve that are played down onto Irena's nervous system, will it achieve anything like the same movement in her hand? When she feels pain in one finger, due perhaps to excessive pressure, will I feel the same sort of pain? Indeed is it roughly the same in men and women? If she gets excited (as in the presence of an attractive young man), what will I feel when the associated signals appear on my nervous system?

We hope to have time to look at phobias and fears. Irena is extremely frightened of spiders. I would like to experience those feelings, to an extent at least. I am scared of being high up in a building. Can we arrange for one of us to be in the UK and the other in the USA – perhaps I can be in the Empire State Building. What will Irena feel when signals from my own nervous system in that situation appear on hers, as she is sitting quietly?

Clearly these experiments are only a start of person to person communication by means of direct nervous system signaling. At this stage we have very little idea as to how far we will be able to take it. Could it be possible in the future, with implants directly positioned in the brain to communicate in the same sort of way. Could we send our thoughts to a computer? Could we think to each other? Could we communicate by thought signals alone? Obviously we will not be able to go that far with our own next experiment. It will be merely a step on the way.

4. Medicine

It is worth remembering that the human brain is an electrochemical entity. In the western world we have, till now, largely concerned ourselves with the chemical aspects of the brain. Chemicals are employed for a number of reasons – to ease a headache, to prevent pregnancy, to help get to sleep or, in the case of coffee, to help wake us up and perform better in examinations. Could anything like the same sort of effects be realized, fairly easily, electronically? If so the potential for e-medicine is enormous. Perhaps electronic signals could be used to provide a viable alternative to cigarettes, without some of the side effects. Indeed electronic signals have already been successfully used to combat the effects of both Parkinson's disease and Alzheimer's disease.

We must however remain rather wary in opening up this field. Just as electronic signals might potentially be used for their positive medicinal effects, they might similarly be used for individuals to get high on a daily, electronic pick-me-up? The field of cybernetics is perhaps just around the corner.

5. Supporting Cases

Much research work is being carried out presently by various research groups around the world which directly supports and influences our own work. For example as recently as 1997 a group at the University of Tokyo attracted a microprocessor directly to the motor neurons of a cockroach, which carried the computing power around as a back pack. Signals from the microprocessor were then used to drive the cockroach around in a planned route. No matter what the cockroach might have itself wanted.

Meanwhile in 1999 it was reported that John Chapin at the MCP Hahnemann School of Medicine in Philadelphia and Miguel Nicolelis at Duke University had implanted electrodes into rats' brains. Initially the rats were taught to pull a lever in order to get a ratty treat. However the implants were positioned such that the rats merely had to think about pulling the lever and these signals, when transmitted to the computer, were enough to cause the treat to be electronically released. Interestingly the rats soon learned that they didn't have to actually pull the lever, merely thinking about it was sufficient. As far as humans are concerned, several groups are experimenting with computers linked to the nervous system. Ross Davis' team at the Neural Engineering Clinic in Augusta, Maine have been developing technology to attempt to treat patients whose central nervous system has been damaged by an accident or a disease such as multiple sclerosis. They have obtained excellent results in regaining muscle control by means of computer generated (as opposed to brain generated) signals.

Perhaps the most stunning research so far though is that carried out by Philip Kennedy and his team at Emory University in Atlanta. There they have implanted an electrode directly into the brain of a paralyzed war veteran, Johnny Ray. He is paralyzed from the neck down and hence cannot control or move any part of his body below that point. A functional MRI scan was used to detect brain activity when Johnny was asked to think about moving his arms and hands. The implant was positioned in an area of the brain seen to be active under such circumstance.

With the implant in place Johnny was able to move a cursor around on a computer screen thereby spelling out words and constructing sentences, merely by thinking about it. The electronic signals in his brain which relate to thoughts, about certain movements, are transmitted to the computer by a radio signal in a similar way to our own implants. What is incredible though is that not only can Johnny, in this way, communicate by means of his thoughts alone but also that his working brain has actually readjusted to its newly found power. His own neurons have grown into, and strengthened the link with, the implant.

6. Cybernetics

All of this research is very much at the heart of what cybernetics (a term originated by Norbert Wiener of MIT) is all about: humans and technology acting together as an overall system. One key element of this is consideration of the human brain as just another, albeit extremely important, physical organ in the human body. The human brain has no magical properties over and above its physical working. A brain's consciousness is merely a function of its operation, it is not some remote entity that exists elsewhere in the ether. Thoughts are merely as a result of particular states of the brain, dependant on a set of electrochemical signals in the brain at that time.

On average a human brain has, something like, 100 billion individual cells. It is a complex network, each cell connecting with thousands of others to produce its own operation. It is extremely difficult, at the present time, to unravel and hope to fully understand its actual operation. It is certainly not a parallel processing device however.

The range of capabilities of, and intelligence associated with, humans is dependent on our brain cells and the way they are connected together. However if we enable implants to link our brain directly with a computer then anything that computer can connect to could potentially operate for us. Not only could doors open and lights switch on automatically, as they did even for my first implant, but we might be able to drive a car or fly a plane merely by thinking about it. I feel that once some rudimentary trials have been carried out we would rapidly learn how to expand our abilities and operate the whole system more effectively.

But communicating from brain to computer and ultimately from human brain to human brain, in terms of thought signals alone opens up new questions. Why would we need to speak? Will language and the culture as we now know it, disappear completely or will it still have a small role to play, perhaps in the development of babies. As humans evolve to this new level so telephones become obsolete. If we communicate by thoughts perhaps we will become less open and learn to control our feelings and emotions more. Indeed a simple evolutionary step would suggest that those who could better control their feelings might be more likely to succeed in the new world.

7. Immediate Uses

Implant technology does though offer some more immediate potential uses. Dependent on the position of an implant, certain body states can be measured, or inferred, e.g. blood pressure, temperature and pulse. The relevant values can then be transmitted to a computer which gives an overall conditional indicator. Whilst this could be useful for athletes and other sports people, it would have a direct impact in patients undergoing constant monitoring. In these cases electrodes repeatedly placed on the skin surface can cause deep sores and much bleeding after a while. The implant alternative is, I feel, worthy of investigation.

But the real potential appears when brain implants are considered. Computer based machines are rapidly becoming more intelligent, perhaps in a complementary way to humans. Linking a human brain to such technology, creating a cyborg seems to be a natural way ahead, simply upgrading the human form. In most cases though the computer brain would not be operating in stand alone, but rather would be part of a network, with mixed intelligence and capabilities. The question then needs to be asked as to how the human fits into that. In that way a cyborg would not be an individual but would themselves be a node on the network. Away from the network your capabilities are limited to the poor performance of humans, connected into the network and you are merely part of a considerably greater whole.

With my first implant it did not take long before I mentally considered the implant to be part of my body, part of me. However the computer was linked to the implant, hence it was linked to me. We were not separate, yet complemented each other. When the implant was removed, on the one hand I felt relieved that any potential medical problems, such as infection, were behind me, however I also felt that I had lost a friend, in that myself and the computer were not longer an item!

With the new implant including a nervous system connection, such feelings of affinity can only get stronger. When brain links are involved they will be stronger still. As a cyborg would you have the same morals and ethics as those of a human? I would think not. Sure the cyborg started in human form and hence human values probably play a part, however I would guess that as a cyborg it would be cyborg morals and ethics that would be in evidence.

8. The Future

We must be careful as we investigate further into the use of implants. Until now they have been mainly for helping out something in the human body that is not functioning correctly, as is the case with a heart pacemaker or a cochlea implant. However implants in general open up the possibility of giving humans extra capabilities. In the short term this may mean we can think about repairing, to a certain extent at least, a nervous system break, and hence get people moving again. Possibly we'll also be able to bring about extra senses and apply complex electronic signals to help both physical and mental illnesses.

When we link human brains and computer brains together though, we are going a stage further. By creating such mental cyborgs we are doing something more. We will change the basic nature of ourselves. We will give ourselves much more powerful means of communication, and the ability to think about problems in many dimensions. Those without an implant, i.e. those that remain as mere humans, will become very sorry individuals unable to compete. They will, roughly speaking, occupy the position that chimpanzees are in today.

If you were to ask me whether I would wish myself to go for the unknown and unchartered cyborg future, I do not have to think twice to answer. No way, under any circumstances do I want to belong to a chimpanzee-like sub species. It's a cyborg life for me.

Acknowledgement

The author wishes to thank Nortel Networks and Computer Associates for their financial assistance. He also wishes to thank the staff of Stoke Mandeville Hospital, Aylesbury, UK – it is only through their expertise that this is becoming a reality.

I would also like to acknowledge the input of the team at Reading, in particular Brian Andrews, William Harwin and Mark Gasson. Finally my sincere thanks go to Ali Jamous from Stoke Mandeville Hospital for his medical expertise.

References and further reading

[1] S. Greenfield, 'The Private Life of the Brain' Penguin 2000
[2] S. Griffiths (ed)., 'Predictions'. Oxford University Press, 1999
[3] A.Scammell (ed.)., 'I in the Sky', Aslib Press, 1999
[4] K. Warwick, 'In the Mind of the Machine', Arrow, 1998
[5] K. Warwick, 'Cybernetic Organisms – Our Future?', Proc. IEEE, Vol. 87, No. 2, pp 387-389, 1999.
[6] K. Warwick, 'Cyborg 1.0', Wired, Vol. 8, No. 2, pp. 144-151, Feb. 2000
[7] K. Warwick, 'QI: The Quest for Intelligence', Piatkus, 2000.
[8] N. Wiener, 'God and Golem Incorporated' Chapman & Hall, 1964

Future of Health Technology
R.G. Bushko (Ed.)
IOS Press, 2002

Affective Medicine: Technology with Emotional Intelligence

Rosalind W. Picard, Ph.D.

*Director, Affective Computing Research Group, Massachusetts Institute of Technology
Media Laboratory, Cambridge, MA, US*

Abstract

For a long time people have kept emotions out of the deliberate tools of medicine and science; scientists, physicians, and patients have often felt and sometimes expressed emotion, but no tools could sense, measure, and respond to their affective information. A series of recent studies indicates that emotions, particularly stress, anger, and depression, are important factors with serious and significant implications for health. This paper highlights research at the MIT Media Lab aimed at giving computers the ability to comfortably sense, recognize, and respond to certain aspects of human emotion, especially affective states such as frustration, confusion, interest, stress, anger, and joy. Examples of recently developed systems are shown, including computer systems that are wearable and computers that respond to people with a kind of active listening, empathy, and sympathy. Results are reported for computer recognition of emotion, for teaching affective skills to autistics, and for having computers help users manage emotions such as frustration.

1. Introduction: Frustration, Irritation, Stress and Health

Perhaps the most common emotions people feel in interacting with today's technology are frustration, irritation and other feelings related to stress. We've been doing experiments in our lab where we bring in people, give them a task on the computer that mildly or strongly frustrates them, and measure how they behave. Our aim is to try to teach the computer how to recognize when the user is frustrated, irritated, annoyed, stressed or otherwise in some significant emotional state, and then to equip the computer so that it can do a better job of serving people, ideally not causing them so much stress. It's recently become a joke in the lab when some piece of equipment fails or causes aggravation – "is this one of Picard's affective computing experiments designed to irritate me?"

What could technology do if it could sense that the user is frustrated or otherwise in some unusual emotional state? Could the system change or be changed, so as to reduce frustration in the future, or could it help the user then and there to feel less stress? Our research has focused on both approaches: identifying components of computer interfaces that could be improved by designers, as well as having the computer help users manage strong negative emotions better. This is all part of our effort in "affective computing," computing that relates to, arises from, or deliberately influences emotion [18]. This article will focus the topic further -- on some recent findings about emotion and medicine -- together with examples of new affective technology we are developing that has potentially interesting and important implications for health.

Stress is increasingly recognized as a medical problem. A recent Blue Cross Blue Shield survey in New England cited the number one health concern of members in this part of the United States to be stress – rated above cancer, AIDS, high blood pressure, and other medical conditions. Dan Goleman, in Chapter 11 of his book Emotional Intelligence [7], cites a number of studies pointing to important roles in health and medicine for emotions – particularly states of stress, anxiety, chronic anger, and depression. Following are just a few of the examples that he includes:

Stress/distress: Studies of the physical manifestations of stress reveal many measurable changes caused by stress in the human body, influencing not only immune system functioning but also heart rate variability, blood pressure, and other important bodily functions. Several studies have been conducted examining the impact of stress on immunity. For example, Sheldon Cohen, a psychologist at Carnegie-Mellon University exposed people to a cold virus after assessing how much stress they were experiencing in their lives. Of course, a robust immune system usually resists a virus, so mere exposure doesn't mean you will get sick. Cohen found that 27% of the low-stress subjects came down with a cold while 47% of the high-stress people came down with the cold. In another study of married couples who kept daily logs of hassles and upsetting events, a strong pattern emerged: three or four days after an especially intense marital fight or other upset, they came down with a cold or upper-respiratory infection.

Depression: In work cited by James Strain, where 100 patients received bone marrow transplants, a follow-up study was conducted of the 13 who had been depressed vs. the other 87. Of the 13 who had depression, only 1 was alive a year later; of the other 87, 34 were still alive two years later. Another study, by Howard Burton et al., associated early death of dialysis patients with depression: depression was found to be a stronger predictor of death than any medical sign. Similarly, heightened risk of death from heart disease has been correlated with an ongoing sense of despair and hopelessness. The effect of depression on heart attack survivors is as great as that of major medical risks such as left ventricular dysfunction or a history of previous heart attacks.

Anger: Dr. Redford Williams at Duke University found that physicians who scored highest on tests of hostility while they were in medical school were seven times as likely to have died by the age of fifty as those who scored low on the hostility tests – their tendency to get angry was found to be a stronger predictor of early death than were factors such as high blood pressure, high cholesterol, and smoking. Findings by Dr. John Barefoot at the University of North Carolina show that scores on a test of hostility correlate with the extent and severity of coronary artery disease in heart patients undergoing angiography.

The studies above are but a few of the many that reveal emotion to be a measurably important health factor. Note that none of the studies show that emotions *cause* medical illness – rather they contribute to decreases in immune system functioning and to other physical factors that may significantly prolong or exacerbate an illness. It is foolish to

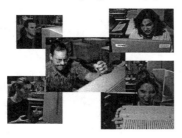

frustration, irritation, ...STRESS

- Number 1 health concern
- links found between immune system cells and nervous system and hormone system..field of psychoneuroimmunology (PNI)
- people with chronic anxiety, depression, hostility, ...were found to have double the risk of disease (see Chap 11 of Goleman's Emotional Intelligence)

Figure 1. Stress is a significant factor in health; it arises in many forms when interacting with technology.

think that "positive thinking" or "making yourself happy" can prevent all illness; it is also foolish to continue to think that emotions have no significant effect on health – the truth appears to lie somewhere in the middle, with emotions playing not the only role, but an important measurable role that has typically been ignored.

In the Affective Computing group at MIT, we are particularly interested in the intelligent handling of affective states commonly expressed around computer systems: frustration, confusion, disliking, liking, interest, boredom, fear, distress, and joy. Computers and other forms of technology are interacting with people in more ways than ever before – beyond desktop, laptop, and palmtop, technology is now embedded into appliances, clothing, jewelry, implants, and even pills we can swallow. With all these new forms, technology has the opportunity to detect physical and physiological expressions of many human emotional states. With additional sensing and processing, the expressions of emotional state can be associated with other events – such as what the person is doing when they get angry or stressed, what else is happening in their body concurrent with episodes of depression, (perhaps related to their heart functioning or their physical activity level) or what the interface (if the person is interacting with one) may have just done [19].

The rest of this paper is divided into four areas: (1) Sensors that enable the user to communicate information related to emotion in a way that is physically and psychologically comfortable; (2) Progress in computer recognition of emotion; (3) Tools for helping people learn affective skills, including a system for autistic kids; (4) Respectfully handling emotions, such as reducing user frustration.

2. Comfortable Sensing of Signals

Emotions often involve both thinking and feeling – both cognitively experienced events and physical changes in the body. Although there is no technology that can truly read your thoughts, there are a growing number of sensors that can capture various physical manifestations of emotion -- video recordings of facial expressions and posture or gesture changes, microphone recordings of vocal inflection changes, skin-surface sensing of muscle tension, heart-rate variability, skin conductivity, blood-glucose levels, and other bodily changes, and (if invasiveness is allowed), swallow-able or implant-able sensors or means of capturing bodily fluids for analysis. These are just a few of a growing number of possibilities.

Our research efforts include building tools to facilitate multiple forms of emotion sensing, not to force this on anyone, but to allow for a larger space of possibilities for those who want to communicate and better understand affective information. The tools include new hardware and software that we have developed to

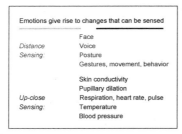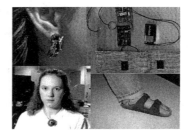

Emotions give rise to changes that can be sensed	
	Face
Distance	Voice
Sensing:	Posture
	Gestures, movement, behavior
	Skin conductivity
	Pupillary dilation
Up-close	Respiration, heart rate, pulse
Sensing:	Temperature
	Blood pressure

Figure 2. Emotion influences many changes in the body. These patterns of change can be sensed by various new wear-able or swallow-able technologies.

enable certain machines not only to receive emotional expression, but also to recognize meaningful patterns of emotional expression. In particular, we have integrated several physiological sensors into clothing and jewelry – a blood volume pressure sensor in an earring, skin conductivity in a shoe and a glove, respiration in a sports bra, and more [19] (See some examples in Figure 2). These sensors communicate with new wearable computers that can control peripherals such as a wearable music player/DJ [8] or a wearable camera [10]. For example, the wearable camera system we built saves video based on your arousal response tagging the data not just with the usual time stamp, but also with information about whether or not it was exciting to you, as indicated by patterns it detects in your skin conductivity [10]. The same system could potentially be modified to detect and communicate health-related variables to you and your physician, perhaps for monitoring and analyzing patterns of stress, anger, or depression.

With any wearable system there are design issues regarding not only what is to be sensed, but also how the sensing system can be made comfortable and robust to noise that arises from activity unrelated to the signal being measured. The key source of noise when measuring emotion from ambulatory patients is artifacts that arise from physical activity. Heart rate, for example, can increase significantly with physical exertion or with sneezing, as well as with anger and other affective states. Inferring the source of a change is easier if you can independently detect the change – such as via context sensors that indicate the person's movement or activity.

One of the physiological sensing systems we built that is robust to motion artifacts is the "Conductor's Jacket," one version of which is shown in Figure 3. This highly expressive wearable system, created by Teresa Marrin, associates patterns of muscle tension and breathing with expressive gestures that the conductor uses to shape the music. Seven electromyogram (EMG) and one respiration sensor are included in the version shown here. The EMG's are attached with custom-fit elastics sewn into the shirt, so that they remain snug without strong adhesives, and yet do not move as the arms are moved. This wearable system was designed first to measure how professional and student conductors naturally communicate expressive information to an orchestra. After analyzing real conducting data from six subjects, Marrin found around thirty significant expressive features (largely related to muscle tension changes that signaled interesting musical events) [16]. She has subsequently developed a version of the jacket that transforms natural expressive gestures of the wearer into real-time expressive shaping of MIDI music [17]. A professional conductor, Marrin is currently using the jacket both for live performance and for helping educate student conductors, providing precise feedback on timing, tension, and other important aspects of expressive technique.

In addition to the goal of making wearable sensing devices robust and physically comfortable, we have been concerned about the psychological factor – how do these sensors feel from a personal comfort standpoint and within a social setting? We do not

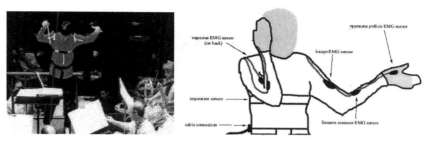

Figure 3. The "Conductor's Jacket" used both for gathering physiological changes related to expression and for controlling MIDI output.

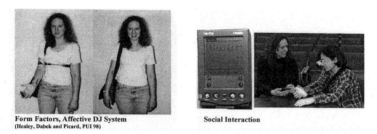

Figure 4. Wearable systems can be increasingly hidden in ordinary clothing; their form factor can be modified to not impair social interaction.

believe there is a one-size-fits-all answer, but rather we find that people like to exercise choices; in many cases, these choices include hiding the sensors, so that they are not visible (although a notable exception was one of the professional conductors we worked with – we took him a sensor jacket with almost everything hidden under the tuxedo, and he asked us to redo it "in red, with the wires in silver on the outside for all to see.") We found that when we integrated sensors with the "lizzy" wearable (Figure 4, at right) that the private eye output display was an impediment to social interaction, and the input device (chording keyboard) took too long for subjects to learn. Consequently we modified a Palm Pilot to serve as an input/output device to the wearable, allowing the Palm to display physiological signals and receive annotations for them. Although a palm device is not hands-free like a heads-up display, it is more comfortable for many people in social settings.

Emotions modulate not only the modes shown in Figure 2, but also many others, including hormone and neurotransmitter levels. The latter are currently not easy to sense without drawing saliva or blood or using other invasive procedures. Presently, none of these procedures provides instantaneous wireless access to the changing levels. However, new implant-able and swallow-able sensors are being developed by many researchers, exploiting strides in nanoscale technology, and giving access to internal bodily signals previously unavailable in real time (e.g., Figure 5, courtesy of Prof. Scott Manalis at MIT).

Sometimes, social-psychological concerns such as privacy make one form of sensing preferable to another. For example, although one person might be comfortable communicating facial expressions to a computer using a video camera, another might be concerned about the identifying information that the camera would see. In distance learning and in intelligent tutoring systems, there is an opportunity for the student to

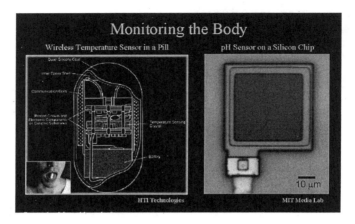

Figure 5. New forms of sensing enable real-time wireless readout of internal bodily signals such as temperature or pH.

transmit signals such as confusion or interest in real-time, without having to stop and click on anything that interrupts their attention [22], and without giving away their identity. One means of accomplishing this is via a wearable sensing system designed and built by research assistant Jocelyn Scheirer, the "expression glasses" described in the next section.

3. Computer Recognition of Emotional Expression

One of the wearable-computing platforms we built includes a small A-to-D with eight channels for physiological sensing. We have developed algorithms that run on the wearable system, extract features from the physiological signals, and relate these to a deliberately expressed emotion. Short segments of four physiological signals for two emotions are shown in Figure 6. Although the segments here look different for each emotion, this was not always the case; in general, the variations within the same emotion from day to day exceeded the variations in different emotions on the same day. Using a variety of methods of pattern recognition and baselining, we have obtained recent results of 81% recognition accuracy in selecting which of eight emotions was expressed by an actress, given 30 days of data, eight emotions per day, and features of the four signals: respiration, blood volume pressure, skin conductivity, and muscle tension. (See Healey and Picard (1998) and Vyzas and Picard (1999) for details of the data collection and the recognition algorithms [9], [25].) The eight emotions investigated were: neutral, hatred, anger, romantic love, platonic love, joy, and reverence. These are the best known results to date for emotion recognition from physiology, and they lie between machine recognition results of affect from speech and of affect from facial expressions.

It should be noted that these results are for a single user, and they are obtained by a forced selection of one of the eight categories; hence, these results are comparable to recognition results in the early days of speech recognition, when the system was re-trained for each speaker, and it knew that the person was speaking one of eight words, although there could be variation in how the person spoke the words from day to day. Much more work remains to be done to understand individual differences as well as differences that depend on context – whether developmental, social, or cultural. I expect that, like research in speech recognition, this work will gradually expand to be able to handle speakers from different cultures, of different ages, speaking (or expressing) continuously, in a variety of environments.

Figure 6 (right) shows a computer task and data-gathering system we designed that was intended to induce negative stress and collect data synchronized with the stress-eliciting events [21]. We gave the user a goal with incentive: race through the task as quickly as possible, obtain the best score (a mix of accuracy and efficiency) and

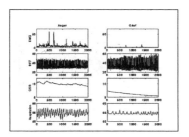 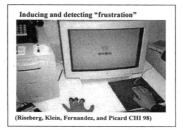

Figure 6. Examples of four physiological signals sensed during different emotional states.

win a $100 prize. Along the way, we had the system freeze up as if the mouse was not working, delaying their progress. We continuously measured two physiological signals—skin conductivity and blood volume pressure—then compared patterns in these signals when all was going smoothly vs. during the episodes of unexpected delays. Although we cannot determine whether these episodes corresponded to true feelings of frustration or non-frustration, we did find that in 21 out of 24 subjects, the patterns detected by our Hidden-Markov-Model based approach were able to significantly discriminate these two kinds of episodes [5]. However, the recognition results were still far from perfect, indicating that although this information is helpful, it must be combined with other signals for a more confident decision.

Stress is sometimes a by-product of feelings such as confusion, which a person may choose to communicate by furrowing his or her brow. The furrowing of the muscle can be detected by a camera if lighting and head position is carefully restricted (otherwise current computer vision techniques are inadequate) but these restrictions, coupled with the recording of identity, can make some subjects uncomfortable. An alternative sensor to a camera is a pair of wearable "expression glasses" (Figure 7) that senses changes in facial muscles [22]. These glasses have a small point of contact with the brow, but otherwise are considered by some users to be less obtrusive than a camera in that the glasses offer privacy, robustness to lighting changes, and the ability to move around freely without having to stay in a fixed position relative to a camera. The expression glasses can be used *while concentrating* on a task – the wearer does not have to stop and think about how to communicate a facial expression. The glasses can be activated either unconsciously or consciously. People are free to make false expressions, or to have a "poker face" to mask true confusion if they do not want to communicate their true feelings, but if they want to communicate them, the glasses offer a virtually effortless way to do so.

Why wear expression glasses, instead of raising your hand or pushing a button to say you're interested or confused, as was implemented decades earlier [23] by Sheridan and his colleagues? The answer is not that there should be one *or* the other; both kinds of feedback offer advantages. Sometimes people miss the subtlety of this point: affect is continuously communicated while you are doing just about anything. When you pick up a pen, you tend to do so very differently when you are angry vs. when you are joyful. When you watch somebody, your eyes behave differently if you are interested than if you are bored. *As you listen* to a conversation or a lecture, your expression gives the speaker feedback, unless, of course, you put on a poker face. In contrast, if you have to think about pushing a button to communicate your feelings, or to raise your hand to say you're confused, then you have to interrupt your concentration to take such an action. Self-report is important, but it is no substitute for the natural channels of largely non-verbal communication that humans use *concurrently* while engaged in conversation, learning, and other activities.

One of the important domains for analyzing stress is with drivers, especially

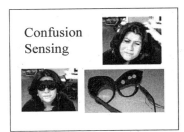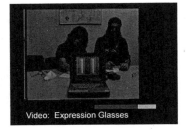

Figure 7. Expression glasses sense facial muscle changes and detect furrowing of the brow, a signal sometimes used to communicate confusion.

drivers trying to do more than drive. We have conducted experiments measuring the impact of low and high cognitive load tasks on drivers talking over a telephone headset while driving in a simulator. We placed drivers under different load conditions (fast or moderate speed, and fast or slow questioning with simple arithmetic problems like "12 + 14") while otherwise keeping the driving task the same. The drivers were occasionally exposed to signs labeled "brake" or "continue" and were instructed to brake as soon as they saw the brake message. Most drivers braked within 0.7-1.4 seconds after the message; however, there were a number of incidents where braking took place 1.5-3.5 seconds after the brake message, or not at all. In almost all of the latter cases, the subject was talking on the phone. On average, the drivers talking on the phone had reaction times to brake messages that were 10% slower than when they were not on the phone; more importantly, the variance in their braking times was four times higher – suggesting that although delayed reactions were infrequent, when delays happened they could be very large and potentially dangerous. The fact that they didn't happen often could furthermore create a false sense of security. Although physiological data gathered in these experiments was limited, our analysis indicated a potential for recognizing patterns that might indicate whether or not a driver was likely to respond with a slowed reaction or not [24].

We are beginning to analyze affect in speech, an area in which humans perform at only about 60% accuracy (on roughly eight emotion categories, when the content of the speech is obscured). Our initial focus is on speech from drivers, taken from the experiment above, examining if the driver's vocal characteristic under different load conditions shows reliable indications of stress [6]. As manufacturers put more gadgets in cars, such as talking navigation systems and restaurant guides or grocery reminders triggered by GPS-sensed location, there is increased potential that the driver might be interrupted at a stressful time that could diminish safety. Another human passenger would be able to sense if the timing was good or not and make a safer decision about interrupting the driver; however, the systems being put into cars are currently oblivious to these factors. If the driver is conversing with one of the car systems, he or she may be distracted at a bad time, compromising safety. We are trying to give the system the ability to sense stress pattern changes in the driver's speech (as well as responsiveness patterns in the driver's behavior, per above) so that the car can be more sensitive to the safety factor.

Our research is developing means of recognition of physiological patterns related to stress in many different natural environments. We have recently moved outside the world of simulators and equipped a car to examine driver behavior features joint with physiological information. One such sensor set-up is shown in Figure 8 (right). In a recent set of experiments we induced stress in a dozen drivers by having them drive around Boston under four stress-eliciting conditions while we recorded

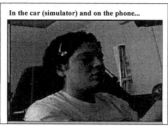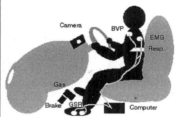

Figure 8. Stress was measured from vocal intonation and from driving behavior when drivers were given tasks over a phone headset (left). We designed and integrated a physiological sensing system into a Volvo for measuring bodily signals related to stress among Boston drivers out on the road (right).

electrocardiogram, skin conductivity, respiration, blood-volume pressure, and electromyogram signals, together with video and other information about the driver's behavior and context. Knowing how stressed somebody truly became is hard to assess; therefore, we used three different methods of assessment: self-report of the driver, driving condition (rest, busy city, easy highway, tolls/turn-around), and third-party coding of complexity level based on number of events each minute during the driving situation. Our analysis of patterns of driver physiology, led to an average stress recognition rate of from 89-96% accuracy depending on which of three methods was used for labeling the "true" stress level of each subject [11].

An increasing amount of human-human communication takes place through machines. In many cases it would be helpful if the machine would simply facilitate the transmission of affective cues. An example of a system designed to expand human-human communication capabilities via computer is the TouchPhone, developed by Jocelyn Scheirer in our lab (Figure 5). The TouchPhone augments regular voice communication with pressure information indicating how tightly the speaker is holding the phone. For example, if you routinely talk to an elderly parent by phone, this would enable you to not only hear their voice, but also to see how they were holding the phone: Is it the same as most days? Or today does their grip seem weaker, tense, or more fidgety? The pressure is continuously mapped to a color seen by the person on the other side – calibrated to blue if light pressure is applied – and to red if strong pressure. The computer performs no interpretation of this signal; the color signal is simply transmitted to the conversational partner as an additional low bit-rate channel of information.

I met with four of my students for four hours of TouchPhone conversations and the results, while anecdotal, were interesting and were consistent with experiences we have had with other emotion-communication technologies. I found that each of the four students had a nearly unique color pressure pattern, which was distracting until I moved the pattern into my periphery where it became ambient, adding a flavor of background rhythm to the conversation. For one student, the pattern changed very slowly, becoming stable red when I started asking some research questions. I thought nothing of it, because he could have simply been squeezing the phone more tightly by shifting his position. However, even though he knew that I could not tell his feelings from the color, he expressed to me that he wasn't trying to squeeze it tighter at all and he thought it was red because he was stressed about a question I asked him. The student was a non-expressive male engineer who had never revealed such signs of stress to me in the years of conversations we had had prior to this TouchPhone conversation. The technology thus facilitated opening up a greater range of emotional communication – by his choice – it did not impose this, but simply made it easier for him. The color did not give away how any of the students was truly feeling. However, the system provided a new channel of non-verbal communication that, in turn, could and did sometimes open up a new line of verbal communication.

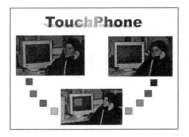
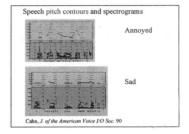

Figure 9. System that senses how phone is being held (left.) Examples of intonation changes in annoyed and sad speech (right).

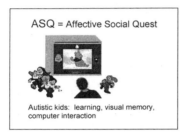
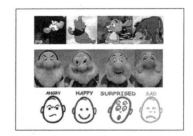

Figure 10. The "ASQ" Computer system shows video clips to autistic kids and prompts them to choose the stuffed dwarf that expresses the emotion appropriate to the video scene. The system senses the child's response and rewards accordingly.

4. Helping Build Human Emotional Skills

Computers just "don't get it" when it comes to practicing many of the social-emotion skills that most of us take for granted. Although autism is a complex disorder, and some of the comments here will not apply to all autistics, there are nonetheless some intriguing characteristics that many autistics share with computers. Both tend to have difficulty with social-emotional cues. Both tend to be poor at generalizing what they learn, and learn best from having huge numbers of examples, patiently provided. Both can be fabulous at certain pattern recognition tasks. Autistics, like computers, also may have very good visual memories. Many autistics have indicated that they like interacting with computers, and some have indicated that communicating on the web "levels the playing field" for them, since emotion communication is limited on the web for everyone.

Because many of the issues we face in giving computers skills of emotional intelligence are similar to those faced by therapists working with autistics, we have begun collaboration with these experts. Current intervention techniques for autistic children suggest that many of them can make progress recognizing and understanding the emotional expressions of people if given lots of examples to learn from and extensive training with these examples.

We have developed a system—"ASQ: Affective Social Quotient"—aimed at helping young autistic children learn to associate emotions with expressions and with situations. The system plays videos of both natural and animated situations giving rise to emotions, and the child interacts with the system by picking up one or more stuffed dwarfs that represent the set of emotions under study, and that wirelessly communicate with the computer. This effort, led by my student Kathi Blocher, has been tested with autistic kids aged 3-7. Within the computer environment, several kids showed an improvement in their ability to recognize emotion [1]. More extensive evaluation is needed in natural environments, but there are already encouraging signs that some of the training is carrying over, such as reports by parents that the kids asked more about emotions at home, and pointed out emotions in their interactions with others. Despite these successes, this work is only one small step; the difficulties in teaching an autistic to appropriately respond to an emotional situation are vast, and we will no doubt face similar difficulties for a long time in trying to teach computers how to respond appropriately.

5. Respectfully Handling Emotions

Not only do many people feel frustration and distress with technology, but also they show it. A widely publicized 1999 study by Concord Communications in the U.S. found that 84% of help-desk managers surveyed said that users admitted to engaging in "violent and abusive" behavior toward computers. A survey by Mori of 1250 people who work with computers in the UK reported that four out of five of them have seen colleagues hurling abuse at their PC's, while a quarter of users under age 25 admitted to having kicked their computer. It seems that no matter how hard researchers work on perfecting the machine and interface design, frustration still occurs. In fact, even if computers were as smart as people, they would still sometimes frustrate people; the same is true in human-human interaction: even the most intelligent people sometimes frustrate others. Hence, there is a need to address frustration at run-time – detecting it, and responding to it.

This need is particularly important in light of the impact of stress on health, and the important role of computers in increasing interacting with patients. In some cases, patients prefer giving information to a computer instead of to a doctor, even when they know the doctor will see the information: computers can go more slowly if the patient wishes, asking questions at the patient's individual speed, not rushing, not appearing arrogant, offering reassurance and information, while allowing the physician more time to focus on other aspects of human interaction [3] [2]. Also, in some cases, patients have reported more accurate information to computers; those referred for assessment of alcohol-related illnesses admitted to a 42% higher consumption of alcohol when interviewed by computer than when interviewed for the same information by psychiatrists [15].

Suppose that a computer could detect patient stress or frustration with high confidence, or that a person directly reports frustration to the machine so that some kind of response by the machine might be appropriate. How should the computer respond? Based on theory that human-computer interaction largely follows the rules of human-human interaction [20], it is germane to explore how a successful human would respond and see if we can find a machine-appropriate way to achieve a similar effect. "It looks like things didn't go very well," and "We apologize to you for this inconvenience" are example statements that people use in helping one another manage frustration once it has occurred. Such kinds of statements are known to help alleviate strong negative emotions such as frustration or rage. But can a computer, which doesn't have feelings of caring, use such techniques effectively to help a user who is having a hard time? To investigate, we built an agent that practices some skills of active listening, empathy, and sympathy, according to the following strategy:

Goal:
Reduce user frustration once it has occurred

Strategy:

1. Recognize (with high probability) that the situation may be frustrating, or that the user is showing signs of frustration likely due to the system
2. Is user willing to talk? If so, then

Practice **active listening,** with **empathy** and **sympathy,** e.g.,
"Good to hear it wasn't terribly frustrating"
"Sorry to hear your experience wasn't better"
"It sounds like you felt fairly frustrated playing this game.
Is that about right?"
Allow for repair, in case computer has "misunderstood"
In extreme cases, the computer may even apologize:
"This computer apologizes to you for its part in .."
3. Polite social closure

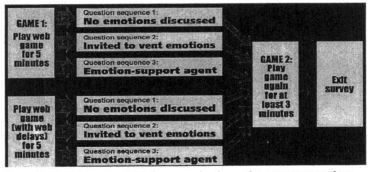

Figure 11: The 2x3 experimental design, comparing the emotion-support agent and two control conditions in both a low-frustration condition and a high-frustration condition.

In developing this system, we avoided language where the computer might refer to itself as "I" or otherwise give any misleading implications of having a "self." The system assesses frustration and interacts with the user through a text dialogue box (with no face, voice, fancy animation or other devices that might provoke anthropomorphism.) The only aspect of the interaction that evokes another person is the use of language, which although cleansed of references to self, nonetheless was made deliberately friendly in tone across all control and test conditions, so that friendliness would not be a factor in this study.

The emotion support agent was tested with 70 users who experienced various levels of frustration upon interacting with a simulated network game [14]. We wanted to measure a strong behavioral indication of frustration, since self-report is notoriously unreliable. Thus we constructed a situation where people were encouraged to do their best while test-playing an easy and boring game, both to show their intelligence, and to win one of two monetary prizes. Half of the subjects were exposed to an especially frustrating situation while they played (simulated network delays, which caused the game to freeze, thereby thwarting their attempt to show their intelligence or win a prize). Afterward, subjects would interact with the agent, which was designed to help them reduce their frustration. Finally, they would have to return to the source of their frustration and engage again with the game, at which point we measured how long they continued to interact with it. Our prediction was based on human-human interaction: if somebody frustrates you, and you are still highly frustrated when you have to go back and interact with them, then you will minimize that interaction; however, if you are no longer feeling frustrated, then you are likely to interact with them longer. The 2x3 experimental design is shown in Figure 6, where thirty-four users played the game in a low-frustration condition, while thirty-six played the same game with simulated delays.

We ran three cases for each of the low and high frustration conditions. The first two cases were controls, text-based friendly interactions having essentially the same length as the emotion-support agent. The first control (*ignore*) just asked about the game, ignoring emotions, and the second control (*vent*) asked about the game, but then asked questions about the person's emotional state and gave them room to vent, with no active listening, empathy or sympathy. After interacting with one of the three (*ignore, vent,* or *emotion-support*), each player was required to return to the game, and to play for three minutes, after which the quit button appeared and they could quit or play up to 20 minutes more. Compared to people in the *ignore* and *vent* control groups, subjects who interacted with the *emotion-support* agent played significantly longer, behavior indicative of a decrease in frustration. People in the *ignore* and *vent* cases both left quickly, and there was no significant difference between their times of play. We also analyzed the data to see if there were any significant effects with respect to gender, trait arousability, and prior game playing experience; none of these factors were significant. (For more details regarding this system, experiment, and findings, see Klein (1998) [13]).

These results suggest that today's machines can begin to help reduce frustration, even when they are not yet smart enough to identify or fix the cause of the frustration. Our findings further indicate that it takes very little time to help the user reduce stress – the emotion savvy agent took no more time than the two controls, and all of the interactions took around 4-6 minutes. This time included not only addressing the person's feelings, but also asking several questions about the game. In other words, less than a few minutes of addressing the emotion were sufficient to provide a significant behavioral change in the user.

Today, physicians usually have so little time with patients that they feel it is impossible to build rapport and communicate about anything except the most obviously significant medical issues. However, given findings such as those highlighted at the start of this paper, emotional factors such as stress, anxiety, depression, and anger can be highly significant medical factors, even when the patient might not mention them. Although our findings of a computer's ability to reduce stress were only based on one kind of stress-provoking situation, the strong behavioral effect we obtained in just a few minutes of addressing the emotion, suggests that perhaps something significant can be done by physicians to address emotions related to health, even within the limits of a brief office encounter. If a computer in a few minutes can produce a significant behavioral effect, how much more effect could a truly sensitive and caring emotion-savvy person have in the same amount of time?

6. Concluding Remarks

This paper has highlighted several research projects in the MIT Media Lab's Affective Computing Research group. The selected projects are believed to be relevant for future health because they advance the state of the art in physiological sensing, in recognition of emotional signals, in development of emotional skills, and in use of computers to help people manage emotions. Based on the growing number of studies showing that emotions such as anger, anxiety, depression and stress are significant medical factors, helping people better manage these emotions becomes a key form of preventive medicine. As computers assist in gathering information from patients, in helping medical patients communicate with one another and with care-providers, and in disseminating information to patients, the need grows for affective intelligence in the computer interface. Patients who have their feelings properly addressed are more likely to leave satisfied, are less likely to return as often, and are less likely to incur legal cost [7]. These effects translate into dollars saved, so that respecting and responding to patients' emotions is good medicine and good business.

Research into the development of affective technologies is relatively new, and many other labs have recently started similar projects, so that it would take a much longer paper to overview all the research in this area. There are also many exciting findings relating affect and cognition, such as those of Isen and colleagues showing a significant impact of a mild positive state on medical decision making – facilitating efficiency and thoroughness in medical diagnostic reasoning [4], with a number of other benefits [12]. Readers who are interested in related work are encouraged to visit the references of the papers cited at the end of this document, which contain over a hundred pointers to related research conducted beyond our lab.

Over the years, scientists have aimed to make machines and technologies that are intelligent and that help people be intelligent. However, they have almost completely neglected the role of emotion in intelligent interaction, leading to an imbalance where emotions are typically ignored. Similarly, emotions have been largely ignored in the general medical community, with the exception of many recent investigations that have measured their impact and found emotion to be a significant factor in health recovery and in disease prevention. I do not wish to see the scale tilted the other way, where machines twitch at every emotional expression, or where physicians treat emotion and not the accompanying medical problems. What is needed is a reasonable balance. The aim of new affective technologies for medicine should be to help medical care givers attend to patients' full health needs – both emotional and non-emotional–in a balanced, respectful and intelligent way.

References

[1] Blocher, K., "Affective Social Quotient (ASQ): Teaching Emotion Recognition with Interactive Media & Wireless Expressive Toys," MIT SM Thesis, May 1999.

[2] Card, W. I. and Lucas, R. W., "Computer interrogation in medical practice," *Int. J. Man-Machine Studies,* **14**, 49-57, 1981.

[3] Dove, G. A. W., Wigg, P., Clarke, J.H.C., Constantinidou, Maria, Royappa, B. A., Evans, C. R., Milne, J., Goss, C., Gordon, M. and de Wardener, H. E., "The therapeutic effect of taking a patient's history by computer," *J. of the Royal College of General Practitioners,* **27**, 477-481, 1977.

[4] Estrada, C. A., Isen, A. M., and Young, M. J. "Positive affect facilitates integration of information and decreases anchoring in reasoning among physicians." *Organizational Behavioral and Human Decision Processes,* **72**, 117-135, 1997.

[5] Fernandez, R. and Picard, R. W., "Signal Processing for Recognition of Human Frustration," *Proc. IEEE ICASSP '98,* Seattle, WA, 1997.

[6] Fernandez, R. and Picard, R. W., "Modeling Drivers' Speech under Stress," *Proc. ISCA Workshop on Speech and Emotions,* Belfast, Sep 2000.

[7] Goleman, D. , *Emotional Intelligence,* Bantam Books, New York, 1995.

[8] Healey, J., Dabek, F. and Picard, R. W., A New Affect-Perceiving Interface and its Application to Personalized Music Selection, *Proc. 1998 Workshop on Perceptual User Interfaces,* San Francisco, CA, 1998.

[9] Healey, J. and Picard, R.W. , "Digital Processing of Affective Signals," *Proc. Int. Conf. on Acoustics, Speech, and Signal Processing,* Seattle, WA, May 1998.

[10] Healey, J. and Picard, R. W. , StartleCam: A Cybernetic Wearable Camera, *Proc. Intl. Symp. on Wearable Computing,* Pittsburgh, PA, 1998.

[11] Healey, J. A. "Wearable and Automotive Systems for Affect Recognition from Physiology," *Ph.D. Thesis, Dept. of Electrical Engineering and Computer Science*, May 2000, MIT.

[12] Isen, A. M., Positive Affect and Decision Making, in Handbook of Emotions, Eds. M. Lewis and J. Haviland, Guilford Press, NY, 2000.

[13] Klein, J., "Computer Response to User Frustration," MIT SM Thesis, Media Arts and Sciences, June 1998.

[14] Klein, J., Moon, Y, and Picard, R. W., "This Computer Responds to User Frustration." *CHI 99 Short Papers*, Pittsburgh, PA. A longer version has been accepted for publication in *Interaction with Computers*.

[15] Lucas, R. W., Mullin, P. J., Luna, C. B. X., and McInroy, D. C., "Psychiatrists and a Computer as Interrogators of Patients with Alcohol-Related Illnesses: A Comparison," *Brit. J. Psychiat.*, 131, 160-7, 1977.

[16] Marrin, T. and Picard, R. W. , "Analysis of Affective Musical Expression with the Conductor's Jacket," *Proc XII Col. Musical Informatics*, Gorizia, Italy, 1998.

[17] Marrin, T., "Inside the Conductor's Jacket: Analysis, Interpretation, and Musical Synthesis of Expressive Gesture," MIT PhD. Thesis, Media Arts and Sciences, 1999.

[18] Picard, R. W., *Affective Computing*, MIT Press, Cambridge, MA, 1997.

[19] Picard, R. W, and Healey, J., Affective Wearables, Personal Technologies 1, No. 4 , 231-240, 1997.

[20] Reeves B. and Nass, C. (1996). The Media Equation, Cambridge University Press; Center for the Study of Language and Information.

[21] Riseberg, J., Klein, J., Fernandez, R. and Picard, R.W., "Frustrating the User on Purpose: Using Biosignals in a Pilot Study to Detect the User's Emotional State, " *CHI '98 Short Papers*, Los Angeles, CA. A longer version of this paper has been accepted for publication in *Interaction with Computers,* 1998.

[22] Scheirer, J., Fernandez, R. and Picard, R.W., "Expression Glasses: A Wearable Device for Facial Expression Recognition," *CHI '99 Short Papers*, Pittsburgh, PA, 1999.

[23] Sheridan, T. B., "Community Dialog Technology", *Proc. of the IEEE*, 63, No. 3, March 1975.

[24] Vyzas, E. "Recognition of Emotional and Cognitive States Using Physiological Data," *Mechanical Engineer Thesis,* June 1999, MIT.

[25] Vyzas, E., and Picard, R. W. , "Online and Offline Recognition of Emotion Expression from Physiological Data," *Workshop on Emotion-Based Agent Architectures at the Int. Conf. on Autonomous Agents*, Seattle, WA, 1999.

Future of Health Technology
R.G. Bushko (Ed.)
IOS Press, 2002

The Future of Medical Computing

Blackford Middleton, M.D., M.P.H., MSc, F.A.C.P., F.A.C.M.I.

Associate Director of Clinical & Quality Analysis for the Partners Healthcare System, and Assistant Professor of Medicine at Harvard Medical School

Abstract

The practice of medicine is inherently dependent upon health technology. Clinicians use a wide variety of technologies in diagnosing, treating, and assessing the care of their patients [1]. In this book, The Future of Health Technology, many different aspects of health technology are discussed in detail. Considering this breadth of coverage, it is challenging to ascertain what remains to be discussed in this chapter on "the future of medical computing". Given this considerable coverage, this chapter will open with a brief vision of the future of medical computing from three perspectives – the Patient, the Ambulatory Provider, and the Hospitalist. Discussion follows on the current and future driving forces for change in healthcare technology, and an overview of the unresolved issues that must be addressed. Necessarily, this chapter will not provide more than an overview of these topics and issues. Rather, it is the author's intent to present several visions of the future of medical computing and outline the issues, which must be overcome to achieve the vision.

1. Visions of the Future

A chapter on the future of medical computing must begin with visions of the future. Three different visions are presented to portray the perspective of the patient, the ambulatory practitioner, and the hospitalist. In the four decades since Ludley and Lested's paper, which may be said to have launched the field of clinical informatics, medical computing has come quite a long way [2]. Since that time, healthcare, like much of society in the western world in general, was radically transformed by the application of computing technology. In addition, the pace of change in computing technology has accelerated throughout that period. Should this pace of change continue, and should we see continued progress in the thorny issues surrounding the application of computers in healthcare, the next few decades should be equally remarkable indeed.

1.1 Patient Perspective

John, a 68-year-old retired autoworker awoke feeling well rested and refreshed. Seeing that his wife Mary was still sleeping, he rose and headed toward the bathroom. At the sink, he reviewed a schedule of the day's activities in the information panel on the wall by the mirror, and was reminded that he had a doctor's visit in the afternoon at 2:00PM. Pills for his high blood pressure, diabetes, and osteoarthritis were dispensed in the smart pill case, which kept track of his medications. After he used the smart commode, he was informed that his weight was up 1-¼ lbs from last week, and that he should increase the roughage in his diet, and decrease fat intake. He got green lights for all his vital signs when he checked them back at the sink with the sensor sleeve he slipped on his arm. Today was a day for him to have his long term sugar control tested at home. He stuck his finger in the machine where this was determined along with his other basic chemistries without drawing blood. These results were immediately displayed back on his information panel and again he got all green lights -- he was feeling good. He asked for a quick check on today's weather to decide what to wear today, and he checked the predicted pollution index and pollen counts because he knew when either of these were up it gave him a runny nose. Lastly he checked the city maps for predictions on traffic problems, construction, civic events, and other population density problems. No red lights so he decided to drive himself to work. Taking his personal digital assistant and pill case, he was ready to go.

John spent most of his day volunteering at the local library. Throughout the day, he loved to periodically check his personal digital assistant for news and sports updates, and responded to reminders about taking his medicines. As John was in a trial for a new medicine to control his nagging low back and knee pains, he was prompted to complete a short symptom survey mid day, and entered new symptoms whenever they arose. What he liked best about his personal digital assistant, however, was the ability to conveniently communicate with his doctor's office and get information about his healthcare, the drugs he was taking, and information on his wife's healthcare conditions and drugs. Prior to going to the doctor's office today, John received an alert that Dr. Smith wanted him to fill out a questionnaire before coming in. John did this on his PDA while taking a break at the library and sent it back wirelessly to the doctor's office.

When John arrived to Dr. Smith's office, he checked himself in, and reviewed his health records at one of the kiosks in the waiting room – it was a bit easier to read the information here than on his PDA; he liked the large type option, and if he wanted he could slip on headphones and have it read to him as well. He felt confident using this system since he was sure it knew him after reading his finger print, and it was a lot easier and faster than waiting for the front desk receptionist! His records looked up to date and he was interested to read some additional information about the drug study he was on, and new research pertaining to his wife's conditions. He indicated to the system that this was a routine visit but he had a couple of additional issues he wanted to raise with the physician. He was prompted with a number of new questions about these new conditions by the system that he easily answered. He slipped on a sensor sleeve, one a bit more elaborate than the one he had at home, and it made a variety of measurements in preparation for his visit with the doctor. He also took time to review his wife Mary's chart on the kiosk. He decided to take a new picture of himself while waiting to see the doctor, and for fun reviewed the pictures of himself from past years. As usual, he had time to spare waiting for the doctor, so he played some of the medical games on the system – they were fun, and helped him understand his body better.

When the doctor called him in, he and John reviewed the information in his health record. Everything looked up to date, Dr. Smith discussed John's new issues, reviewed the sensor sleeve readings, quickly looked him over, and together they decided what to do next. Dr. Smith ordered some labs, and was reminded by his record system to order one special blood test for the investigational drug study, and ordered an image of John's left knee, which seemed to be slightly swollen and warm. After finishing with Dr. Smith, John checked himself out and had all his laboratory and x-rays done in the same facility. All of this was made easy by the fact that everywhere he showed up they were expecting him, ready to go, and he just confirmed his identity with his health card, and fingerprint. On the way home, John called Mary, and they agreed on the movie they would order that night to watch on the home entertainment system.

1.2 Ambulatory Practitioner

Dr. Smith's workday began at home while he was eating breakfast. As he was on call for his group, and he received a beep on his personal digital assistant indicating a patient wanted to speak to him. The PDA looked up the record of the caller, and presented the patient's health summary information to Dr. Smith. The patient had chronic pain syndrome probably due to complications of her multiple sclerosis so Dr. Smith spoke to the patient briefly after reviewing her record, adjusted the patient's existing medications, and ordered a new pain pill. While he had his PDA out, he reviewed the schedule for the day. After hospital rounds, he had a morning full of patients in the clinic, teaching medical residents over the noon hour, patients in the afternoon, and then his research conference for the drug trial he was participating in at 3:00PM. As he looked at the schedule of clinic patients, the PDA indicated that two were new patients, and for these he was given permission to access their summary online health records from encounters with other physicians to review, and permission to add to his own records for the new patients to their online health records.

On two of his chronic care patients, the device informed him that there was new research pertaining to their health conditions that might be of interest to him. For one other, he was informed that there was a clinical trial this patient might be eligible for. Lastly, he scanned his information retrieval agents to see if there were any other new articles of interest to him; three did look interesting and he asked to have them downloaded to his inbox for later review and addition to his personal knowledge management system. Lastly, he checked the PDA to see when and where his professional society's clinical meetings were this year, and checked on how many continuing education hours he had accumulated so far this year to help decide if he should go. He scanned his secure email inbox to see if there any work items or messages he could address right then and there: he did answer a couple of quick emails, did 3 prescription refills and authorized 1 patient referral request. After a quick check of the news headlines, sports, and his stock portfolio, and goodbyes to his wife and kids, he headed off to work.

At the clinic, checked in and put on his security and tracking badge, and sat down at his clinical workstation in his office. The badge was the greatest invention ever in his mind: all he had to do was have it on and any workstation he approached recognized him and launched his favorite applications. All he had to do was type in a password. The clinical workstation in his consultation office gave him an extended display of all the information presented to him on his PDA, and more. He looked again at the day's schedule, reviewed his inbox and work list items, and scanned several of his hospital and clinic patient's charts for a quick read on their health status. He did this by looking at the visual indicator summary for each chart online: this summary data visualization allowed him to review many health parameters pertaining to that patient's health problems at a glance, and was linked to all the textual information online. He had learned to recognize the data patterns in the graphical display at a glance. The same displays, when switched to the inpatient review mode, allowed him to check on the handful of patients he had in two of the local hospitals being cared for by his hospitalist colleagues. For one, he added two new parameters to the visual display for things he liked to follow on patients with their problems. Things seemed to be going pretty well for most of his patients in hospital, so he turned to his schedule of morning patients. The ability to do these virtual rounds certainly made follow up on his patients when discharged easier, and kept things working smoothly with his hospitalist colleagues.

As patients arrived to the clinic, the clinical workstation informed him of the workflow status throughout his clinic. He could tell when patients were in the waiting room, or in the exam rooms, and what was happening to them along the way. Patients were given security-tracking badges, too, in his clinic. It allowed the information system to keep track of where they were in the clinic and how long they were waiting! All the clinical staff wore them, too, so Dr. Smith could see who was where. This system allowed him to be sure patient care was moving along, and informed him which medical assistant was caring for his patients so he could send orders to the right person.

That afternoon, when he saw that John had arrived, one of his favorite patients, he reviewed John's chart, and the visual summary presented to him in the display. John's problems seemed to be under fairly good control: the trends for his important clinical indicators and parameters, and his clinical risk management prediction indices for John's conditions, all looked pretty good. Dr. Smith looked over the issues raised by John in the dialogue he had had with the kiosk in the waiting room, and he reviewed the system's suggestions for additional questions he might ask, and the differential diagnosis suggested by the patient history so far. It was helpful to have this in mind as he talked with the patient further and examined him. He likes to play a little game with the system and kept track of how often its suggestions made him think of something he hadn't considered. Happily, it looked like there was nothing new to worry about except a sore knee probably related to his osteoarthritis, but Dr. Smith always liked to ask a few questions himself of the patient to get an idea of the patient's progress. Just before walking into the exam room, Dr. Smith reviewed John's progress on the investigational new drug trial: the sore knee could be an important observation to report to the clinical study data center. He noted the study would pay for the costs of an image of the knee if he thought it was clinically important.

In the room with John, Dr. Smith reviewed the patient's progress using displays from the clinical workstation in the exam room. John was doing pretty well, but appeared to be having a gradual decline in functional status. He had reported a new symptom possibly related to the drug trial, and wasn't having a good result with the drug (although Dr. Smith didn't know if he was on placebo or not in this double blinded trial). Dr. Smith reviewed the research protocol for his patient, as well as the disease management guidelines and intervention suggested by the system for his other health problems. He was reminded of the labs due for both disease management and the new drug research protocol. After examining John, they returned to the information system and Dr. Smith used it to share what might be going on in his painful knee. Dr. Smith used the system to quickly show a picture of the anatomy of the knee to discuss why it might be swollen, and sent a care agent to John's PDA which would instruct him how to care for his knee. Dr. Smith reviewed the investigations suggested by the system and agreed with all but one. He and John discussed the use of a new medication to provide additional pain control for his knee, and Dr. Smith sent a medication agent to John's PDA that would help him learn about the medication, use it appropriately, give him reminders about when doses were due, and provide him a way to report any new symptoms on this drug. John left feeling better, headed toward the labs, and Dr. Smith finished his clinical documentation before he left the exam room. He dictated his comments to the system using the on screen structured dictation guide. When he was finished, he was immediately presented with a complete document online to review and sign electronically.

The information he recorded was instantly routed to laboratory, billing, the clinical research organization, and the population data service that Dr. Smith subscribed to and used. Dr. Smith wasn't completely sure about what was going on with John's knee so he launched an agent that would send a set of anonymous data from John's chart to the online clinical decision support service Dr. Smith used. If he was willing to share anonymous clinical data from his practice with the service with his patients' consent, the service gave him in return many reports and analytic services he found very helpful. In John's case, he would get an analysis of the case with a differential diagnosis, a clinical management risk prediction agent he could add to John's chart, and a list of all the relevant clinical evidence for John's case later that day. He enjoyed this service because it gave him a sense of confidence that he wasn't missing anything, and if he answered the few questions that came back from the service, he got CME as well!

1.3 Hospitalist

Dr. Jones awoke in the call room early in the morning. It had been a rough night, but he loved it. In the hospital environment, he felt he was able to do whatever it took to make his patients well. He never missed seeing patients in the clinic, but counted on a good relationship with those doctors, and access to their information system to understand the patients who came to the hospital better. First thing he did sitting up was to review the clinical workstation in his call room: this gave him a quick overview of all the patients in his charge in the hospital. The highly summarized graphical display showed of a large number of important clinical parameters and allowed him to quickly access each patient's status. He then flipped to his schedule for the day, and reviewed the work items, and procedures, expected that day for each of his patients. He reviewed the critical alerts and reminders for all of his patients, and the message queue in his inbox. He then reviewed the news headlines, and sports scores as he got up. He checked to see that his medical computing tablet was charged up and confirmed that the clinical workstation display was replicated on his medical tablet. Dr. Jones remembered the days when he carried around a clipboard in the hospital as a medical student before medical tablets became widely available. He liked to think of his medical tablet as his "electronic clipboard."

Dr. Jones joined the multidisciplinary team for rounding in the hospital after eating a bagel at the nurse's station, and checking his patients in the critical care unit. This month he not only cared for his own patients but also served as a teaching attending for the university service in his hospital. Before rounds began, he reviewed all of his information retrieval agents to see if there was new information that might apply to any of his patients, or new critical results from the lab, or alarming trends in any of his patients' clinical indicators and clinical risk management indices. On two of his critical patients he was alerted about worrisome trends in their status, and on one he saw there was a critical alert in the night that his nursing colleagues had dealt with themselves. Thank goodness he had considered this possibility and had selected the standing orders for this contingency in the clinical system. On three other patients, potentially relevant new articles had come out matching the search parameters of the information retrieval agents he had created for each patient, that he wanted to discuss with the care team. He had the articles sent to his inbox as well as to every member of his team.

Seeing each patient, Dr. Jones reviewed the summary graphical display on the bedside clinical workstation in each room, talked with and examined the patient, and used his medical tablet to dictate his note, and capture orders for that patient. Everything he did on his medical tablet was immediately updated on the clinical workstation in the room. The team reviewed all the patients' health parameters, and their predicted risks for adverse events and inpatient mortality outside of the room. In addition, they reviewed the patient's resource consumption compared to expected resource consumption for similar patients in the hospital's clinical data repository. The hospital participated in the national hospital data repository project, so Dr. Jones was immediately able to compare the clinical indicators and clinical risk management estimates with those derived from a sample of similar patients from similar hospitals across the country. The hospital seemed to be always on a drive to control costs, but Dr. Jones liked the ability to see instantly whether his patients were 'sicker' than the sample drawn from the national repository. If they were sicker, he felt justified in going 'all out' for his patients, and he knew the hospital wouldn't suffer financially because of the new risk-adjusted national reimbursement plan the government had come up with. He also knew that when the system's futility score for a patient exceeded threshold, he could reasonably focus his efforts on palliative care.

The team reviewed the alerts and reminders on their medical tablets for each patient and the suggested interventions as they went from room to room. As he rounded throughout the morning, he made sure summaries of all his notes and the patient's clinical data were sent automatically to the consultants co-managing the patients with him, as well as the patient's primary physician in the community. On one of the new patients with a strange hematological malignancy, Dr. Jones reviewed the progress the patient had with new pharmaceutical agents designed using all that was known about the malignancy's biological properties, and the patient's genomic sequence. The things there were doing today with 'designer drugs' he could not have even imagined five years ago.

2. Driving Forces for Improved Clinical Information Management

"Necessity is the mother of invention."   George Farquhar. 1678-1707

In the past half century, healthcare in the Western world has seen more change than at any previous time in history. What are the current driving forces for change in healthcare and how will advances in medical computing be affected by these forces, or, more probably, result from these driving forces? In this section, several driving forces and their impact on medical computing are discussed.

In the modern era, Western healthcare has seen a dramatic expansion in services, technology, and costs. Fueled by the largest economic expansion in history, healthcare became the largest component of the US economy, exceeding 13% of the GDP, and $1 trillion in expenditures before the end of the 20th Century. As the baby boom began, spending on healthcare research stimulated the development of many new technologies. With these successes, and the expansion of healthcare services, hospitals, and physicians, healthcare became perceived as a "right" for every member of US society. Concurrently, with the expanding economy, and the advent of worker's unions, and tax incentives for the purchase of healthcare insurance, the costs of healthcare shifted to employers, and healthcare became an employee benefit. Employees, therefore, became insensitive to the cost of healthcare and demand for healthcare services skyrocketed [3].

As healthcare costs began to spiral out of control, public and private payers began to seek ways to find relief. To date, these financial pressures for cost containment have been the major driver for healthcare computing. Concomitantly, however, other pressures bore down on healthcare: medical errors [4], and patient safety [5], better risk management, organizational upheaval, and new pressures from the healthcare consumer. There is a 'technological imperative' in healthcare that has itself been a driving force for change. US healthcare has always adopted the latest and greatest technology without fully considering costs associated with new technology because providers and healthcare delivery systems were largely insensitive to cost.

All of these forces arising together, cost containment, reimbursement reform, organizational upheaval, patient safety, and consumerism, place acute pressures on the healthcare delivery system to produce data that would document not only the costs, but also the safety and efficacy, of services rendered. While many other industries have adopted modern information management technology, healthcare – for a variety of reasons – has been slow to adopt these tools. In this author's opinion, it is the need for data, primarily the data to drive financial processes, but also more recently the data to document and improve the safety and efficacy of healthcare that will finally drive modern medicine into the Information Age.

3. The Future of Medical Computing

To achieve the vision outlined at the beginning of this chapter several critical issues must be resolved for the successful application of computing technology to information management in healthcare [6].

3.1 Healthcare Data Standards And Attributes

One of the most challenging issues in healthcare information technology is development of healthcare data standards that facilitate not only interoperability between heterogeneous information systems, but also aggregation and interpretation of pooled data from multiple sources.   The NCQA defines the information space in healthcare as including all information pertaining to a patient's healthcare experience. Information may come from hospital environments clinical environments, the patient's workplace, home, and elsewhere. Data from these various environments is coded and structured to a varying degree depending upon the information source system from which it comes. Progress is being made on developing a universal healthcare information model that would allow information system developers to model their own data structures in a way that would be consistent with a universal healthcare information model. The most notable effort in this area is the HL-7 Reference Information Model [7, 8].

Development of a reference information model alone, however, is not sufficient to address all the needs for robust data integrity and interoperability between disparate healthcare information systems. A reference information model must be complemented by a reference terminology that allows modeling of surface forms related to canonical terms in a reference terminology for the user interface, or localization to other languages in other healthcare settings [9]. Progress is being made in this area with the SNOMED RT (reference terminology) effort [10].

In addition to these efforts, however, the future of medical computing will depend upon definition of new data attributes to support these modeling efforts and account for healthcare information coming from anywhere within a patient's infosphere. Such new attributes will include delineation of source of data, creator of data, temporal aspects of the data, data criticality, and information to support both textual and numeric data normalization across systems. For example, with respect to normalization it is mathematically feasible to normalize quantitative information from multiple laboratory systems each with a unique reference range for a particular laboratory result. More challenging is the notion of normalizing terminology strings as entered by a user of a healthcare information system to a referenced canonical form as defined by a reference information model and reference terminology [11].

3.2 Privacy, Confidentiality, And Security

As technical work proceeds on healthcare data standards and attributes, another issue for the future of medical computing centers on healthcare information privacy, confidentiality, and security [12]. Recently released regulations from the US government help to define privacy standards for healthcare information. These rules, arising from the Healthcare Information Portability And Accountability Act of 1996 [13] define who are responsible parties in healthcare for protecting information security, what information is protected, how healthcare information may be used, and requirements for informed consent from patients for the use of their individually identifiable healthcare information. In addition, these regulations establish civil and criminal penalties for inappropriate disclosure of healthcare information.   While these regulations provide many new protections for healthcare information, many other fundamental issues remain to be resolved.

For example, fundamental issues about data ownership in healthcare remain unresolved. It is generally accepted that patients are the "owners" of their personally identifiable healthcare information, but healthcare delivery systems and providers who create healthcare records based upon patient healthcare information have limited property rights to that information when instantiated in their record keeping systems. Tensions still exist between these personal privacy rights of healthcare consumers and the rights of healthcare delivery systems and providers [14].

Another aspect of the privacy and confidentiality debate centers on how protections of healthcare information confidentiality and security can be maintained when information is exchanged between multiple parties in the healthcare delivery chain. For example, information collected at a doctor's visit is potentially exchanged with many other parties for reimbursement purposes, quality analysis, risk management, research, and public health reporting. The new federal regulations describe the need for "chain of trust" agreements between healthcare delivery system partners who share or exchange personal healthcare information. How such agreements will be enforced, and what liabilities associated with these agreements when a breech occurs somewhere along the chain of partners, remains to be resolved. The technical implications for maintaining healthcare information security may in fact call for new data attributes that can be used to assess and monitor information security.

3.3 Data Monetization

Another critical issue for the future of medical computing and the appropriate use and exchange of healthcare information centers on how healthcare data will be valued, or the "Monetization" of healthcare information. In the absence of clear-cut ownership guidelines for healthcare information it is impossible to determine how to monetize healthcare information, or information transactions. Is personally identifiable healthcare information of value beyond the immediate care delivery process? Or, what is the value of personal healthcare information when anonymous in aggregate data sets after appropriate de-identification? Currently, value is attached to both aggregate and individually identifiable information on the Internet [3]. The value chain as it is currently operating, however, does not typically return value to the creator or owner of the data. That is, if a patient provides personal healthcare information to a clinical data repository, what value should be returned to that patient? If data were treated as property then the well-established economic, legal, and regulatory framework, which exists for other property, could be readily applied to healthcare data.

3.4 Internet Effects In Healthcare

An equally interesting issue arises, however, when considering whether Internet effects in healthcare will lead to freely substitutable inputs to the healthcare services production function, or a distribution of healthcare activities and services that previously were centralized in a healthcare delivery system. Healthcare services are at risk of becoming increasingly a commodity product if patients and healthcare consumers can go online and compare all providers and all services easily, and freely choose between them. At the local level, healthcare services will essentially become commodity products that are relatively freely exchangeable in a local medical marketplace. Patients will have access to clinician performance information online, and will use this information to make healthcare purchasing decisions. This will also potentially result in a redistribution of the inputs to healthcare as expensive services or providers are replaced with less expensive services and providers judged to have an equivalent value from the healthcare consumer's perspective. Patients may shop far and wide on the Internet for healthcare products and services they used to receive in their local marketplace. Healthcare decision-making may be distributed also; patients may seek virtual second opinions from remote providers or centers of excellence. Patients may assume more responsibility for their own care, and manage more of their care at home. Thus, in local marketplaces, physician's assistants may replace physicians, and many hospital services already replaced by ambulatory surgical centers, in some cases may ultimately occur in the home environment.

3.5 Healthcare Ethics And The Internet

As medicine enters into the information age a wide variety of ethical issues arise to impact upon the future of medical computing. Clearly, data security and personal privacy issues as described above will call for widespread adoption of improved information security management policies and technology to support them. Patients and healthcare providers will essentially need to adopt "universal information precautions" similar to the universal HIV precautions adopted during the HIV epidemic. The impact of this evolution on healthcare delivery costs, the doctor patient relationship, and the information economy through data monetization in healthcare, remain to be seen.

Fundamental questions arise as to who may disclose what healthcare information to whom, and who is in control of personally identifiable healthcare information. These questions will persist until clear ownership and property attributes are defined for personal healthcare information. Historically, healthcare information has been created and validated by providers. As information technologies are applied in healthcare, and continued substitution effects as described above proceed, the "locus of control" for information management may move dramatically toward the individual. Yet, this raises an important clinical question, and a question for the validity of aggregated healthcare data: If an individual is creating and maintaining her own personal healthcare records, how will the validity of that data be assessed for clinical care, or population research?

A related issue arises around the notion of partial disclosure of personally identifiable healthcare information. In the traditional medical model, a physician strives to have as complete a picture of a patient's healthcare information as possible. Particularly in primary care disciplines, providers make every attempt to have a complete record of all the patient's problems, medications, and key historical information. If the locus of control moves toward the healthcare consumer, who has the right to control disclosure of healthcare information to healthcare providers, what guarantee can healthcare providers give that their clinical decision-making has been informed by a complete picture of the patient's status? The implications of such partial disclosure in terms of legal liability, malpractice, and clinical decision-making are difficult to assess but likely to be important.

4. Potential Impact And Implications

Medical computing of the future will have a significant impact on the practice of medicine, and considerable implications for the nature of that practice, the physician, the healthcare services organization, and the patient herself. We will see a new healthcare consumer, a new healthcare provider, and a new healthcare delivery organization.

4.1 The New Healthcare Consumer

As in many other service sectors, healthcare has seen the rise of the empowered consumer – one who is demanding fast and convenient service, choice of physician, access to 'lifestyle drugs', and soon to come 'designer drugs' based on individual genomic attributes, and access to traditional and alternative therapies that previously were not often viewed as medically necessary [15]. Consumers were enjoying the advent of the Internet in many other sectors of the modern economy, and began to 'go online' in droves to seek healthcare information on the Internet before the end of the last century [16, 17]. The consumer also began to assume greater responsibility for healthcare decision-making as employers began to shift their healthcare benefit costs from a defined benefit program toward a defined employee contribution program. The aging baby-boomers also find themselves increasingly making healthcare decisions for the generation of their parents as it moves into the senior years. Finally, with the realization of the frequency of medical errors in modern clinical practice, consumers and employers making healthcare purchasing decisions became acutely aware of their need to critically judge the quality of the healthcare they were purchasing and receiving [18].

4.2 The New Clinician

Just as the consumer of healthcare information and services has evolved, so will the clinician and healthcare delivery systems providing healthcare services and information. As medicine enters the information age, practicing clinicians increasingly are called upon to serve as intermediaries and interpreters placed between the healthcare consumer and the onslaught of clinical information available on the Web, and direct to consumer marketing activities. It is not uncommon for patients to present to their physicians with printouts from the Internet pertaining to their healthcare conditions or questions. It is impractical for the clinician to respond to these situations with anything other then a suggestion to the patient that the information can be copied and added to his chart and reviewed by the clinician later. It appears most consumers trust their physician more then most other sources of healthcare information [19]. As clinicians become comfortable with online tools and resources, it will be possible for these clinicians to respond to patient information requests and interest with suggestions of credible online resources and healthcare information portals for the patients to review.

More importantly perhaps for the evolution of the clinician in the information age, however, is that the clinician must necessarily become not only an information broker as described above, but also develop new skills in information management. Future clinicians will have expectations placed upon them for creating valid data that can be used for clinical decision support and outcomes analysis. Data collected by clinicians at the point of care will be used to drive decision support systems in real time, and will contribute to population databases used in outcomes analysis and data-mining for best practices [20]. Thus, clinicians must become expert in not only acquiring and synthesizing information as has been done for years, but also translating that information and syntheses with an information management system, for example a smart electronic medical record [21, 22].

As these online tools and resources evolve, and as large numbers of patient records become available in aggregate form, clinicians will also be called upon to provide patients realistic estimates of outcomes and risks based upon best evidence and analysis of large populations. The notion of shared decision-making between physician and patient will take on increasing importance as consumers have access to clinical performance data online, and develop the expectation of improved risk assessment and discussion of clinical interventions with their physicians [23]. Much research still needs to be done in this area, but it is likely a new breed of clinician will evolve, perhaps even a specialty discipline, which can address these decision-making and analytic questions as a consultative service.

The most important clinical evolution which will occur with the advent of the information age in healthcare is the rise of accountability in clinical practice. Already, consumers going online, and healthcare purchasers in certain markets, are gaining access to clinical performance data that help them make healthcare service choices and purchasing decisions. Clinicians will be increasingly called upon to supply healthcare information from the practice environment, and even the point of care, to support reporting on patient safety, medical error, and other outcomes reports. Such accountability in healthcare is novel and will drive healthcare delivery systems to automate information management to support the data needs for analysis.

4.3 The New Healthcare Delivery Organization

Another aspect of the evolution of the clinician in the information age in healthcare is that the traditional Internet effects of disintermediation and mass customization will have powerful effects on the organization of healthcare services. Tertiary and quaternary care expertise will tend to become localized at high volume centers, to which patients will be referred for specialty services. Centers with such localization of specialty expertise will serve as consultative resources through both in person referrals, but also increasingly through telemedicine-type services and simple asynchronous consultations. For example, cardiac care centers performing many procedures may draw patients from the local region as well as nationally, and may provide remote operative assistance through telepresence surgery [24, 25]. Primary and acute care, and emergency services, will remain widely distributed, and remain a feature of local healthcare delivery markets. Healthcare services will ultimately be most widely distributed when the consumer herself is an active participant in her own healthcare, or even directing certain discretionary parts of her care.

Healthcare delivery organizations will look much more like 'virtual' organizations in other industries: geographic proximity will matter less than affiliations established and maintained with connectivity supporting efficient management and information flow. Healthcare will never lose the important element of 'hands-on' care, and the fact that healthcare consumers tend to receive their healthcare goods and services from a local marketplace will not change. What will change, however, is that the providers of in person services will increasingly be ancillary healthcare providers working with remote clinicians, remote clinicians will have ever expanding panels of virtual patients, and their healthcare consumer will assume a greater role in their own healthcare. The patient will consume greater amounts of self-directed care, and play a greater role in managing their own chronic conditions through improved consumer oriented decision support tools, tools for collaborative chronic disease management between the patient and remote providers, and remote monitoring capabilities to the home, and to the workplace.

5. Conclusion

The visions of the future of medical computing presented here will come to be sooner than might be expected given the issues to overcome. Progress is being made, however, on the thorny technical problems described above. Perhaps the greatest challenge to progress is in developing the appropriate enabling local and national policies to address the societal issues described above as well.

References

[1] Shortliffe, E.H., et al., eds. *Medical Informatics: Computer Applications in Health Care.* 1990, Addison Wesley: Menlo Park, CA.

[2] Ledley, R.S. and L.B. Lusted, *The use of electronic computers in medical data processing.* IEEE Trans Med Electron, 1960. 7(31).

[3] The Institute of the Future. *Health and Health Care 2010: The Forecast, The Challenge.* 2000, San Francisco: Jossey-Bass Publishers.

[4] Kohn, L.J., J.M. Corrigan, and M.S. Donaldson, *To Err is Human: Building a Safer Health System*, ed. Institute of Medicine Committee on Quality of Health Care in America. 2000, Washington, DC: National Academy Press. 312.

[5] Institute of Medicine Committee on Improving the Quality of Health Care in America. *Crossing the Quality Chasm: a New Health System for the 21st Century.* 2001, Washington, DC: National Academy Press.

[6] Committee on Enhancing the Internet for Health Applications. *Networking Health: Prescriptions for the Internet*, ed. E.H. Shortliffe. 2000, Washington, DC: National Academy Press.

[7] Bakken, S., et al., *Toward vocabulary domain specifications for health level 7-coded data elements.* Journal of the American Medical Informatics Association, 2000. 7(4): p. 333-42.

[8] Beeler, G.W., Jr., *On the Rim: the making of HL7's Reference Information Model.* MD Computing, 1999. 16(6): p. 27-9.

[9] Blair, J. and S. Cohn, *Report on Uniform Data Standards for Patient Medical Record Information.* 2000, National Committe for Vital and Health Statistics.

[10] Spackman, K.A., K.E. Campbell, and R.A. Cote, *SNOMED RT: a reference terminology for health care.* Proceedings / AMIA Annual Fall Symposium, 1997: p. 640-4.

[11] Ricciardi, T.N., F.E. Masarie, and B. Middleton, *Clinical Benchmarking Enabled by the Digital Health Record.* MEDINFO, 2001.

[12] Committee on Maintaining Privacy and Security in Health Care Applications of the National Information Infrastructure. *For the Record: Protecting Electronic Health Information*, ed. Computer Science and Telecommunications Board. 1997: National Research Council. 1-288.

[13] *Health Insurance Portability and Accountability Act.* PL104-191, 104th US Congress, August 21, 1996.

[14] Goldman, J., *Protecting privacy to improve health care.* Health Affairs, 1998. 17(6): p. 47-60.

[15] Barrett, M.J., et al., *Personalized Medicine.* 2000, Forrester Research, Inc.: Cambridge, MA. p. 1-20.

[16] Mefford, B. and M.R. Bard, *Consumer Demand for Provider Connectivity.* Cyber Dialogue: Cybercitizen Health, 2000. **Yr 2000**(5): p. 1-7.

[17] Cain, M.M., J. Sarasohn-Kahn, and J.C. Wayne, *Health e-People: The Online Consumer Experience.* 2000, Institute for the Future: San Francisco. p. 1-73.

[18] Greene, J., *Quality improvement movement--jump start from the Leapfrog Group [news].* Hospitals & Health Networks, 2000. 74(7): p. 14.

[19] Given, R. and S. Haiges, *Taking the Pulse: Physicians and the Internet.* 2000, Deloitte Consulting/CyberDialogue: New York.

[20] Bohren, B.F., M. Hadzikadic, and E.N. Hanley, Jr., *Extracting knowledge from large medical databases: an automated approach.* Computers & Biomedical Research, 1995. **28**(3): p. 191-210.

[21] Committee on Improving the Patient Record. *The Computer-Based Patient Record: An Essential Technology for Healthcare.* Revised edition, ed. R.S. Dick, E.B. Steen, and D.E. Detmer. 1997, Washington D.C.: National Academy Press. 1-234.

[22] Sujansky, W.V., *The benefits and challenges of an electronic medical record: much more than a "word processed" patient chart.* Western Journal of Medicine, 1998. **169**(3): p. 176-83.

[23] Kassirer, J.P., *Patients, Physicians, and the Internet.* Health Affairs, 2000. **19**(6): p. 115-123.

[24] Satava, R.M. and S.B. Jones, *Medicine beyond the year 2000.* Caduceus, 1997. **13**(2): p. 49-64.

[25] Satava, R.M., *Virtual reality and telepresence for military medicine.* Annals of the Academy of Medicine, Singapore, 1997. **26**(1): p. 118-20.

Future of Health Technology
R.G. Bushko (Ed.)
IOS Press, 2002

Intelligent Agent Software for Medicine

Henry Lieberman, Ph.D.

Research ScientistMedia Laboratory, Massachusetts Institute of Technology, Cambridge, MA, US

Cindy Mason, Ph.D.

Assistant Research Engineer, University of California, Berkeley, CA, US

Abstract

An important trend for the future of health technology will be the increasing use of *intelligent agent* software for medical applications. As the complexity of situations faced by both patients and health care providers grows, conventional interfaces that rely on users to manually transfer data and manually perform each problem-solving step, won't be able to keep up. This article describes how software agents that incorporate learning, personalization, proactivity, context-sensitivity and collaboration will lead to a new generation of medical applications that will streamline user interfaces and enable more sophisticated communication and problem-solving.

1. Why Agents?

Medicine is fast becoming a science of information. Information about patient history, symptoms, functions and lifestyle; information about diseases, diagnostics, drugs, and treatment methods play an ever-increasing role. But there can be too much of a good thing.

The dilemma faced by doctors, patients and medical administrators is to find and utilize the relevant information at the right time. Computers, of course, help manage information, but the current generation of computer interfaces can't keep growing at the same rate medical information is growing. We can't keep piling on new applications, adding new icons to our screens and new choices to our menus. Sooner or later, our software will have to work smarter, not just add more features.

Intelligent Agent software [2] is a new paradigm of computer software that aims to bring human-like capabilities to software -- such as learning, proactivity, inference, heuristic problem solving, goal-based action and communication. This doesn't necessarily mean that we can make the computer as smart as a person -- that goal is not yet achievable -- but it is a profound change from today's software, which mostly acts like a passive tool, performing fixed data-manipulation functions only on demand.

Interface agents are agents that act directly as assistants to the user of an interactive graphical interface. Like a secretary, travel agent, stockbroker, or medical assistant, they can provide suggestions and help lessen burdens on those that employ them. The best ones provide personalized assistance, remembering past interactions, and using them to infer the user's preferences. They automate commonly performed tasks, constantly improving their behavior and being always on the lookout for opportunities.

Collaborative agents can also work behind the scenes as well as directly in the user interface. Collaborative agents take information from many different sources and locations. They collaborate when multiple agents act as a team in analyzing data and solving problems, bringing multi-perspective and multi-expertise capabilities to bear in solving problems.

Collaborative agents communicate using *agent communication language*. These languages, unlike simple protocols that simply transfer data, contain complex social interactions that reflect a community of agents – providing help or asking for it, providing and requesting opinions and perspectives, organizing, monitoring, and so forth. Collaborative agents' interactions and dynamic groupings often model the flow and function among systems and people they are intended to help, providing a natural example of form following function and coincidentally, a model of information flow among the organization(s) in which they operate.

The premise of the collaborative agents paradigm is that legacy systems are leveraged as much as possible. Collaborative agents are thus an important enabling technology for rapidly integrating and prioritizing diverse data sources in large, complex distributed information systems. The compositional stance of the paradigm also provides an operational design for growth, allowing hospitals to evolve newly deployed support systems alongside pre-existing information structures, thus ensuring scalability for future information system requirements.

2. Connecting the personal with the public

One of the most intriguing areas for the use of agents in medicine is in helping to make connections between personal information and public information. Example of personal information in medicine would be information specific to a particular patient, health-care provider, or facility, such as patient history and treatment records, test results, a physician's personal notes, and hospital records. These records are usually stored in private databases. Examples of general information would be medical reference books, medical Web sites (either for the physician or the patient), the medical research literature, and public health statistics. These are stored in databases which are public, or intended for a large audience.

Right now, these sources of information are completely separate, and the task is left to people to explicitly establish these connections. Which medical references pertain to a specific person's condition? Which Web sites should a particular patient look at? Which journal articles help a hospital decide which piece of equipment to buy for their needs?

Integrating private and public information is difficult, because nobody has the time or energy to monitor and consider all sources of potentially relevant information. What people really want to know is "What in this is relevant to me and to my current situation?". We can delegate to the agent the job of at least trying to guess what might be relevant and bring it to our attention, thus potentially saving us time and trouble.

One of the strengths of agents is that they can synthesize partial information that comes from different sources to present an integrated view to the user. Tools like search engines help find information, of course, but everyone who types the same phrase into a search engine receives the same hits, so a search engine cannot deliver personalized results. The software has got to know something about you.

We'll present some examples of how agents can perform the function of connecting personal and public information. The first will be oriented toward the patient, addressing the question of providing relevant assistance to the ever-increasing number of patients who educate themselves on personal medical topics via the Web. The second scenario, more oriented towards physicians, will show how the physician's immediate context can be used to facilitate semi-automatic annotation and retrieval of images from a database of medical images. The capabilities demonstrated in the patient scenario could, of course, be equally valuable in some circumstances to the physician, and vice versa. Both scenarios are rough, of course, but we hope this will illustrate the potential and power of agent software.

3. Interface agents can discover serendipitous connections

Search engines are great when you know exactly what you want, but people never quite know exactly what they want, and what they want to know keeps changing with changing conditions, interests and what they discover. Sometimes the most interesting information pops up via *serendipitous connections* -- when two seemingly unrelated pieces of information turn out accidentally to have a strong link.

Medicine is full of cases where finding unexpected relationships between diverse pieces of information is important. Drug interactions is an obvious example -- patients may be taking two different drugs for totally unrelated conditions, but if the two drugs have a bad interaction, knowing that can mean the difference between life and death. Some rare diseases are characterized by an unusual combination of symptoms that most harried physicians might not think to check for.

It is hard to imagine a traditional search engine that could find serendipitous connections automatically, but we have developed a browsing assistant agent, *Letizia* [4], [5], [7] that does just that.

Letizia records the user's choices in a standard Web browser, then reads and analyzes each page that the user sees. It compiles a user profile, a weighted list of keywords, that represents the user's interests. Letizia "follows you around" on the Web, updating this profile dynamically,

Then, when the user is viewing a particular page, Letizia initiates an incremental, breadth-first search starting from each link on the page. That is, it looks first at every page one link away from the user's choice, then two links away, and so on. Every so often, it filters the pages searched through the user's profile and delivers the best one so far as a recommendation. When the user jumps to a new page, so does Letizia's search. This process is illustrated below.

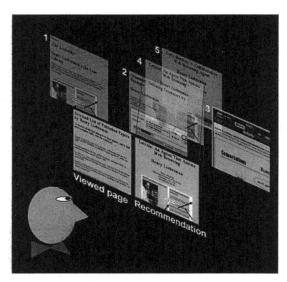

Figure 1. Letizia's search. The user is looking at the page on the left marked "Viewed Page". Linked to it directly are pages 1, 2, and 3. 4 and 5 are two and three links away, respectively. Letizia chooses 4 as best fitting the user's interest, and recommends it.

How does this process discover serendipitous connections? User browsing tends to be "chunky" in the sense that users look at several pages covering related topics for a certain interval of time, punctuated by topic shifts. Just because they change topics doesn't mean that they cease to be interested in the old topic, and so Letizia has the job of maintaining the user's "persistence of interest". When a topic happens to satisfy several of the user's interests simultaneously, even if they are seemingly unrelated, Letizia will award it a high score. That will bring up pages of high interest even if they are a few links away. Let's look at an example.

Suppose we have a female user who likes to browse about health topics on the many Web sites devoted to health. She is a smoker, and would like to quit. She browses several sites that give advice about quitting smoking. From that browsing pattern, Letizia would infer keywords such as the following:

Smoking, tobacco, nicotine, patch, Nicorette, emphysema, cancer, counseling, group, addiction...

Much later, perhaps in a different session, she would examine an unrelated topic, birth control methods. Looking at Planned Parenthood, and other sites, she happens upon articles concerning the pill. The profile would now also contain:

Birth control, condom, pill, diaphragm, estrogen, prostaglandin,...

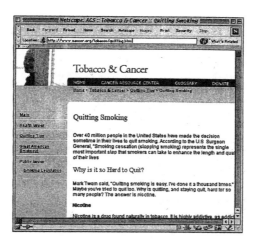

Figure 2. A patient browses Web sites concerning different topics. Letizia learns an interest profile that includes keywords from both these topics.

Now, again much later, and perhaps during a different session, the user visits a general site containing Medical news, here Healthlink, maintained by the Medical College of Wisconsin. It contains news items on a wide variety of medical topics.

At first glance, none of the headline articles might seem of interest to our user. However, while the user is scanning the headlines, Letizia is busy searching the subsidiary links from the Healthlink home page, without any explicit action on the part of the user. After a short while, Letizia brings up an article it found several links away in the Q & A section, one that warns about the risks of birth control pills to smokers, which our user might not have known.

Of course, had she typed "smoking birth control pollen allergies ACL injuries...", and all her other health interests into a search engine, she might have found the same article, but she probably wouldn't have thought to do that. Because smoking and birth control were in her Letizia interest profile, we can bring up the "news she can use". Some sites let you select topics of personal interest via questionnaires, but the problem is people often forget to update them as their interests change. Should our user succeed in quitting smoking or switch birth control methods, static questionnaires wouldn't reflect such changes.

In contrast to a search engine, which might retrieve pages from anywhere on the Web, Letizia's search is localized, starting with the current page and widening over time. In our example, though there might be many pages about the smoking-and-birth-control-pill issue on the Web, Letizia is much more likely to retrieve the Medical College of Wisconsin's article rather than one from an arbitrary source. Because Letizia tends to keep a user "in the neighborhood", sources are most likely to be those with which the patient is already familiar and trusting.

Letizia is an example of how agents that learn personalized information from watching the user's actions, and make suggestions proactively, can help users connect personally relevant information with information that is aimed at a general audience, such as on the Web.

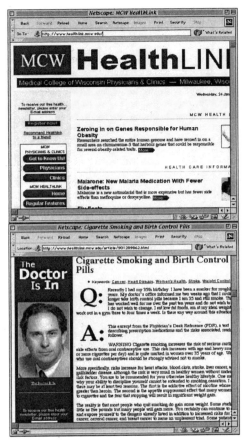

Figure 3. When the user arrives at the news page, Letizia automatically retrieves an article about birth control and smoking, two topics of high personal interest to the user.

4. Interface Agents can use context to associate metadata with data

Another function that an interface agent can assume is to use the *context* of the user's work to assist in problem solving. Most of today's applications do not make any significant use of context; your text editor and your spreadsheet don't communicate, even if you are using them both on a common task where they might profitably share information. This is because the current paradigm of software is based on the notion of "applications" -- that each piece of software is a world unto itself and transfers of information occur only via files and cut and paste. This is silly.

A full discussion of the importance of context in user interaction can be found in [6]. In this article, we'll show how agents that help with context can assist in a task of annotation and retrieval of medical images. As the fidelity and accessibility of computer graphics and digital cameras increases, imaging has become more and more important in medicine. Pictures can communicate in a way that words alone cannot. Doctors and hospitals maintain enormous collections of patient images, and soon patients will manage their own collections of their own medical images.

Like any image library, medical images are useful only if you know what they mean, and can retrieve them as needed. Annotating images with metadata information about data, in this case information about the images such as patient identification, time, place, equipment, diagnostic information, etc. is tedious and time-consuming. Similarly tedious and time-consuming is using query applications to retrieve or browse collections. Thus many opportunities to use images are lost.

Our idea was to integrate the annotation and retrieval of images into a single, integrated application, and entrust a software agent, Aria [8] with the job of detecting opportunities for annotation and retrieval of images in the context of the user's everyday work. Aria stands for Annotation and Retrieval Integration Agent.

Aria is composed of a text editor that can be used to compose e-mail messages or Web pages and a photo library, the Shoebox. When the user types in the text editor, Aria is continuously analyzing the text typed and extracting keywords, which are automatically used to retrieve images from the image database. The query is recomputed at every keystroke.

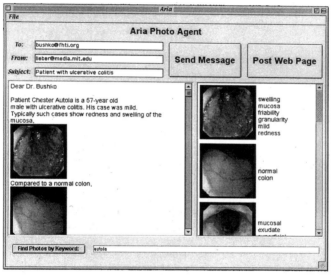

Figure 4. As the physician discusses a case, Aria automatically retrieves relevant images, and uses keywords from the discussion to annotate the image in the database.

Thus as soon as the user types a word, he or she sees the picture column recomputed, ordering the pictures from most relevant top to least bottom. The user can simply drag an image into the text to include it.

Dragging the image into the text also directs the system to scan the surrounding text, and use those keywords as annotations that automatically go back into the database, without any user action necessary.

In the example above, as soon as Dr. Lieberman types "57-year old male with ulcerative colitis" into the e-mail message, pictures from a relevant database were retrieved by Aria. The words "ulcerative colitis" were typed not as a query to a search engine, but to communicate these words to the e-mail correspondent. This "recycling" of user input reduces the total number of user interactions necessary. Why should we retype a query for "ulcerative colitis" when we already told the computer we're interested in it?

Similarly, typing "redness" brings up an image that displays that characteristic, which the doctor inserts to illustrate his point. But he also types "swelling of the mucosa" to describe that picture, so the keywords "swelling" and "mucosa" are automatically associated with the image. He can, of course, edit out annotation that the system gets wrong. The next time he or a colleague types a description of ulcerative colitis with swelling of the mucosa, that image will automatically appear. To make his point, he would like to contrast the patient's colon with a normal colon, and as soon as the words "normal colon" are typed, a picture of a normal colon appears.

Contrast this interaction with unwieldy conventional annotation and retrieval applications. We were able to complete the interaction with:

- No dialog boxes
- No filenames
- No saving and loading files
- No cut and paste
- No queries typed to a retrieval application
- No annotation application

Agent software holds great potential to streamline the user interface by allowing agents to pick up information from its natural context, avoiding the explicit user interactions that would otherwise have to take place.

The previous scenarios all concerned a single agent assisting a single user. We'll now move to consider a broader picture where multiple computer agents, distributed over time and space, assist multiple people working together in an organization. This scenario is supported by the technology of collaborative software agents.

5. A Night in the Life of a Hospital Agent

The emergence of collaborative agent teams will enable new ways to manage diverse distributed data sources, saving valuable patient and hospital time and reducing potential for errors in tedious procedures. In the following hypothetical scenario, we project how a team of collaborative agents might work through the night in a Los Angeles hospital. Although we have not implemented this particular scenario, the collaborative agent technology behind it is real, and we predict that it will become the future of integrating software in hospitals.

Agents assigned to computers in diagnostics, x-ray, and other testing labs are working around the clock with other agents in the hospital to ensure data integrity, consistency and efficient use of hospital and staff resources, improving patient care and reducing anxiety and conflicts among staff and family members.

What are these agents doing? As afternoon rounds wind to a close, Dr. Brown stops in on his last patient, Betty, who is scheduled for transplant surgery in the morning. Dr. Brown holds Betty's hand and describes what will happen next. Dr. Brown communicates a series of tests to be performed to Hal, the agent in Betty's wristband that listens while Dr. Brown visits with Betty.

Hal's job is to ensure all procedures and interactions related to Betty go as smooth as possible while she is here. Betty received the wristband when she was admitted and will wear it until she is released. Hal knows a lot about Betty because he's already talked to the other agents that are down in the pharmacy and in Dr. Brown's office. Hal also knows other agents that might be of use if anything goes wrong with Betty during the night. Hal will know because the agents assigned to monitor her wearable computing devices are working for him. As Hal begins the task of creating the orders, reports, requests and schedules to fill Dr. Brown's order, he consults his knowledge base regarding the surgery and Betty's history. He reasons that before issuing a request for a blood draw at the 2pm rounds, it would be a good idea in this situation to check with the agents in lab records to determine if these tests has been done before on Betty and retrieves any notes or other relevant information regarding the tests.

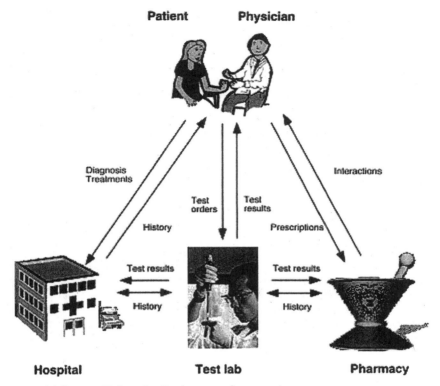

Figure 5. Partial diagram of information flow between software agents

While Hal is waiting for the reply from records to arrive, he also requests information from the pharmacy agent regarding any medications that could interfere with the tests he is about to order and checks these against the ones he knows Betty is on. Hal notices the returned information from the lab, and places a note for the scheduling agent that blood should be taken from Betty's right foot, as her veins have a history of collapsing and there has been difficulty drawing Betty's blood lately.   All of the preliminary checks appear in order, so Hal begins tending to other tasks.

Around 3:20am, as results from automated data analysis complete and arrive in Hal's data repository, Hal begins to examine the incoming results, looking to see if there is anything unusual to raise an alarm about.

He notices the CBC sed rate is rather unusual, and requests the test be repeated. The agent down in the lab has received over a dozen requests to repeat this test, so it does a self-monitoring test and realizes its own meter is not functioning. It raises an alarm with the lab attendant who manages to correct the situation and re-start the lab computer. Hal runs a few other routine checks and looks at the trends in monitoring data that were collected during the night before disseminating results and patient status. Hal shares the results with agent managing the patient chart, the agent collating and prioritizing the PCP's morning reports, and the surgery room. Hal's agent protocol ensures the chart agent, the badge agent, and PCP agent pass an identifier consistency check as the patient enters the surgery room at 5:30 am as morning rounds begin.

6. Collaborative Agents

Notice how different the above scenario is from the way today's medical information systems are organized. Typically, patient records, lab tests, hospital administration records, pharmacy systems, etc. would all be implemented in separate computer systems and the job is left to people to get information in and out of the systems when needed, and fill out forms, translating between different formats when necessary. It has been estimated that over 30% of a physician's time is consumed with routine information entry and information seeking tasks. In our scenario above, these tasks are largely accomplished autonomously by software agents themselves. But to do that, the software agents need to reason about goals, methods, resources, and communication strategies.

The fields of Multi-Agent Systems and Distributed Artificial Intelligence [1, 3] study the principles of communication and processing for collaborative agent problem solving. A focus of research in this area is *agent communication languages*, which express higher level concepts than today's data transfer protocols. These languages allow agents to communicate not only simple transfers of data, but also concepts such as goals and methods, or asking particular agents about their capabilities. Agent toolkits [10] provide general facilities for things like how to find out which agents are capable of solving a given problem, keeping track of which agents are working on which problems, where and when goals are satisfied, sharing partial results, etc. Analysis of agent communication patterns can yield valuable strategic information such as how to manage the tradeoff between expending effort in advance to determine which agent can solve a problem, or letting several agents try and integrating the results [9].

7. Conclusion

The new paradigm of intelligent agent software holds great promise in helping medical practitioners and patients deal with the problems of "information overload" that result from both the explosion of available medical information and the complexity of conventional computer software. By helping to connect personal information with public information, utilize information that is implicit in a user's context, and perform collaborative problem solving, software agents might be just what the doctor ordered for the next generation of medical software.

References

[1] Bond, Alan H. and Les Gasser (Editors). Readings in Distributed Artificial Intelligence. Morgan Kaufman Publishers. 1988.
[2] Bradshaw, Jeffrey, ed. Intelligent Agents, MIT Press, 1996.
[3] Ferber, Jacques, Multi-Agent Systems : An Introduction to Distributed Artificial Intelligence, Addison-Wesley, 1999.
[4] Lieberman, H. Letizia: An Agent That Assists Web Browsing, International Joint Conference on Artificial Intelligence IJCAI-95, Montréal, August 1995.
[5] Lieberman, H., Autonomous Interface Agents, ACM Conference on Computers and Human Interface CHI-97, Atlanta, May 1997.
[6] Lieberman, Henry and Ted Selker, Out of Context: Computer Systems that Learn From, and Adapt To, Context, IBM Systems Journal, Vol 39, Nos 3&4, pp.617-631, 2000.

[7] Lieberman, Henry, Christopher Fry and Louis Weitzman, Why Surf Alone? Exploring the Web with Reconnaissance Agents, Communications of the ACM, to appear, 2001.

[8] Lieberman, Henry, Elizabeth Rosenzweig and Push Singh, An Agent for Integrated Annotation and Retrieval of Images, forthcoming.

[9] Mason, Cindy, Introspection as Control in Result-Sharing Assumption-Based Reasoning Agents, International Workshop on Distributed Artificial Intelligence, Lake Quinalt, Washington, 1994.

[10] Mason, Cindy, ROO: A Distributed AI Toolkit for Belief-Based Reasoing Agents, International Conference on Cooperative Knowledge-Based Systems, Keele, England, 1994.

Future of Health Technology
R.G. Bushko (Ed.)
IOS Press, 2002

Speech and Language Technologies, Intelligent Content Management and Intelligent Assistants

Jo Lernout

Abstract

This chapter focuses on Speech and Language Technologies, Intelligent Content Management and Intelligent Assistants. It describes impact of these technologies on healthcare assuming a 10-year scope.

1. Definitions:

Today's speech and language technologies, combined with artificial intelligence enable individuals to communicate more easily, across language barriers, with other people and with the machines that surround us in our daily lives. What technologies are currently available in this field?

1.1 Speech Technologies

a) Computer programs, which enable human speech to be recognized: What words are spoken? *(STT, Speech-to-Text* conversion) What is the (semantic) meaning of the spoken words? (Natural Language Understanding) Who is speaking? Speaker verification: Is the speaker the one she/he claims to be? (as verified against pre-stored patterns) Speaker identification: Amongst many possible speaker profiles identify who is speaking.

b) Computer programs to *compress speech,* store it and forward the speech files, and decompress the speech upon demand. Speaker's profile, gender, intonation, etc... are kept intact in this process.

c) Computer programs to synthesize text-to-speech *(TTS).* Current state-of-the-art program reproduces speech in a humanlike voice, inclusive prosody (the rhythm, sign and dance of natural human speech).

d) Computer programs to conduct a spoken *dialogue* driven interaction between humans and machines. The aim is to allow a user to express her/himself in a natural and very intuitive way, in order to give the machine commands to be executed by the machine, or in order to query the machine in search of information to be found by the machine.

Above mentioned speech technologies are usually and currently available on many different types of digital devices: PC's, servers, mobile phones, automotive dashboard devices, PDA's (Personal Digital Assistants) and run on different types of operating systems: Windows®, WinCE®, Linux®, Sun Solaris®, etc...

Speech technologies are using a combination of statistical analysis <u>pattern recognition</u> algorithms (Analysis of the speech pattern spectrum, FFT, Fast Fourrier Transformation, Hidden Markov Models or HMM's, Artificial Neural Networks, ANN's, etc.), and <u>computational linguistics</u>, such as rule based systems (if-then rules) and sentence parsers to analyze the sentence, extract the meaning, generate TTS prosody and pronunciation rules, etc...

Today, large vocabulary STT systems are most of the time based on SLM's (Statistical Language Models) to guess the relationship between spoken/recognized vowels and consonants and the most likely word candidates these utterances represent. SLM's are usually based on text bases of at least a couple of hundred million words, most representative for a particular language or dialect thereof and most representative for a particular domain, such as business memo's, newspapers, radiology reports, civil law texts, etc...

1.2 Other Language Technologies

Computational linguistics (modeling the relationships between speech utterances and the potential word candidates, modeling the morphology of words, describing all terminology, describing the meaning of words in sentences, parsing the sentence, syntax, grammar, etc...) are applied to the above mentioned speech technologies, but are also applied in:

e) *Automatic Machine Translation (AMT):*
Translation of text from one (natural) language to another, executed by computer programs. When ① proper analysis of each sentence of the source language is done, and when ② proper re-generation is done in another (target) language, and when ③ special lexica (words that have a particular meaning in a particular context) are called from pre-stored lexicon bases and when ④ TM's (Translation Memory) are used, as a pre-processor to call frequently asked terms, bodies of text, idioms which were once programmed and already translated in the TM by human translators, <u>then</u> the quality of the AMT is substantially high, and in some very technical text oriented cases, can reach today the quality of human translators. AMT is run on most off-the-shelf computer systems: PC's, servers, even PDA's.

f) *Natural Language Understanding (NLU) and Natural Language Query (NLQ):*

Using some of the computational linguistic components described in 2.a., and certainly when supplemented with concept networks (CN's), complete analysis and understanding of spoken, typed or scribbled sentences is achieved; then the analysis can be used to give parameters to other programs of the computer device, to automatically execute the requested command, or the analysis is converted automatically into structured data base query statements, such as Boolean SQR statements, avoiding for the user the burden to deal with such difficult Boolean query language. CN's (concept networks), also called SN's (semantic networks) are extensive libraries of descriptions of the many different concepts humans are dealing with in the broad concept of the world we live in, or in a narrow domain of a particular profession (medical, legal, etc.) or a particular company. CN's describe the world in nested concepts, such as the relationship between a bike and its parts, the verb "biking", the sports that have to do with racing, biking, the fuzzynyms (such as related vehicles), the synonyms, etc...

A CN will vastly enhance the NLU to extract the real meaning and essence of what the user really wants when a question is expressed: a dialogue between user and machine can either help the user to broaden his/her question or narrow the question. Multilingual CN's or SN's describe the world's concepts simultaneously in different natural languages.

g) *Intelligent Content Management (ICM)*

Applying all of the above mentioned computational linguistic components, and combining this statistical text analysis algorithms (tagging words in text, measuring their frequency in a text body against this relative usage frequency in the language of that text body, etc.), ICM applications will automatically read a body of text, extract and sort by frequency the most relevant topics, automatically classify the text, automatically make summaries in a user specified number of sentences of words. ICM systems allow users to search by speaking or typing queries in full natural sentences, then understand the meaning of the query, then browse all available text or structured database bodies, and present the user summaries and topic overviews of only the relevant-to-the-query text bodies, then allow the user to go directly down to the paragraph and word level which contains the answer to the query (relevancy ranking).

Cross-lingual ICM systems allow search in one natural language to find answers in text bodies in simultaneous different languages, and present topic extraction, overviews and summaries to the user in the language of the query.

A special version of ICM is Audiomining®, which allows the user to type in a query, and if the answer is contained in a body of an audio base (a call center registered call, a broadcast of radio, television, or in a music CD or DVD, a stored voice-mail), then using ICM and STT (Speech-to-Text), the system will allow to find the matching portion and present it to the user. The ICM solutions mentioned here are currently available as applications running on PC's and servers.

Optically scanned and bitmapped stored bodies of text can be converted via OCR (Optical Character Recognition) into ASCII-format and then "ICM'd" via the above mentioned ICM technologies.

When visualization techniques are applied such as VR (Virtual Reality) representation of links between data-elements (data elements could come from structured databases, text bodies, audio-bases, optically stored documents), then users can query with NLU, and literally *see* the links between different data types, represented almost in 3D on a CRT or flat panel screen. Touching icons at the end of each link, allows the user "dig deeper" into the info-soup, to retrieve gradually more detail at the tip of each link by clicking on the icon representing the type of data and further links "behind" the icon.

3. Intelligent Assistants (IA's):

IA's combine all the technologies mentioned in 1) and 2) and act as automatic "servants" to the user. IA's can be general in nature: they gradually "learn" (today mostly via if-then rule programs) the behavior patterns of their "masters/users", store other personal info and preferences of their users and then gradually serve their "master" better and better: e.g. automatic loading of the user's speech profile for better STT, automatic adaptation to the acoustical environment, automatic setting of preferences (i.e. first present the summaries of the urgent e-mails from a specific list of senders), faster browsing through the dialogue-preferences, etc...

Specialized IA's will be equipped to both adapt to their "regular master's" wish list, but at the same time they are specialized in a particular task: e.g. unified messaging, radiology-reporting, etc...

4. Current Applications in Healthcare

How can speech technologies combined with artificial intelligence contribute to a healthcare environment? What are the advantages to merge those technologies in present day healthcare?

4.1 STT (Speech-to-Text)

The current state-of-the-art STT is permitting doctors, nurses, and other medical staff to generate a medical report by simply dictating the report into a special "Dictaphone®" device or other similar digital device (specialized PDA, PC,...) or even into a phone (landline or cellular). Current STT will convert the dictated text with 95 to 98% accuracy on word level into text. The user only needs to train a few (10 to 15) seconds her/his voice for the specialized medical program, by reading 2 sentences of sample text, and the system is user ready. The productivity gain is substantial, the cost for medical transcription drops sharply and the user doesn't notice a big difference when comparing the habits and user-friendliness of previous "old age" non-digital recorder systems.

The speech recognition accuracy is improving constantly, because previously recorded dictation, after being transcribed and verified, yields many useful acoustical data elements (such as voices and utterances from many different speakers), which can be recycled to improve the recognition quality.

The services and applications for STT in the healthcare market are offered as standalone systems on PC's, clustered client server based systems for doctor practices sharing the resource, specialized transcription/correction/ verification workstations for medical assistants, and finally web-based services packages allowing the doctor to dictate, send the file over a protected and secured intranet to a service of transcriptionists, and receive the correct text.

Turnaround time to go from dictation to finalized medical reports is in all cases drastically reduced, and so are the costs to get a correct text i's dotted and t's crossed.
(Example: L&H Radiology package, Powerscribe, existing in different language versions and available today)

4.2 ICM-based applications in Healthcare

Intelligent Content Management applications are applied to medical records for:

- Automatic categorization, filing and summarization

- Automatic linking to structured databases containing info about patient, disease, doctor, etc...

- Automatic coding for healthcare insurance purposes

All medical ICM applications rely intensively on the statistical and linguistic analysis of patient records, and work best when specialized CN's (Concept Nets) are developed per medical area

Automatic coding yields great potential for cost savings: the manual coding process is to be done by specialized personnel, and is often prone to errors of both "undercoding" (causing less insurance money to be paid back) or "overcoding" (causing risks for penalties when independent audits show overcoding).

Finally, ICM's greatest potential in the near future lies in the massive cross-lingual, multimodal natural language query based info-extraction from all recorded medical records. This will allow to "find the needle in the multilingual/multimodal healthcare haystack".

For example: healthcare professionals, granted privileged but secured access to this "haystack" (being all accessible but anonymous recorded patient/ doctor/ disease/ treatment/ anamnesys/ diagnose/ prognosis/ final results from treatment/ etc... whether they are stored in voice files, text files, structured databases, videotapes) will be capable to ask questions in full natural language, and these users will not have to know where the data is stored, nor in what file, nor under what header, classifier, etc...

All cross-linking is done on the fly on request. The ICM system will find the data that is relevant to the question, give the main topics, give summaries, translate on the fly from one language to another, and will allow the user to browse directly to the relevant paragraphs or detailed data elements (cf. the needle in the haystacks). Specialized programs can be written on top of that to recognize particular patterns or trends, add-up results, take averages, etc... For example, an English query can be launched in the following style:

"Give me the overviews of all the records about male patients older than 55 years, treated in the USA for senile diabetes, with insulin-type XXX!"

The ICM query system will search across all files, whatever type of file, even audio-recordings, and gather all relevant data, even if the data are in another language than English, and present topic-ranging, relevant rankings, overviews and summaries, in English, to the querier.

Such ICM technology is available today in component format, but could be built as a complete application in less than 2 to 3 years from now. Already today, Natural Language Query by voice, even over the phone, or typed queries, allow doctors to access patient records and time schedules, in a dialogue between user and info-system. With Realspeak®, L&H's high-quality Text-to-Speech, patient records or other info is read in a clear spoken voice to the doctor.

5. Future Trends: What can be expected in 2 to 10 years?

The 21st century promises even greater advances in both the technology and the medical sector. What evolutions may we still expect that could enhance the quality of our lives?

5.1 Speech-to-Text and Intelligent Content Management:

These technologies and their derived applications, will gradually, but constantly, improve in terms of speech recognition accuracy, using additional technologies such as: "face recognition", "lip reading", "gaze tracking", etc... These image recognition technologies will become widely available, since PC's and PDA's (certainly PDA/cellular phones equipped with digital camera's, UMTS broadband wireless technologies and powerful processors) will all be delivered with built-in digital video camera, probably in less than 2 to 3 years from now. These image technologies will enhance video conferencing between PC-users and PDA-UMTS-users, but they will also contribute to enhance STT performance. Face recognition will automatically identify and verify the user, load appropriate user and speech profiles and secure data access via enhanced biometric verification such as a combination of fingerprint, face recognition and speaker verification technologies. But face and gaze tracking, combined with lip reading will also be combined with STT to free the user from close talk/headset microphones, and allow the user to "point & click" just by "gazing" at the point of interest on the display, and then express commands by spoken NLU (Natural Language Understanding).

ICM will gradually improve by self-learning statistical pattern tracking techniques, so that the precision to find the needle in the "healthcare haystack" will gradually be enhanced. Additionally the amounts of healthcare data to be gathered and browsed will gradually increase, which will both provide more relevant data and the statistical interpretation. Buyers of that info will be many healthcare professionals, pharmaceutical companies, and bioengineering companies, the NIH etc...

5.2 Healthcare Intelligent Assistants:

By 2005, the info-assistants will have the look and feel of Intelligent Assistants, which will consist of all the here mentioned multimodal NL-based user interfaces, and which will conduct intelligent searches with growing precision. To that will be added, probably supported by expert systems, Intelligent Assistants that will become helpful resources to the doctor in diagnosing various kinds of diseases.

By 2010, diagnosis and health monitoring Intelligent Assistants, profiled to each individual patient, will conduct semi-automatic diagnoses and semi-automatic monitoring, reachable at home, in the office and even on the move. Such Intelligent Healthcare Assistants will be linked to all kinds of sensors to measure blood pressure, ECG, and quick diagnose tools such as personalized protein identifiers leading to early detection of a disease.

By 2010, DNA identification will probably be part of the remote "sensory" leading to a very precise diagnosis and treatment progress monitoring. These personal Intelligent Healthcare Assistants will have a major positive impact in terms of reducing Healthcare costs, since early detecting means better prevention, and since remote sensory and monitoring will reduce costs of visits to medical centers for most ambulant healthcare matters.

5.3 Bio-Engineering Research Tools, Bio-Informatics:

The point where bio-engineering and genetics meet ICM and other Information Technologies will lead, (and have already led today) to supercomputers which will greatly speed up gene sequencing and proteomics ("the hunt for proteins"), which is actually the hunt for the relationship between healthy and defaulted genes and their relative protein folding causing specific cells to be what they are, or causing specific cells to become faulty, i.e. sick in one or another way.

Coupling gene sequencing, genetics, proteomics and targeted search for related literature in all kinds of scientific publications is called the field of Bio-Informatics. Many large computer companies (e.g. Compaq, IBM, Sun Microsystems) have engaged in multi-million joint R&D programs with biotech companies (e.g. Celera Genomics) to develop this next generation of bio-informatics supercomputer, to be ready by 2005. The info they provide is vital for the whole healthcare community, and will kick-start a whole new range of targeted and personalized drug developments, and will also boost the very promising stem cell approach to healthcare.

Interestingly enough, new gene sequencing techniques, analyzing spectral representations of the molecular weight of C, T, A, G relies on some of the speech pattern recognition technologies such as FFT and HMM. Therefore, the cross-section of pattern recognition technologies, supercomputers, ICM and genetics, i.e. the bio-informatics, will revolutionize in less than 10 years many areas of the healthcare industry.

Advancing Global Health
Information Infrastructure

Future of Health Technology
R.G. Bushko (Ed.)
IOS Press, 2002

Developing the Health Information Infrastructure in the United States

Mary Jo Deering, Ph.D.*

Director of Health Communication and eHealth, Office of Disease Prevention and Health Promotion (ODPHP), U.S. Department of Health and Human Services (HHS) & Lead HHS Staff for the Work Group on the National Health Information Infrastructure of the National Committee on Vital and Health Statistics

Abstract

Consumers, patients, and their families; health care providers and managers; public health professionals and policy makers need integrated multi-function health information structures that allow them to locate and apply information when and where they need it to make better decisions about health. The National Committee on Vital and Health Statistics (NCVHS), which advises the Secretary of Health and Human Services (HHS) on health information policy, is promoting a comprehensive vision of the National Health Information Infrastructure (NHII). The NHII is defined as the set of technologies, standards, applications, systems, values, and laws that support all facets of individual health, health care, and public health. It is not a unitary database. The broad goal of the NHII is to deliver information to consumers, patients, professionals, and other health decision-makers when and where they need it. The NCVHS' Interim Report presented three overlapping "dimensions" of the NHII: the personal health dimension, the health care provider dimension, and the community health dimension, to highlight the functions and value of information linkages from various perspectives. The content of an NHII includes clinical, population, and personal data, practice guidelines, biomedical, health services, and other research findings; and consumer health information. This data is, and will likely remain, stored in many locations. To succeed, such an effort will require coordinated, collaborative action. The NCVHS' final report to the HHS Secretary will include recommendations for Federal leadership and for other relevant stakeholders, including public health agencies; health care providers, plans and purchasers; the IT industry; standards development organizations; and consumer groups.

1. The Opportunity

Healthy People 2010, the nation's disease prevention and health promotion agenda for the next decade, has two goals: increase the quantity and quality of years of healthy life, and eliminate health disparities. [1] Extensive knowledge about how to extend years of healthy life already exists, but it often does not reach the right people when, where, and how they need it. Research findings on improving quality of life and reducing health disparities will not bring parallel increases in good health without better ways of collecting, synthesizing, and distributing them. Consumers, patients, and their families; health care providers and managers; public health professionals and policy makers need integrated multi-function health information structures that allow them to locate and apply information when and where they need it to make better decisions about health.

All who share an interest in good health can benefit from having the right health information, at the right time, at the right place, or connecting efficiently to one another when needed. The resources to make information available and provide these interconnections seem tantalizingly close at hand. Dramatic developments in information and communication technologies point toward a comprehensive framework that could link users to knowledge and each other more effectively, with benefits for all. But, like the sorcerer's apprentice, we risk permitting this near-magical assistance to be fragmented--even counter productive–through our own failure to act intelligently, energetically, and in a coordinated manner.

Many building blocks of an effective health knowledge support system already exist; countless construction crews are already hard at work. If they don't talk to each other, build to common standards, collaborate on cross-cutting components, and secure adequate financing, their projects will collapse or never connect. Two scenarios suggest the alternate paths we could take. They illustrate the shared concerns and overlapping interests of different people confronting one health issue.

1.1 Supporting Health in 2010: The present course. John H., aged 66, diabetic

John: I know I'm supposed to be managing my diabetes. My doctor scares me enough with the possibility of amputation if we don't stay on top of my condition. But it's hard to remember everything I'm supposed to do. Often I forget to check my glucose. Living on my own, I don't have much motivation to eat right or be more active. I don't know how to shop for or cook the kind of food I should. It's real hard for me to make my appointments since the doctor's office is way across town and I can't drive anymore. I pester the nurse by calling a lot, but she always has to get the doctor to call back.

John's doctor: John isn't following up on his diabetes self-care. I have no way to give him helpful reminders about his every day care. He forgets his appointments even when we send him a postcard in advance, so he's missing some important screenings for secondary and tertiary prevention. I think he's seeing more than one doctor, and I have no way to regularly compare clinical notes. There might be some new drugs to help him, but I haven't seen a useful synthesis of the recommendations. I can't be sure that he has told me all the medications he's taking, so I can't check for potentially dangerous interactions.

Medicare Official: The cost of care for diabetics is rising sharply as the population ages. We have evidence that scientifically and economically justified prevention programs are not being used routinely in daily clinical management. We can't track quality of care by providers or plans at the level we'd need to in order to make strategic interventions. We know we have a significant problem with continuity of care due to turnover in plans and providers and with the increasing geographic mobility of older people. This has serious adverse health and economic consequences in diabetes.

Public Health Official: We're not making much headway against diabetes. We don't have good information about where it may be affecting specific groups in local communities, urban or rural, so we can't target our diabetes prevention and control programs at the level where they would be most effective.

1.2 Supporting Health in 2010: The way it could be. John H., aged 66, diabetic

John: Thank heaven for the health alert system that my doctor gave me. It's real convenient and helps me feel reassured. My system printed out a simple diet and exercise program for me. It also shows me daily reminders. When I do my home glucose test, it can trigger an alarm for me and my doctor if there's a problem. I don't have black out spells anymore because the program can suggest a change in my insulin dose, which the doctor's system can okay. I can email the doctor and get self-care tips from her Web site. I feel like she's giving me better attention and care.

John's doctor: John's diabetes is under control. When his blood glucose drops, the home monitoring system catches it and recommends the appropriate insulin adjustment. The system's reminders for self-care and appointments seem to help. I initiated a request that he get his annual eye and foot exams; the system can do the scheduling with his other doctors online and provide the pertinent information to them from his records. I can consult easier with his other doctors. Now the drugs he's taking are all in my medication checker and I get automatic alerts about interactions. Our structured email system helps him get his questions answered and his prescriptions refilled. I feel I can manage his care with less hassle.

Medicare Official: Our diabetic care is improving and costs per patient have dropped–as with other diseases-- since we adapted models from the Government Computer Patient Record project and DoD's unified health portal. Continuity across plans and providers is much better; we're capturing better quality information. Since HIPAA implementation finally kicked in, administrative costs are down.

Public Health Official: Our expanded local data system is helping us do a better job of identifying areas with high rates of diabetes. We've been able to develop special education and outreach programs for communities that need them; we've expanded our Spanish-language efforts in a number of places that showed large groups of high risk Hispanic people.

Many elements of an NHII exist already; many others–and some not yet imagined–are likely to appear. However, they are developing in haphazard fashion, often incompatible with each other or in proprietary vertical stovepipes. While HIPAA made health *insurance* portable, health *information* essential for continuity of care is not easily carried between providers of competing systems. Virtually no market-driven systems provide for the integration of information across a community. Achieving the equivalent of the "Golden Spike" meeting of transcontinental railway lines will require the participation of government, the health care and technology industries, voluntary and philanthropic organizations, and the people it is intended to benefit.

Several authoritative bodies have made recommendations about the infrastructure requirements for the NHII and opportunities for Federal leadership [2, 3, 4]. The Work Group on the NHII of the National Committee on Vital and Health Statistics (NCVHS) is currently developing recommendations for Federal action on the NHII that address the need for leadership and coordination.

2. Setting Strategic Goals For an NHII

Since 1998, the National Committee on Vital and Health Statistics (NCVHS), which serves as the public advisory body for the Secretary of Health and Human Services on national health information policy, has been envisioning the rational evolution of a National Health Information Infrastructure that would address consumer, health care provider and public health information needs. NCVHS created a Work Group on the National Health Information Infrastructure, whose official Charge defines the NHII:

The "NHII" is a set of technologies, standards, and applications that support communication and information to improve clinical care, monitor public health, and educate consumers and patients. It is not a unitary database. The broad goal of the NHII is health knowledge management and delivery, so that the full array of information needed to improve the public's health and health care is optimally available for professionals, policy makers, researchers, patients, care givers, and consumers. The NHII as a system should seek to improve and enhance privacy and confidentiality of personal health information.[5]

In October, 1998, the Work Group presented a Concept Paper to the Department of Health and Human Services. [6] It stressed that content of an NHII would be diverse, reflecting the multiple purposes stated in the Work Group's Charge. It also emphasized that the development and maintenance of an NHII would involve public agencies, health care and research institutions, professional and standards organizations, consumer organizations, and the telecommunications and computer industries.

In June 2000, the Work Group elaborated on these concepts in an Interim Report, "Toward a National Health Information Infrastructure" [3] As envisioned in this paper, the NHII is the set of technologies, standards, applications, systems, values, and laws that support all facets of individual health, health care, and public health. The broad goal of the NHII is to deliver information to individuals – consumers, patients, and professionals - when and where they need it, so they can use this information to make informed decisions about health and health care. [7] The content of an NHII includes clinical, population, and personal data, practice guidelines, biomedical, health services, and other research findings; and consumer health information. The NHII is not a unitary database. This data is, and will likely remain, stored in many locations. An NHII would seek to connect that information where links are appropriate, authorized by law and patient permissions, and protected by security policies and mechanisms. [8]

The report presented three "dimensions" of an NHII, the personal health dimension, the health care provider dimension, and the community health dimension, to highlight the functions and value of information linkages from various perspectives. The dimensions are not envisioned as unitary "records," stored in any single place, but as virtual information spaces. The personal and provider dimensions each include electronic health records which are overlapping but distinct. Each includes specific information from the community health dimension that is pertinent to the individual, such as local environmental hazards. The community dimension includes carefully selected information from the provider dimension–anonymous health data for monitoring trends and, with strict safeguards, personally-identifiable information that is required to be transmitted to public health agencies by law.

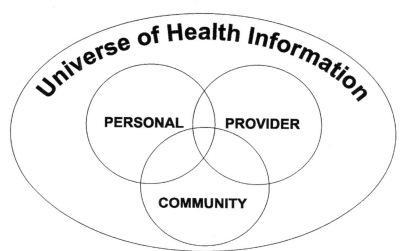

Figure 1. Dimensions of the National Health Information Infrastructure

The Personal Health Dimension (PHD): This dimension supports the management of individual wellness and health care decision-making. It encompasses data about health status and health care in the format of a consumer health record, but also other information and resources relevant to personal health. It makes possible convenient, reliable, secure, and portable access to high quality individual health and wellness information to improve decision-making by individuals and their health care providers. The PHD will encompass information supplied both by the individual and by his or her health care providers. The information will be protected by mechanisms to ensure the confidentiality and security of personal health information. [9]

The Health Care Provider Dimension (HCPD): This dimension encompasses information to enhance the quality and efficiency of health services for each individual. The HCPD includes information captured during the patient care process and concurrently integrates this information with clinical guidelines, protocols and selected information that the provider is authorized to access from the personal health record, along with information from the Community Health Dimension that is relevant to the patient's care. The HCPD centers on the individual's health care patterns. The information is typically encounter-oriented and protected by mechanisms to ensure the confidentiality of each individual's health care information. The HCPD would be relevant in physicians' offices; hospitals; ambulatory care, long term care, and mental health facilities; and home care sites to facilitate continuity of care. [10]

The Community Health Dimension (CHD): This dimension encompasses a broad range of information, including population-based health data and resources, necessary to improve public health. The CHD will include statutorily authorized data in public health systems and the Health Care Provider Dimension. Anonymous data could be used for research or other public health purposes. The CHD will have strict legal and technological safeguards, including appropriate security and permissions, to protect the confidentiality of data from other dimensions. [11]

The importance of the linkages across all three dimensions is illustrated in the following scenario: *A vacation emergency in the not too distant future by Joyce P.*

When I turned 66 last month, my sister and I took a camping vacation out West. One day as we marveled at a chain of waterfalls, I got severe stomach and chest pains. Luckily, I've subscribed to the Portable Medical Alert System since my first bout of angina five years ago, so I wear patch sensors on my chest and a wrist transmitter with a built-in positioning system. My PMAS sent emergency messages to the closest paramedic team and to my own cardiologist in New York. They both got my vital signs and location. The communications system also linked my doctor to the emergency team. By the time the paramedics reached me, my doctor had sent them relevant parts of my medical history, including previous EKGs. Once at the emergency facility, Dr. Smith took over. She asked my permission to access my online personal health record to get information on previous stomach problems, which didn't show up in my cardiologist's record. I agreed. After a thorough evaluation, including a new EKG for comparison, Dr. Smith told me I probably had viral gastroenteritis. We updated my personal health record at the same time Dr. Smith did hers, and then she discharged me in my sister's care.

The next day I felt much better, but I had lost the written follow-up instructions. No problem. I logged onto my mobile phone and found them where Dr. Smith had entered them the day before: on my personal health home page. My regimen was simple: lots of fluids and watch my diet. The next three days passed without incident, unless you count the elk on the trail.

The day we left, the local paper noted lots of other campers had become sick too. It turns out the local health department has an automated surveillance system that collects anonymous patient data from local health care providers. This system recognized a cluster of tourists with similar symptoms in one part of the park. After a little detective work, they found the culprit. A construction crew had punctured a sewer line, which in turn contaminated a number of wells providing water to park restaurants and other facilities. Come to think of it, my sister and I noticed that the drinking fountains in the park hadn't been working, so I guess park management got the alert. [12]

The Work Group held four regional hearings on the Interim Report in 2000 and January 2001 to hear opinions from experts and the public on the issues it raised. [13] Speakers validated the report's vision and agreed that NCVHS was headed in the right direction. They addressed the barriers to achieving the objectives described in the report, including financial and technical barriers, and made recommendations for actions that the Federal government could take to overcome them. They also highlighted consumer interests and the role of principal stakeholder groups in achieving the NHII vision. The next step, it was agreed, would be to enlist all key stakeholders in the development and implementation of a blueprint–or, more accurately, coordinated blueprints–for long-term action. Federal leadership was deemed essential.

3. Next Steps

In the words of Don Detmer, former Chair of the NCVHS and of its NHII Work Group, we need "a road map to get us there, a budget, and designated drivers" [14]

The NHII Work Group is now drafting its final report, which will be completed toward the end of 2001. The report will reflect public testimony, studies and recommendations by authoritative bodies such as the National Research Council and the President's Information Technology Advisory Committee [2,4], and the foundations already laid by HIPAA and other standards efforts [see, for example, 15, 16] The report will include recommendations for HHS leadership of a comprehensive, collaborative effort to develop an NHII. It will identify opportunities for improved coordination of internal and Federal-wide NHII-related policy, programs, research and technology activities; and for expanded support of cost-benefit studies, pilot projects, and standards development. It will suggest legislative and budgetary initiatives for Congress to promote interoperable linked systems and health-related information flows across plans and providers. It will identify opportunities to improve health data flows among public health agencies at the federal, state, and local levels, and for better linkages between these agencies and health care providers. It will suggest opportunities for health care membership and trade organizations to take greater leadership on NHII-related issues and suggest actions for providers, plans, and purchasers to accelerate NHII development. It will suggest ways in which standards organizations, the IT industry, consumer and community organizations can be involved.

This approach reflects several key assumptions. First and foremost, while technology is an enabling foundation of the NHII, developing our NHII is not primarily an IT enterprise. Hardware, software, and standards for both of these and for the information they deliver are vital, but they are neither the drivers of the effort nor the greatest barriers to its achievement. Second, the greatest barriers are likely to be in the attitudes and practices of individuals and institutions, including government. Until they see the value of exchanging information (with all appropriate safeguards) beyond their current connections, the necessary linkages will not be created and decision-enriching information will not reach those who need it. Third, the privacy issue may be both a bigger and smaller barrier than is often imagined. It is bigger because assurances of confidentiality and security of personal health information are absolutely essential for beneficial information exchange to occur. It may be smaller because, as legal and technical safeguards are strengthened, it will be easier for people to decide that the potential benefits of electronic information exchange significantly outweigh potential risks. Finally, while cost–however it is determined–must be addressed, it should be shared among all the parties who stand to benefit. Not all benefits can be monetized, but government, health plans and providers, employers, industry, consumers and patients will all reap rewards.

To succeed, such an effort will need to involve stakeholders from consumer health, health care, and public health. Above all, it will have to build trust among all users that the knowledge system is both valuable and safe. The rapid evolution of technology ensures that many individual components of the NHII will exist well before the end of the decade. But if the system is a disconnected patchwork, and it is not equitably distributed, then the value of the end result will be limited. Achieving the two broad goals of Healthy People 2010 will require a coordinated national health information infrastructure that links those who need to be connected and delivers quality content to everyone who needs it.

*The views expressed are those of the author and do not necessarily represent the views of the U.S. Department of Health and Human Services or the National Committee on Vital and Health Statistics. The author thanks Cynthia Baur for her thoughtful comments on the text.

References

[1] U.S. Department of Health and Human Services, Healthy People 2010, 2nd Edition in two volumes. U.S. Government Printing Office, Washington, D.C., 2000. http://www.health.gov/healthypeople

[2] National Research Council, Committee on Enhancing the Internet for Health Applications: Technical Requirements and Implementation Strategies, Computer Science and Telecommunications Board, Commission on Physical Sciences, Mathematics, and Applications. Networking Health: Prescriptions for the Internet. National Academy Press, Washington, D.C., 2000.

[3] National Committee on Vital and Health Statistics, Toward a national health information infrastructure. Interim Report, June, 2000. U.S. Department of Health and Human Services, Washington, D.C.. http://www.ncvhs.hhs.gov/NHII2kReport.htm

[4] President's Information Technology Advisory Committee, Panel on Transforming Health Care. Transforming Health Care Through Information Technology. Report to the President. Washington, D.C., February, 2001. http://www.ccic.gov/pubs/pitac/pitac-hc-9feb01.pdf

[5] National Committee on Vital and Health Statistics, Executive Subcommittee, Work Group on National Health Information Infrastructure. Charge. Washington, D.C. February 4, 1999. http://www.ncvhs.hhs.gov/nhichrg.htm

[6] National Committee on Vital and Health Statistics, Assuring a Health Dimension for the National Information Infrastructure. A Concept Paper by the National Committee on Vital and Health Statistics, presented to the U.S. Department of Health and Human Services Data Council, October 14, 1998. Washington, D.C. http://www.ncvhs.hhs.gov/hii-nii.htm

[7] National Committee on Vital and Health Statistics, Toward a national health information infrastructure. Interim Report, June, 2000. U.S. Department of Health and Human Services, Washington, D.C., p. 1.

[8] National Committee on Vital and Health Statistics, Toward a national health information infrastructure. Interim Report, June, 2000. U.S. Department of Health and Human Services, Washington, D.C., p. 8.

[9] National Committee on Vital and Health Statistics, Toward a national health information infrastructure. Interim Report, June, 2000. U.S. Department of Health and Human Services, Washington, D.C., p. 9.

[10] National Committee on Vital and Health Statistics, Toward a national health information infrastructure. Interim Report, June, 2000. U.S. Department of Health and Human Services, Washington, D.C., p. 16.

[11] National Committee on Vital and Health Statistics, Toward a national health information infrastructure. Interim Report, June, 2000. U.S. Department of Health and Human Services, Washington, D.C., p. 23.

[12] National Committee on Vital and Health Statistics, Toward a national health information infrastructure. Interim Report, June, 2000. U.S. Department of Health and Human Services, Washington, D.C., p. 3

[13] National Committee on Vital and Health Statistics, Joint Hearings of the Work Groups on: National Health Information Infrastructure and Health Statistics for the 21st Century, July 10, 2000, October 30, 2000, November 20, 2000, and January 11, 2001. Transcripts. http://www.ncvhs.hhs.gov/lastmntr.htm

[14] National Committee on Vital and Health Statistics, 50th Anniversary of the National Committee on Vital and Health Statistics, June 20, 2000. Unedited transcript. http://www.ncvhs.hhs.gov/ncvhs50tr.htm

[15] U.S. Department of Health and Human Services, Administrative Simplification Web Site . http://aspe.hhs.gov/admnsimp/Index.htm

[16] National Committee on Vital and Health Statistics, Uniform Data Standards for Patient Medical Record Information. Report to the Secretary of the U.S. Department of Health and Human Services. Washington, D.C., July 6, 2000

Future of Health Technology
R.G. Bushko (Ed.)
IOS Press, 2002

The Future of Telemedicine

Meg Wilson

Instructor, MSSTC Program, IC(2) Institute, University of Texas, Austin, US

Abstract

Despite a decade of tremendous advances in telemedicine, it still has potential far beyond current reality. New technologies are making the use of telemedicine ever more compelling and cost and payment barriers are being tackled so fewer barriers will impede the broad adoption of a now-proven cost-saving delivery of a variety of health care services. Adoption of telemedicine will accelerate with the aging of the Baby Boomer generation and globalization forces will broaden adoption and drive cost down.

Introduction

The healthcare world is divided into two camps: risk-takers and the risk-averse: those who readily adopt new technologies and those who don't. Telemedicine has been developed and used by risk-takers but its wholesale implementation responsibility now resides with the risk-averse. The future opportunity in telemedicine is to move it from a risky endeavor to one that becomes a common tool of healthcare.

Technology is no longer the key issue in the future of telemedicine. The technology of today is impressive. The technology of the future will be extraordinary: it will be too effective not to use on a routine basis. But the ever-present barriers of entry cost, acceptance of service and uncertain regulation have the potential of muffling what should be a revolution in health care provision.

1. Brief History of Telemedicine

Telemedicine had its birth 30-35 years ago, led by pioneers such as Dr. Jane Preston, who believed that television-based technology could fill an essential gap of lack of expertise in underserved and hard-to-serve areas. Over time, these creative risk-takers have tackled innovative applications for telemedicine despite immature technology, cost, reimbursement and acceptance of service barriers.

One late 80s-early 90s project, developed in Central Texas by a telecom R&D consortium, Project Bluebonnet, set up an extensive test of service delivery, absolute cost of delivery, comparative cost of service and total benefits of innovative service. The Austin Diagnostic Clinic had several doctors who would travel 1.5 hours each way to take care of dialysis patients. The doctors' services were key during the beginning and end of the process and little needed in the hours between. The travel time and downtime during dialysis were non-productive and expensive. The test included setting up a high-speed connection between Austin and the renal clinic in Giddings, Texas and setting up a teleconferencing system at each site. A state-of-the art wall screen was put into Dr. Jack Moncrief's office in Austin. He could be "present" when the staff hooked patients up at the beginning of dialysis. He could be visually and audibly "on call' during dialysis, and he could be present at the conclusion of dialysis. He could do "rounds" periodically to check on each patient. No travel time was required and he could see his regular Austin patients while being on call. The project's conclusions: the service was good and appropriate, the videoconferencing system was adequate, the telecommunications costs were prohibitively expensive, and the overall productivity gains almost covered the telecom costs.

Other early adopters include the military, the correctional system, rural regional healthcare providers, and public health providers. The Army and Navy as two examples, had a driving need and enough resources to invest in technology development as well as innovative service delivery systems. Thus we see Brooke Army Medical Center working with Ft. Hood to provide Ob/Gyn and Dermatology services and the USS Carl Vinson Aircraft Carrier providing full scale medical care for a floating city with the backup of a 24x7 wireless real-time telemedicine system available for specialist consultation and care.

Prison officials understood early in the technology's shakeout that they had a problem with a large captive patient population who were dangerous and expensive to transport for medical care. They could afford, through the stability of their physical plant, the subsidization of state and federal funding, the cooperation of publicly supported teaching hospitals, and the policy concern for the security of their charges, to be early adopters of telemedicine for consultations, patient diagnosis and ongoing patient care.

Regional health providers such as Texas Tech Health Science Center, the Mayo Clinic, and the Eastern Montana Telemedicine Network were risk-taking innovators in the face of demand and used all available tools to serve rural populations in need of public health, regular medical care and specialist services. Telemedicine services range from emergency in-flight care to nurse-doctor consultations and medical education.

2. The State of Telemedicine: Millennial Pulse

Telecommunications costs continued to be a factor throughout the 90s. Only now with the advent of ISDN, fiber, cable modem, Ethernet, T1, T3 and Internet-based systems and the potential of extensive and reliable wireless systems, are telecommunications costs no longer a dominant cost barrier to telemedicine. Initiatives to develop the Next Generation Internet will play a large part in further reducing access costs for telemedicine. In the U.S., a recent study by the National Academies' National Research Council found that using the web to its full potential for health services would require advanced technical capabilities currently not available. To reach widespread and effective use of the Internet by the medical community, the following areas need to be addressed:

- research, development and deployment of technologies needed to support health-related applications of the Internet;
- demonstration and evaluation of health applications on the Internet;
- education programs to help health organizations and their employees adopt Internet applications and develop effective policies for doing so; and
- efforts to resolve policy issues that impede use of the Internet for health applications
  The National Research Council also recommended that:

- the health community ensure that new networking initiatives, such as the Next Generation Internet, support health and biomedical applications;
- the U.S. Department of Health and Human Services (HHS) fund pilot projects that link multiple organizations to the Internet to exchange information;
- federal agencies with large programs associated with health care (Department of Defense, Department of Veterans Affairs, and HHS) take the lead in harnessing Internet applications. [1]

The primary barriers to telemedicine development and adoption are no longer technical – they are cost, risk-aversion, policy and legal barriers. Continued efforts are being made to address unresolved policies issues such as professional licensure and Medicare reimbursement policies. A number of US federal agencies are engaged in the development of policy regarding telemedicine including the Health Care Financing Administration (HCFA), the governmental body that sets standards and policies for services covered under Medicare and Medicaid. On January 1, 1999, HCFA began Medicare payments for teleconsultations in rural health professional shortage areas only. This first-ever national policy on Medicare reimbursement for telemedicine services was the result of the Balanced Budget Act of 1997. [2] Other involved agencies include the Office for the Advancement of Telehealth which is dedicated to the diffusion of telemedicine technology, the Joint Working Group on Telemedicine, and the Food and Drug Administration.

A 1997 national survey of 80 telemedicine programs, undertaken jointly by Telemedicine Today and the Association of Telemedicine Service Providers, found that reimbursement was identified as the most important of nine barriers to program sustainability. [3] Providers of telemedicine networks are addressing a number of issues, which if solved, will open the way for broader adoption of telemedicine, including: [4]

- Confidentiality of patient information: The increased use of the Internet has lead to major concerns about confidentiality and privacy. Currently, the lack of uniform legislation on privacy and confidentiality negatively affects the health care industry and particularly the tele-info part of the industry. Improved internet privacy, encryption and related security technologies can and will provide sufficient protection of private information – it is up to the policy makers to establish the minimum standards and profile of security – the technology industry can respond appropriately but without cohesive policies, they will only be shooting fish in a barrel.

- Licensure of providers in other states: Since telemedicine facilitates the practice of medicine across state lines, several states have enacted restrictive laws to keep out health professionals with out-of-state licenses.

- Medicare and Medicaid reimbursement: Several states including California, Oklahoma, Texas, Louisiana and Hawaii require private insurance carriers to pay for long-distance health care. Others, like Georgia, have negotiated arrangements with Medicaid and the insurance industry. As of August 2000, 150 private providers were reimbursing for most telemedicine services in Georgia. [5]

- Private pay reimbursement: Research shows that some insurance providers balk at paying for services not conducted in the traditional face-to-face doctor/ patient model. However, the same national survey cited above found that "when they're efficient and well-run, telemedicine programs that are not dependent on HCFA for reimbursement can make their own way quite nicely. This is especially true in managed and capitated care environments". [6]

- Malpractice standards
- Antitrust limitations
- Federal and state fraud and abuse laws
- Telecommunications contracting.

"During the last decade certain telemedicine applications, such as video-consulting and teleradiology, have matured to become essential health care services. Others, such as telepathology, remain the subject of intensive research effort". [7] Research shows that, in the U.S., health providers are using telemedicine in a growing number of specialties including dermatology, oncology, radiology, surgery, cardiology, and mental health. Teleradiology was one of the first uses of telemedicine to receive full reimbursement under U.S. Medicare and is the single most widely deployed use of telemedicine in the country.

Telehealth or telecare covers distance nursing, traditional concepts of public health and community support. "It is relevant to both the primary and secondary medical sectors, as well as having application to the veterinary field", and includes many aspects of these emerging fields. [8] Equestrian care of Olympic contenders is dependent upon telemedicine!

Patient monitoring is a major use of telecare – remote patient monitors observe patients' conditions via audio and video monitors, as well the telephone and computer while the patient remains at home. Cardiac monitoring, fetal monitoring, and pulmonary monitoring are the largest uses of remote patient monitors. Major insurance plans usually covers all three areas. The technology for such monitoring is well developed and the prospect now, is for increasingly expanded and innovative uses of such monitors.

As an example, HCFA announced in March 2000 that it has chosen a group headed by Columbia University to conduct a demonstration project that will use advanced computer and communications technology to bring higher quality health care to diabetics living in isolated rural and inner-city areas. The units in patients' homes will allow video conferencing, access to information and medical data inter-change. Computerized devices will check blood pressure, read blood sugar levels, take pictures of skin and feet for signs of infection and screen for other factors that affect diabetes management. The Clinical Information System will provide storage for clinical data to be used in the development and application of patient care guidelines and clinical standards. The project will use home telemedicine units linked to a Clinical Information System maintained by Columbia Presbyterian Medical Center. The project is targeting African American and Spanish-speaking Medicare beneficiaries. Columbia is the lead in this consortium and will be joined by 10 other hospitals and associations. [9]

There are a number of countries that are establishing projects that use telemedicine in a variety of ways. Throughout the world people in rural and remote area struggle to access quality specialty medical care in a timely manner due to an inadequate health care delivery system and a shortage of trained specialists. [10] The US military has used current telemedicine capabilities for emergency care services in Bosnia and as a stopgap until more normal services can be reestablished in war-torn communities.

Canada's Office of Health and the Information Highway (OHIH) believes tele-homecare systems have an enormous capacity to enhance the delivery of home health care and thereby increase the quality of care, while reducing cost. As the result of a study completed two years ago by the Advisory Council on Health Infrastructure, Canada has launched an $80 million dollar program, called Canada Health Infrastructure Partnerships Program. This project will support development and implementation of large-scale, collaborative model projects as well as some smaller projects with broad potential in the areas of telehealth and electronic patient records. [11] The study noted that where intellectual property with a potential for commercialization was likely to be developed, return to the parties should be in line with the contributions made and the risks assumed. This is key to the private partners who will help develop new technologies for telemedicine.

Tele-homecare is in its early stages in Canada and has been used primarily for monitoring or consultation following a hospital visit or in lieu of a visit. The OHIH also supports provincial tele-homecare projects and works with the federal health Transition Fund ($150 million Canadian) and the Health Infostructure Support Program ($10 million Canadian). [12]

Many other countries are making significant advances in telemedicine, technologies and applications systems (particularly teleradiology). Globalization factors will drive broad-based application of systems that may be run on a basis that eventually ignores borders and artificial barriers. [13]

3. The Future of Telemedicine

Experts believe that over the next five to ten years, Telemedicine will have a profound revolutionary effect on the delivery of medical care throughout the world. Telemedicine can bring medical services directly to the point of need by making it practical for direct communications between patient and health care provider and physician and specialist. In addition, telemedicine can help sustain the education of the physician by providing a direct link between the general practitioner and the major medical centers. [14]

It is estimated that health care systems are expected to spend as much as $15 Billion on information technologies within the next five years. A key element of that information technology is telemedicine, advanced computerized patient record systems, and decision support systems. [15] Other countries are making similar investments in technologies that will support telemedicine (e.g. EU's Fifth RTD Framework #2 Theme on User-Friendly Information Society, Canada as mentioned, and Australia's diabetes program and their capital and tax incentives for technologies focused on providing both early detection and follow on treatment [16]).

Thus, it is realistic to assume that new technologies and new application concepts are going to propel telemedicine into a higher plane of adoption. They broadly fall into four categories: peripherals, videoconferencing/integrated systems, telecommunications and new service paradigms.

3.1 Peripherals

There is a plethora of data capture tools – audio, analog, digital, video, still image, x-ray, EKG, etc. These include stethoscopes, dermatoscopes, slit lamps, video opthalmo scopes, oto scopes, nasopharyngo scopes, and multiple radiology scopes. The capability for these technologies will increase through lower cost data-capture tools, better resolution, better compression algorithms, effective encryption systems, better transmission options, more bandwidth and more integrated and compatible data sharing systems. Challenging applications such as telepathology will find multi-method data capture systems that allow for appropriate data interpretation on the receiver side.

As noted earlier, there are special efforts underway to monitor diabetics. One technology under development is software to assist in the diagnosis of retinal disorders, such as diabetic retinopathy. It is being developed in conjunction with a clinical study aimed at assessing the sensitivity and specificity of images produced by non-mydriatic cameras of average resolution used for wide-scale detection and prevention of the disease. Tele-medicine options will allow pictures to be processed in remote areas and forwarded to experts if the software alerts to a potential problem making the procedure available to remote populations and those areas with limited resources. The Computer Research Institute of Montreal (CRIM) is currently developing the technology. [17]

3.2 Videoconferencing and Video integration Systems

The cost of videoconferencing systems has dropped by one and two decimal places over the 90s. High-end systems from CLI used to cost over $100,000. VTEL's low-end system cost ~$40,000. Consolidation in the industry has left fewer providers and lower costs overall for all types of systems. PictureTel, one of the consolidation winners has a wide variety of systems for telemedicine use and their costs are down to thousands of $s. [18]. Video streaming capabilities allow for almost full motion video and audio with no jerks or delays. The cost and size of these units will continue to drop while performance continually improves.

Desktop cameras and videophone systems were the dream of 10 years ago and the reality of today. They will be inexpensive and commonplace within another 5 years. Doctor to doctor consultations will become a multi-media phone call.

One of the remaining challenges for telemedicine sits at the video level – the switch between the data-capture peripherals and the transmission or telecommunications link. The integration level still needs improvement, to allow for easier user capture and control of multiple inputs and reliable, intuitive send options. That data and telecom interchange capability is a weak point in the system. Fortunately, standards, better communications and data "munging" software, and intelligent image processing are being developed and will become an integral part of the video/communications system.

3.3 Telecommunications

The dominance of Internet based communications and data sharing will characterize the next decade. The key to a cost-effective future for telemedicine lies in the development of smart buildings. New construction and renovations must be outfitted with scalable infrastructure: not only outfitting the telecom system of choice at the time but proper conduit and drop points to change a building's system and to easily add capability should a room or building section's use change. New assisted living and nursing home facilities should all install the highest capability possible at the time of construction and the conduit and communications panels to handle upgrades and expansions.

The advent of cable modem, ISDN, and DSL and computer camera systems, email and palm-pilot-style downloadable systems for home use means that direct service options will be possible for all but the most sophisticated systems for home monitoring applications.

3.4 New Service Paradigms

Telemedicine has primarily concentrated on rural and special populations. In the future, home care will become a primary application of telemedicine – telehealth care will dominate just by sheer numbers of individuals involved.

As an example of the kind of driver that will enable home-based telehealth care, the HealthHero Network (HHN) has developed a service model and technology to expand this type of care far into the next decade. The HHN remote monitor (Health Buddy Personal Information Appliance) offers a savings of as much as 68% off the average monthly cost of traditional homecare nurse service ($3,100/yr for HHN vs. $9600/yr for homecare nurse). The low cost of setup offers advantages to HHN -- only five years ago, a "typical" telemedicine set-up could cost as much as $300,000. The set-up cost for the HHN is only around $75,000. The HHN monitor requires only a standard telephone line for the patient and Internet access for the healthcare provider – that combination provides rapid transmittal of a patient's health care information to health care providers and allows health care providers to monitor a patient's illness from their offices, while the patient remains in the comfort of his/her home.

The Health Buddy serves as a two-way communications link between the patient and the website and consists of a simple four-button device that plugs into any phone outlet, home or away from home. The device prompts the patient to answer questions. These responses are automatically transmitted to a secure database through a toll-free telephone number and follow-up questions or feedback are sent back to the patient. Using the data collected, healthcare providers perform proactive healthcare management by alerting the caregiver to intervene when necessary to prevent critical situations before they happen. [19] [20]

With the advent of this type of home monitoring system, home health workers can add an additional level of service with add-on features during home visits. CRIM's retinal scanner system could be used this way for diabetics. Juvenile diabetics, who suffer from very unstable insulin levels could get near-real-time monitoring and advice rather than the current system of recording blood sugar levels on paper and faxing them in once a week!

The editor of Telemedicine Today aptly summed up the issue in an August 1998 editorial when he said, "We feel that telecommunications technology can make a real difference to people who have suffered from strokes, fires, post-surgical complications, and catastrophic accidents … the growth of tele-home health services may be impelled by economic forces that are making it harder for home health agencies to make a living. In the past year Medicare has reduced per-visit reimbursements by a national average of 15 percent, and home care payments are under intense scrutiny by insurers. Increasingly, telenursing is seen as the solution to the problem of how to deliver equivalent service at a lower cost". [21]

With the aging of the population in most developing nations, tele-homecare has probably one of the greatest potentials for rapid growth worldwide. The National Association for Home Care estimates that 15,000 providers delivered care to 7 million individuals requiring in-home services resulting from acute illness and long-term health conditions… In Europe, the aging pattern resembles the U. S. trends. Additionally, the rapidly changing demographic characteristics and the (wise) tradition for caring for elders at home creates a challenge and a unique opportunity for the implementation of tele-homecare. [22]

The promise of telemedicine is providing significantly improved and cost effective access to quality health care. Telemedicine is helping to transform the delivery of health care and improve the health of millions of people throughout the world. Nevertheless, significant hurdles remain, including legal and regulatory barriers and acceptance of the use of telemedicine by traditional medical establishments. Successful telemedicine programs often support clinical activities, distance learning and continuing medical education programs across a common infrastructure using a range of technologies.

4. Conclusion

Clearly, the demographics of the baby boomer generation will dictate that the numbers of demanding patients, wanting the latest and best technologies to provide them the latest, best and cheapest services on a real time basis, will overwhelm risk-averse decision makers. Appropriate use of telemedicine in traditional settings will be supplemented by the new paradigm of telehealth in homecare and assisted care. Agencies such as HCFA will be shouted down by the swelled ranks of AARP if they haven't figured out how to read the tea leaves within the next 5 years. The need to hold down healthcare cost without significant loss of service will dictate that *__all__* available strategies and technologies will be used to their maximum capability!

References

[1] Significant Technological Barriers Remain for Providing Health Care on the Internet, The National Academies News, Feb. 23, 2000, www.nationalacademicies.org/news.nsf/
[2] Office for the Advancement of Telehealth, www.telehealth.hrsa.gov/reimbtext.htm#reimb
[3] http://www.telemedtoday.com/mainpages/editorAugust.htm
[4] Advanced Health Systems, Telemedicine Newsletter, http://arentfox.com 8/1/00
[5] [1] Funding and Policy Barriers Plague Telemedicine, http://cnn.com/2000/Tech/computing
[6]] http://www.telemedtoday.com/mainpages/editorAugust.htm
[7] http://www.roysocmed.ac.uk/pub/jtt.htm
[8] http://www.roysocmed.ac.uk/pub/jtt.htm
[9] Medicare Using Telemedicine to Help Diabetics, Fact Sheet, HCFA web site located at www.hcfa.gov/facts/ dated March 20, 2000
[10] Significant Technological Barriers Remain for Providing health Care on the Internet, The National Academies News, Feb. 23, 2000, on the web at www.nationalacademicies.org/news.nsf/
[11] www.hc-sc.gc.ca/english/archives/releases/2000/2000_72e.htm
[12] Canada Health Infoway: Paths to Better Health, final report of the Advisory Council on Health Infrastructure, on the web at www.hc-sc.gc.ca/ohih-bsi/whatdo/achivs/fin-rpt/exsum_e.html
[13] See for example December 1998, http://www.telemedtoday.com/mainpages/pastissues.htm
[14] American Telemedicine Association, Telemedicine: A Brief Overview, http://www.atmeda.org/whatis/whitepaper.html
[15] Advanced Health Systems, http://arentfox.com 8/2/00
[16] Unpublished masters paper, MSSTC, IC2, UT Austin, Technology Assessment for course STC 380, "Retsoft, A Computer-Assisted Ophthalmologic Examination Of The Retina", June 30, 2000, Louis Conrad, Nick Daley, Michael Lamke, Bill Minter. Also, Canada Health Infoway: Paths to Better Health, final report of the Advisory Council on Health Infrastructure, on the web at www.hc-sc.gc.ca/ohih-bsi/whatdo/achivs/fin-rpt/exsum_e.html
[17] Unpublished masters paper, MSSTC, IC2, UT Austin, Technology Assessment for course STC 380/383, "Retsoft, A Computer-Assisted Ophthalmologic Examination Of The Retina", June 30, 2000, Louis Conrad, Nick Daley, Michael Lamke, Bill Minter.
[18] http://www.telemedtoday.com/video/products.htm
[19]]Unpublished masters paper, MSSTC, IC2, UT Austin, Technology Assessment for course STC 380/383, "Ideal Path Analysis for the Health Hero Network Internet-Based System", August 11, 2000, Yvonne Jackson, Anna Hardesty, Kathey Ferland, Lance Weaver. Pgs 7-8
[20] www.healthhero.com
[21] http://www.telemedtoday.com/mainpages/pastissues.htm, August, 1998
[22] unpublished masters paper, MSSTC, IC2, UT Austin, Technology Assessment for course STC 380/383, "Ideal Path Analysis for the Health Hero Network Internet-Based System", Yvonne Jackson, Anna Hardesty, Kathey Ferland, Lance Weaver. pg 10
[23] Telehealth Update, Office for the Advancement of Telehealth, http://telehealth.hrsa.gov/reimbtxt.htm Funding and Policy Barriers Plague Telemedicine, http://cnn.com/2000/Tech/computing, accessed 8/9/00
[24] (US National Library of Medicine web site, Next Generation Internet, www.nlm.nih.gov/research/ accessed on 8/1/00)
[25] http://www.telemedprimer.com/links.html

Future of Health Technology
R.G. Bushko (Ed.)
IOS Press, 2002

Advanced Technology Program: Information Infrastructure for Healthcare Focused Program

Richard N. Spivack[1]

Economist, Economic Assessment Office of the Advanced Technology Program, National Institute of Standards and Technology, US Department of Commerce

Abstract

This paper describes an initiative begun by the Advanced Technology Program[2] in 1994 referred to as the Information Infrastructure for Healthcare (IIH) focused program. The IIH focus program began with an initial exchange of ideas among members of the private and public sectors (industry's submission of "white papers"[3]; workshops conducted by the ATP; meetings held between individuals from both groups) to identify those technologies necessary for the development of a national information infrastructure in healthcare. A discussion of the development of the focus program through a "white paper" process notes differences that existed between what the ATP had hoped to gain through this method and how the private sector responded. A statistical description of the participants as well as a brief discussion of the ATP review and selection process is included.

1. Introduction

The Advanced Technology Program (ATP) at the National Institute of Standards and Technology (NIST) is a cost-sharing program designed to partner the federal government with the private sector to further both the development and dissemination of "high-risk"[4] technologies which offer the potential for significant, broad-based economic benefits for the nation. In this program, industry proposes research projects to the ATP to be judged in competitions for funding based upon both the technical and economic/business merits of the proposal. From 1990 through 2000, the ATP held "General/Open" competitions each year open to all technologies.

---

[1] Richard N. Spivack is an economist in the Economic Assessment Office of the ATP.

[2] The ATP statute originated in the Omnibus Trade and Competitiveness Act of 1988 (Pub. L. 100-418, 15 U.S.C. 278n) and was amended by the American Technology Preeminence Act of 1991 (Pub. L. 102-245)

[3] A mechanism by which industry conceptualizes the problems it is having difficulty addressing, including the kinds of technological barriers that must be overcome

[4] High risk technologies are defined as technical challenges " that should result in a dramatic change in the future direction of technology. Risk may be high in developing single innovations, integrating technologies, or both." *ATP Proposal Preparation Kit*, U.S. Department of Commerce, NIST, November 1999, p. 29.

From 1994 through 1998, the ATP awarded most of its funding through "focused-program"[5] competitions in which a suite of projects was funded to mobilize technology to address a particular problem. Thirty focused program competitions were held, each with a unifying set of project goals. The following is a synopsis of one of these programs, the Information Infrastructure for Healthcare focused program (IIH) which conducted three solicitations in 1994, 1995, and 1997.

The IIH focused program was initiated in 1994 amid a nationwide discussion of the rising costs of healthcare and the quality of care offered. The objective of the ATP IIH focus program was to develop the information infrastructure technologies needed to cut dramatically the 20% of the United States' $1 trillion healthcare cost spent on paperwork, and to improve the quality and flexible delivery of care by faster broad access to better information. ATP awards for research made possible new technological capabilities in firms, allowing them to introduce advanced functionalities into their existing IIH products and to introduce new products. These awards allowed the smallest firms to extend their limited resources and gave them additional ability to overcome research barriers impeding the attraction of private venture capital funding. It encouraged large companies to pursue enabling, high-risk research and development in a time of tight discretionary budgets.

2. ATP and Focused Programs

In response to the ATP's initial request for white papers leading to the development of focused programs, close to one thousand papers covering a range of technologies were submitted and sorted by a technology taxonomy. A subset of this total addressed healthcare issues providing both the scope and technical detail required. Papers were submitted by companies, individuals with companies, associations of companies, university professors, members of other organizations, and private citizens without organizational affiliation. Some were submitted by large consortia offering a comprehensive roadmap for the ATP in developing a partnership with industry. The white paper process provided a place for people to share their ideas and an opportunity for the ATP to more clearly define the goals of the focused program. The white papers submitted to the ATP addressed a set of published criteria including: technical ideas; economic benefit; industry commitment; and, need for ATP funding.

It becomes the responsibility of the designated program manager (PM) to further refine the scope of the proposed program by broadening the relationship already established with the private sector. The PM for the IIH focused program organized a small focus group followed by a public workshop attended by representatives from industry, as well as the non-profit and academic communities.[6] From the resulting general discussion held at the workshop, a consensus developed, identifying infrastructural information technologies as offering the best means to achieve a significant reduction in healthcare costs while at the same time increasing quality of care as well as offering the possibility for a significant positive impact upon the U.S. economy. Information technologies for healthcare also offered one of the most clearly defined areas of technological development requiring the public/private partnership offered by the ATP. The role of the ATP was thus defined as one

---

[5] "Focused programs are defined as multi-year efforts aimed at specific, well-defined technology and business goals. These programs, which involve the parallel development of a suite of interlocking R&D projects, tackle major technology problems with high payoff potential which cannot be solved by an occasional project coming through the general competition. By managing groups of projects that complement and reinforce each other, the ATP can have the greatest possible impact on the economy."

[6] Advanced Technology Program, "Information Infrastructure for Healthcare (94-04)", U.S. Department of Commerce, NIST, 1994, p. 15.

of fostering cooperation and communication and serving as the catalyst needed to bring together the members of the information technology and medical communities to achieve the stated objectives.

Additional interactions were held between the PM and representatives from the private sector complementing the discussions held at the workshop and identifying the increased demands placed upon the U.S. healthcare industry to raise the quality of service, to extend consistent quality between rural and urban areas, to provide accurate measures of success, and to accomplish all of these with lower costs in a timely fashion while establishing national standards for the electronic transfer of patient records and related medical documents. This information, offering quite different notions of technological innovation in this area, fell into three distinct categories: a systems approach to an entire technological field; identification of a technological area purported to offer special promise for significant economic spillovers if "bottlenecks" are addressed; and, specific technical ideas that will, if supported, ultimately result in particular products.

Specific technologies identified in the IIH white papers included, but were not limited to, development of:

- Information tools to automate, validate and distribute clinical practice guidelines for mass use. These could include clinical practice guidelines that capture the current "best practices" for an array of medical situations.
- The tools to enable healthcare providers and quality/cost monitors to browse and to extract data automatically from a multitude of scattered clinical and administrative databases, without requiring changes to the existing databases.
- Tools that facilitate the production of clinical notes and, as a byproduct, gather the codified clinical data and store it in a database system.
- An interoperable open-systems architecture to serve as an interface between independent healthcare information systems.

This input gave impetus to the final scope of the proposed focused program in the development of information infrastructure. As defined here, information infrastructure development includes: the integration, synthesis, and definition of any information that needs to be shared across the enterprise; and, the means by which to transport, store, and access that information in a way that enhances, rather than impedes, user productivity.

3. Information Infrastructure for Healthcare Focused Program

The *ATP Information InfraStructure for Healthcare Focused Program*[7] solicitation kit identified the program's goals as follows:

Technical Goals
To establish the technologies for:
- Reliable storage and retrieval of complex medical information for varied applications;
- Real-time, data-driven medical decisions;
- Real-time data entry by mobile medical personnel;
- Real-time global transport of complex medical records with accuracy, speed, and security;
- Computer-based medical training, diagnostic, and reference tools.

---

[7] Advanced Technology Program, "Information Infrastructure for Healthcare (94-04)", U.S. Department of Commerce, NIST, 1994.

Business Goals
To gain the capability to develop products that will:

- Reduce unit healthcare costs;
- Improve quality of healthcare (higher treatment success rates and avoidance of complications);
- Capture global market share of new and improved products and services.
- Undertake infrastructural development focusing upon 'tools' and prototype systems to enhance the flow of information between existing 'legacy' systems in the healthcare enterprise while being scalable from a single provider's office to a fully integrated healthcare system. Infrastructural development is intended to enable enterprise-wide integration of information among all sectors of the healthcare industry and is expected to encompass the following:

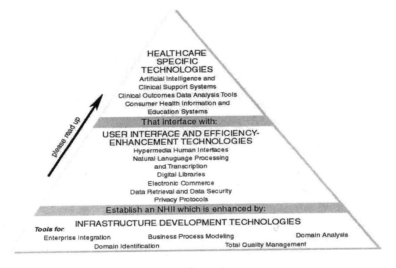

Figure 1

A model of the program, which would result in a portfolio of required technologies, is presented in figure 1 in the form of a "pyramid" consisting of three categories, which should be read from bottom to top: (1) Infrastructure Development Technologies (e.g., tools for enterprise integration, business process modeling); (2) User Interface and Efficiency-Enhanced Technologies (e.g., hypermedia human interfaces, natural language processing, data retrieval & advanced search mechanisms); and (3) Healthcare-Specific Technologies (e.g., clinical decision support systems, consumer health information and education systems).[8] Each level is represented as being distinct from the next with the notion being that development of those technologies in the lower levels should precede development of those above, resulting in a "bottom-up" approach. This logic influenced the announcement of the first and second solicitations whereby only those projects which "fit" into the respective levels were to receive funding. It became obvious, after a period of time, that there was considerable interplay among the designated levels and that components from more than one level may be proposed in any given project. This thinking was

---

[8] Ibid, p. 4.

incorporated into the announcement for the third solicitation recognizing that technological R&D in this industry requires simultaneous development of "infrastructural" technologies throughout the entire pyramid.

4. IIH Focused Program Awardees[9]

Table 1 below provides summary statistical data from the three IIH solicitations held between 1994 and 1997, in which 221 proposals were received and 32 awards were made to 79 participants. R&D funding totaled $295 million, representing a commitment of $146 million from the government and $149 million from the private sector.

Table 1 IIH Focused Program Participation

	1994	1995	1997
Total Number of **Proposals** Submitted	59	68	94
Total Number of **Projects** Funded	16	10	6
Type of Award **Participant**			
Single Applicant	10	7	6
Joint Venture	6	3	
Total Number of **Participants**	43	32	6
Type/Size of Organization			
PS (For-Profit Small Company)	17	12	6
PM (For-Profit Medium Company)	6	4	
PL (For-Profit Large Company)	6	5	
NP (Non-Profit)	7	8	
U (University)	4	3	

A casual observation reveals the dominant role of small for-profit companies (PS) across all three solicitations. These companies participated both as single applicants (SA) as well as members of joint ventures (JV). SA award recipients included start-ups as well as research organizations in medium and large size companies. The JV's were varied consisting of several types of organizational structures in both size and scale, and with different orientations to technology development. They included a diverse group of large and small companies, non-profit organizations, and universities. In some instances, competitors joined to overcome rather complex technical issues. The IIH focused program encouraged the formation of collaborations among computer and medical professionals and organizations to enhance the development of needed technologies.

5. New Format for Proposal Solicitation, Review and Selection

Beginning with fiscal year 1999, the ATP merged the concept of focused program competitions and general competitions, resulting in an "Open" format, combining the best features of previous competition models. Under an open competition a proposal selected for funding that is synergistic with an existing focused program is managed under that

---

[9] The statistical data included in the tables and charts that follow are from the Business Reporting System (BRS) database maintained by the ATP Economic Assessment Office. Begun in 1994, the BRS provides a comprehensive data tool used for tracking purposes on a routine and regular basis and for measuring progress of projects against business plans and projected economic benefits as outlined in the project proposals and updated over the course of the projects.

program. In other cases proposals developing complementary technologies that form a critical mass will be "bundled"[10] together and treated as a virtual focused program managed in a manner similar to that of announced focused programs. In the case of healthcare informatics, proposals which in the past would have been submitted under the IIH focused program competition will be directed towards the Information Technology Source Evaluation Board (SEB)[11]. Those proposals selected for funding will be administered as part of the IIH focused program. ATP continues to work with industry and other organizations to define and update current challenges and opportunities in medical informatics.

In future competitions it is anticipated that those companies wishing to submit proposals which address elements of any of the three levels identified in the pyramid (see figure 1) may do so. Alternatively, companies may wish to submit proposals offering innovative solutions to those technical challenges outlined in the white paper authored jointly by ATP and industry titled, "Initiatives in Healthcare Informatics," and accessible on the ATP web site. New technical areas not addressed in either the IIH focused program, or in the white paper, or in other ATP focused program areas are also encouraged. All proposals submitted to the ATP will be evaluated solely for their scientific and technological merit and their potential for broad-based economic benefits, with parts weighted equally. No longer is there a need to determine whether a proposal falls within the scope of a specific technical program.

The introduction of this new Open Competition is part of an on-going process on the part of the ATP to improve upon its operations, in this case by offering a vehicle by which industry may respond more quickly to common barriers and opportunities without the delay brought about by the development of a focused program.[12]

6. Conclusions

The ATP IIH focused program has contributed significantly to accelerating the development of infrastructural tools as well as the user interface and efficiency-enhancement technology necessary for a National Information Infrastructure for Healthcare. It has encouraged their development from the "bottom up" rather than imposing them in a "top down" fashion, which could have resulted in restrictions on the types of technologies developed. The driving force behind these advances remains the development of open, interoperable, yet secure systems--systems that will provide the medical community with the capability to integrate diverse information and business systems as well as the data necessary to support continuous quality improvement, thus addressing several primary issues of critical importance in today's delivery of healthcare.

The IIH focused program has also acted as a catalyst in establishing collaborations bringing together the stakeholders and providing the opportunity to pursue cross-disciplinary projects, with participation from healthcare providers as well as computer scientists and information technology specialists. In several cases the collaborations that

---

[10] The "bundling" of proposals for the purpose of creating a "virtual" focused program will only occur when a critical mass of proposals in a shared domain has been achieved. Any proposal that does not fall within an announced or virtual focused program is managed independently.

[11] The SEB is the primary means by which all proposals are reviewed. Membership is comprised solely of federal employees possessing technical and business expertise.

[12] Developing a focused program often encompasses a one-to-two year period. A program manager is assigned to a particular industrial sector in response to industry needs and asked to define whether or not ATP has a role. Current focused programs were designed with a finite time horizon. Those programs which were scheduled for multi-year competitions were intended to complete a body of work as established in the program definition or as modified due to changes in the technology environment. Both developing a new focused program and modifying an existing one were lengthy, laborious processes.

were formed included companies that never had nor, under ordinary circumstances, never would have worked together.

These efforts have led to a reduction in the likelihood of closed systems and have increased industry entry opportunities for small to medium-sized companies. For the end-user, this program has accelerated market acceptance and enabled industry to improve medical care while lowering costs.

Today, with rapid changes in both technology and in the delivery of healthcare, there are new challenges in healthcare informatics research. The Advanced Technology Program provides an excellent vehicle by which for government-industry partnerships in this domain will accelerate the development of high-risk technologies with promise of significant commercial payoffs and widespread benefits for the economy.

References

[1] Blum, Bruce I. and Karen Duncan, eds., *A History of Medical Informatics*, Addison Wesley, Reading, MA (1990).

[2] Etzkowitz, Henry, Andrew Webster, and Peter Healey (eds.), *Capitalizing Knowledge: New Intersection of Industry and Academia*, State University of New York Press, Albany, New York (1998).

[3] National Science Foundation, *Comparing National Efforts at Technological Foresight, Science Indicators*. Chp. 6. National Science Foundation, Arlington, VA 1998.

[4] U.S. Department of Commerce, National Institute of Standards and Technology, *ATP Proposal Kit* , November 1999.

[5] U.S. Department of Commerce, National Institute of Standards and Technology, Advanced Technology Program, *Information Infrastructure for Healthcare* (94-04; 95-10; 97-03), 1994, 1995, 1997.

[6] U.S. Department of Commerce, National Institute of Standards and Technology, Advanced Technology Program, *Program Idea Guide*, May 1997.

Future of Health Technology
R.G. Bushko (Ed.)
IOS Press, 2002

Quality Enhancing Conceptual Tools for Medical Decision Making

Graziella Tonfoni, Ph.D.

Professor of Computational Linguistics, University of Bologna, Italy.
Visiting Research Professor, School of Engineering and Applied Science,
George Washington University, Washington D.C., US

Abstract

The scientific and the medical communities are among the first asked both to advance highly specialized knowledge and to make it available to a wider community of users, accessing specialized knowledge and searching for single pieces of information for a whole variety of purposes that require diverse information needs and demands. Health advisors may want to update progress in research in a certain field of medicine, to ask experts the right kinds of questions and, even more fundamentally, to be able to describe those health problems they may encounter in their patients' community with words and expressions that can be both understandable and accurate.

Researchers, physicians and nurses all face the need to share information that comes out of stabilized, or established, research, meaning research that has been accurately tested as opposed to new and untested assumptions, and to thus establish a common code. A common code may be used by experts in the field to communicate, exchange and compare results and to translate some of the results into common sense-based explanations that can be made widely available. In order to circulate new discoveries and highly specialized knowledge in medicine and to disseminate it to a larger community, accurate planning of consistent metaphors and analogies are of crucial help.

Accurate metaphors and analogies come as a result of a skilled art and science; no metaphor or analogy can represent a specific topic within a highly specialized knowledge domain without having first undergone major processes of redefinition. This is precisely what will be explored in this chapter, the added value of both powerful and reliable conceptual tools in the medical field, such as metaphors and analogies, and a commonly shared code to make qualitative reasoning about medical information possible. To improve progress in research and medical care, everyone needs to establish a common language to work with and from. In terms of medical advice documentation, the use of a visual system, CTML, would be instrumental in providing and documenting information. This system can be understood by and thus connect researchers, health care professionals, and patients.

1. Introduction

Today health advice information is available in a variety of different forms and formats, ranging from booklets and brochures to more extended sets of articles and books up to information made available throughout the web. The increasing and continuing complexity and growth that characterizes health advice information and services poses the urgent need to provide medical information experts and medical operators with enhanced conceptual tools, which may help them harmoniously integrate existing literature available in the field and select, discriminate and highlight relevant information coming from web discussions and web groups.

Medical operators need an easy-to-access, easy-to-acquire, easy-to-use consensual system, which may help them process major quantities of data, which may be fuzzy, redundant and overlapping, needing to be updated and upgraded and revised most of the time. The health advice and medical knowledge management system outlined here is meant to be a highly comprehensive system, which makes qualitative reasoning upon medical information possible.

Based upon a well-established specific vocabulary, this system may be integrated easily with a highly specialized mark up language, which provides medical operators with a set of categories meant to help sort out and classify various kinds of health advice information coming both synchronously and asynchronously out of completely different kinds of sources. First, it is most important to be able to understand where a certain kind of health advice document comes from. This is determined by the kind of information it was first generated as and the kind of knowledge it is meant to lead the patient to at that specific time. Specific conceptual tools are therefore meant to provide conceptual mapping to facilitate access to information already available and to allow discrimination among different kinds of knowledge, which may be either immediately needed or useful later.

Enhanced encoding procedures in the form of documentation tagging and labelling, which are part of a highly comprehensive and highly consistent annotation system, will accurately inform health advisors in advance about the nature of information they are likely to find within a certain booklet, book, website etc. Those same encoding procedures will also support accurate conversion of information coming in the form of ongoing web-based conversations and discourse into a more stable format, which may be easily recognized and consistently packaged as additional documentation to be provided.

The mark up language presented here is meant to capture those indications, which are absolutely needed in order to accommodate the various and continuously changing needs for interpreting and retaining information displayed in various forms and formats.

Making decisions about the quantity and quality of information required by each patient is made possible through a set of indications which are meant to help health advisors acquire both the knowledge they are seeking and the knowledge which they do not yet know they need and to pass it along in friendly and effective ways to patients.

Valuable research has been pursued in the field of information [1], supporting evidence of the crucial role of communication skills in establishing trust with the patient and family.

A health advice document may therefore be easily defined as a piece of information which has been either extracted from a reliable source (research books and research literature) or further converted into a more palatable form, after having undergone a set of more or less radical modifications, reformulations and refinements. These alterations or dilutions are meant to make the highly technical terminology accessible and comprehensible in the form of tailored vocabularies, medical text adaptations and abridgments. A health advice document may also have derived from an ongoing and dynamically evolving information flow, such as web-based group conversations that are then converted into a more stable format such as a summary or some kind of compilation and condensation of a more extended text.

Health advice documentation meant to meet the patients' diversified needs may be defined as a derivative product out of a flow of conversation, be it really or virtually carried on between the expert knowledge provider, the health advisors and the patient. Regardless, the patient needs to be facilitated and accompanied throughout the communicative intercourse that originated with his or her first quest for information. Each health advice document, whether in booklet or web-based form, needs to be perceived by the patients as part of an ongoing conversation. Such conversation, carried on either in person, on paper or online, represents for the patient the real reason why the text was produced and displayed.

Patients will proceed toward seeking further information or health advice based upon both the friendliness and effectiveness of these conversations. The quality of the health advice documentation plays a substantial role in the patient's decision to or not to continue their search for health advice.

2. Conceptual Tools for Facilitating Medical Decision Making Processes

Without physical models available, it is difficult to think of new concepts and ways of reorganizing already existing knowledge within a certain scientific domain. Identification of relevant models is therefore important in order to represent problems, uncover hidden facts and name processes that would otherwise remain opaque or even unknown. Since metaphorical reasoning is highly complex, being able to refer to a highly articulated framework for interpretation will result in the development of a useful process meant to facilitate accurate interpretation, particularly in the medical field.

Introducing new concepts for facilitating the interpretation of newly observed facts and phenomena will consequently trigger the need for an accessible and accurate terminology.

Applying metaphorical reasoning means creating a conceptual platform for supporting new definitions with derivative experience coming from other fields, which are well known and therefore more stable [2]. Such a process may be of tremendous assistance in facilitating reasoning once the medical information user's perspective and point of view have been accurately described and defined. It is indeed most important to be able to establish a common background for sharing both expert knowledge and common sense reasoning outputs. Common sense is most relevant for rethinking and reorganizing a specific medical knowledge domain. The domains undergo continuous changes and are monitored by different individuals and groups, which leads into different and sometimes even opposite directions.

Single individual and collaborative group efforts that exchange knowledge must accurately rethink the inner nature of each word and its constant redefinition by introducing and incorporating physical models of reasoning. These models may be consensually shared and may mark a fundamental step toward better coordination.

Accurate observation and interpretation of complex situations through the consistent design of precisely defined metaphors will lead researchers in the field as well as anyone else trying to understand specialized knowledge for practical reasons, as health advisors need to be, to gain a deeper understanding and mastering of a complex knowledge domain, such as the medical domain.

The planning and further designing of consistent metaphors may evolve into an extremely delicate operation, which implies a previous selection process among different possibilities followed by the consistent reinterpretation of relevant aspects and the accurate selection of a technically reformulated lexicon. A specialized lexicon needs to be based upon consistent reconfiguration of just those elements that are relevant and need to be transferred from one well-known domain into a newly established one. There is indeed no need to magnify the complexity of the terminology being used, which may in fact become an impediment to effective understanding. Therefore, each term needs to be accurately redefined; without this previous reconfiguration process, fuzziness and confusion may arise later. More specifically, a metaphor that is produced to support redefinition within a specific field of medical expertise, is a dynamic structure meant to be a reliable cognitive tool for supporting the description of newly defined problems and for designing ways to cope with such problems consistently.

Metaphors are dynamic and are therefore specifically suited for grasping the inherent complexity of the phenomenon or set of phenomena, which they are meant to represent, both synthetically and analytically. Since metaphors are primarily conceived and used as synthetic procedures planned to establish new meaning connections, it may sound contradictory and unusual to think of metaphors as analytic procedures.

By introducing the concept of progressive reconfiguration of a metaphorical structure stage by stage, the possibility of introducing analytical thinking into the planning and designing of precisely articulated metaphors in medical expertise representation becomes real.

In order to better understand which important implications can be derived, let us more carefully consider the nature of a metaphor as the result of a whole process of meaning attribution and progressive redefinition. A scientific metaphor results from the accurate transfer of a certain meaning that evolves from the selection of relevant features from one "old," in the sense that it is a well-established and known domain, into a "new" and less established and still vaguely designed domain.

A new metaphor being introduced into health care documentation is meant to enlighten first and then describe, define and explain an event, fact or set of events or facts. Metaphors not only allow, but also welcome, a whole set of possible interpretations; they are therefore by definition meant to be centrifugal. They entail the expansion of possible meaning attributions toward different directions and paths, departing from the core definition. In order to make sure that a scientific metaphor used in health advice documentation is adequate in conveying specifically that kind of meaning, which is intended to be conveyed by the researcher first and by the physician and health advisor next, it needs to undergo most fundamental changes and become centripetal. This means that different kinds of meaning attribution processes will have to converge toward a very precise core definition.

A metaphor in health care advice is always generated within a relatively stable realm. It comes from a certain region of meaning where different semantic attributions are possible and may in fact occur, but only some may alternatively prevail or dominate and be transferred into newly established conceptual domains. Metaphorical perception in current literature is in fact based on most welcome concurrence of various meanings attributions. If this is precisely what metaphors are good for and are about in poetry or in daily use, the same does not apply to the planning and designing of scientific metaphors, which are meant to facilitate highly specific meaning attribution to avoid undesired meaning accretion.

To be reliable, a scientific metaphor must be conceived as part of a more comprehensive framework. By "framework" we mean a skeletal structure of meaning that has been previously designated, set up and accurately checked in each of its single parts, which are all interconnected and joined together. A scientific metaphor designer needs to proceed toward an accurate and highly specific definition of each of those parts to turn a general framework into a more specific domain, which is a meaning configuration governed by a single overall ruling principle. Only at that point will the metaphorical domain be ready to become an operative tool for more articulated interpretation and understanding of a complex phenomenon or set of phenomena. Through this domain a whole set of problems can not only be synthesized, but also analysed and viewed according to a dynamic and multidimensional perspective, which is first thoroughly explained and then practically approached.

3. On Metaphorical Configurations In Health Advice

Since metaphors and analogies are part of our life and of our communicative intercourse on a daily basis, analogical reasoning may profitably support health advice interactions and conversations. A wide literature has been produced starting in 1980 with Lakoff's analysis [2], a major contribution in the field. In 1983 and 1995, Gentner [3] and Hofstadter [4], respectively, continued with quite extensive and meaningful literature also including Bushko's specific contribution [5]. They have been able to harmoniously link knowledge coming from cognitive science and computer science to studies on reasoning in metaphorical processing and their practical use.

A metaphor often only covers some parts and aspects of a certain domain, whereas an alternative metaphor may cover some others, which would otherwise be missing or just left out. Metaphorical reasoning in health advice applies to a very complex realm, and only a combination of different models for visualizing and expressing various aspects involved allows health advisors to create explanatory maps to hand out to patients. This provides a friendly, and therefore effective, way to distribute information to patients. We may productively distinguish between "large scale metaphors" and "reduced scale metaphors," "operational metaphors" and "narrative metaphors," as to be able to accurately evaluate the degree of approximation they may actually reach in representing and conveying medical expertise.

A process of medical knowledge reconfiguration may reach a high level of accuracy if the consistency of each single word is checked. Each term needs therefore to be redefined according to a preset series of differentiated stages of analysis. In today's world of health advice, we are likely to encounter the following set of contexts in which knowledge is provided:
a) medical knowledge dissemination: the process of distributing expert and stabilized knowledge widely, meaning in small particles among many users showing different information needs;
b) medical knowledge dispersion: the process of spreading information over a wide area of users after selective separation of relevant from non relevant information has occurred according to users' demands;
c) medical knowledge dissipation: the process of spreading information in random ways, which are not controlled by just one single institution, therefore very hard to monitor and check;
d) medical knowledge distortion: the process of altering or twisting information absorbed in random ways and not monitored and verified afterwards;
e) medical knowledge diffusion: the process of deliberately spreading information through newly established channels and media with no further monitoring;.
f) medical knowledge disruption: the process of breaking apart information to make it more accessible; such process may prevent meaning reconfiguration based on common sense to happen, deeply affecting a more comprehensive understanding;
g) medical knowledge distribution: the process of dividing knowledge into smaller information units related to various other units according to different categories that have been preset;
h) medical knowledge dissolution: the process of separation between and among knowledge packages, which may cause loss of connections that were previously present as part of common sense based interpretation;
i) medical knowledge disintegration: the process of separation within the kernel structure of a body of medical knowledge, causing transformations at different levels and at various degrees to occur;

j) medical knowledge distillation: the process of extracting abstract concepts out of common sense-based knowledge causing the formation of new meaningful conceptual links;

k) medical knowledge distinction: the process of separating different information units according to a set of categories;

l) medical knowledge dilution: the process of deliberate reduction of meaningful information quantity and its conversion into plain text with neither technical words nor specialized terminology;

m)medical knowledge dissociation: the process by which a strongly bound combination of words breaks up into current words, which are still understandable; it represents the conversion of a highly specialized content into more friendly expression.

Transferring a word from a previous and well established context of interpretation into a new and dynamically evolving context for interpretation implies that the word will change its meaning too. Nevertheless traces of modifications are left and permit tracking on details of each transformation that has occurred.

Progressively transferring a word from a highly specialized to a less specialized domain may involve a whole set of revision stages at different levels of approximation, until a final meaningful stage is reached. This will result by means of a set of precise operations that have been performed on the same word and document. Proceeding from the expected interpretation toward stages of progressive perturbation will result in a series of radical changes that are very likely to discard meaningful links. A highly consistent reconfiguration will show the specific need for an accurate multifaceted representation of those very specific meaning aggregation processes. These processes cause the overall interpretation to progressively shift and then radically change at the end as a final output result. In order to capture such complexity, only a very articulated and complex metaphorical structure can serve the purpose where words belonging to one main domain may easily be coordinated and referred too.

Packaging of medical expertise is therefore bound to different stages. A careful analysis of meaningful links, which have already been discarded, is an absolute requirement for any researcher and scientist in the medical field today. This analysis allows the researcher to actually understand what changes may have happened and what have been or are the consequences of such changes. Different details of each meaning reconfiguration may be grasped only if the observational point of view is carefully reviewed, just like analysing the same word, which is undergoing multiple changes in many directions at the same time. It will be part of the original decision-making on accurate design and further expansion in the health advice document to include and dynamically visualize those most fundamental changes that have occurred as result of progress in research.

By clearly highlighting the most appropriate points of observation, qualitatively different pieces of medical information can be accessed by a whole variety of users, meeting a diverse set of needs without any misunderstanding or confusion. Without accurate monitoring of the overall process, it would become very hard for any user to discriminate between relevant and irrelevant information within a single body of knowledge. A whole set of indications that are easy to perceive and interpret will be of major help in identifying the most consistent access.

4. On Medical Reasoning By Analogy

Reasoning by analogy within a specific medical knowledge domain to provide advice to patients has to be conceived in terms of harmonious interplay of different kinds of experiences. This requires the consensual sharing of a common terminology and progressive building of a new framework of reference to package knowledge in both consistent and practical ways. Accurate conversion of technical terms into more palatable words becomes a requirement. By tracing the different layers and processes, it will be much easier to share output results based upon a terminology that facilitates the exchange of information and works in progress within a relatively unstable knowledge domain. Medical knowledge, for example, also involves many actors playing different roles.

We may think of an analogy as a whole system that originally has been planned, conceived and designed for a certain set of contexts, which can be defined as "contexts for meaning management" [6]. Not only should categories introduced be consistently checked to allow for new categories to be accessible in different areas of specific knowledge, but also an overall reconfiguration of functions and contexts needs to be progressively reshaped to allow the analogy to become simultaneously "a same structure but different functions system" [7].

According to accurate decision-making, new categories will have to be introduced in a way that proves suitable and "relatively stable" [8]. These decisions are based upon considerations regarding which kinds of specific knowledge domains need to be addressed. Medical knowledge progressive reconfiguration is based upon consensus on newly introduced categories as well as upon agreement about systematically used definitions. Just like a technical term undergoing changes, old meaning concretions that have accumulated will be substituted with new accretions based on consensual decision-making on knowledge that will then be made available more widely. Transitional stages must be foreseen to allow reconfiguration to actually take place based upon accurate verification. The first operation consists of the accurate preparation of a stabilized set of categories and of a stabilized body of knowledge to be organized as the result of accurate decision making by experts within the specific knowledge domain.

The nature of a medical knowledge management system will therefore be "polyhedral," "multifaceted" and "incremental." By "polyhedral" we mean that multiple perspectives will be allowed according to what each user is willing to see through the system, depending on a predefined task or set of tasks which have been assigned. The system will have to be accessed by researchers, physicians and health advisors.

By "multifaceted" we mean that different categories of users are expected or that the same user may be willing to access quantitatively and qualitatively different information at each given time. Such a user may be willing to change his or her role or play different roles at different times by redefining his or her information needs at each given time. The system may have to be accessed by researchers who want to check if physicians are indeed provided with a consistent amount of information. On the other hand, physicians may want to access more specialized knowledge and see if the conversion of knowledge provided to health advisors in general is indeed accurate.

By "incremental" we mean, precisely, that different kinds of medical fields of knowledge and expertise are covered and that different kinds of knowledge are made available at different levels of access and use. In addition, each knowledge packet is subject to both update and upgrade according to information coming in from different sources. Researchers are asked to be very sensitive to the issue in order to make sure that expert knowledge provided is checked, verified and up-to-date.

Appropriate training will have to be provided at many levels and for different purposes. Guidelines and precise directions for those expert users in charge of feeding in new information will also need to be established. These experts will provide information according to particularly relevant experiences, which have been selected and found to be of significance in order to extend reasoning by analogy further. Physicians are asked to input relevant cases, as are health advisors.

Monitoring on the users' side will constitute a guarantee for maintenance according to a predefined set of requirements, though some centralized control will also be needed as to ascertain functionality. Roles and tasks embedded within the originating structure to be performed by the system are, in fact, respected. Explicit use of a shared language may result in a most useful device to allow the different parts and layers of the system to work harmoniously and consistently, especially those that will be dedicated to the team of experts in charge of maintenance.

The concept of a cooperating team of experts in the various medical knowledge domains mostly resides in the identification of commonality of a task. There is obviously a basic need for sharing experience within a certain research community, particularly in a fast and highly consensual way, which in turn needs to be facilitated by a consensual code. A high level of cohesion is required for effective information passing and knowledge packaging through conversational intercourse. There is a distinct need for identification, for the belonging and sharing of a common framework for interpretation and for labelling according to a highly consistent model of reference. In the medical field, this may be most profitably embedded and provided within the system and accurately categorized as "special common knowledge" [9].

As soon as upgrading and updating needs emerge and become progressively more relevant, those very same individual researchers or groups of experts that are involved and willing to participate in the process must analyse in depths the existing body of knowledge. They also must review the way the knowledge was first developed to create the conditions for consistent updating and upgrading.

Diversification of various levels of depth in accessing knowledge as well as skilled capacity of making the same resources available at different degrees according to the users' diverse needs and tasks is one of the most fundamental issues to be addressed. The medical knowledge management system this way will be able to provide qualitatively different kinds of responses. Reasoning by analogy also provides support for diagnosing, searching, learning, solving problems, and keeping expertise up-to-date. According to the complexity of tasks to be accomplished, a medical knowledge management system will serve as an incredibly effective facility.

A very ambitious aim would be to unify geographically-dispersed communities of researchers, physicians and health advisors, therefore establishing a real point of reference for further experiences to be shared, evaluated and selected for consistent reporting and eventual incorporation. By accessing a medical knowledge management system intended also as a learning facility, each researcher will be motivated to collect more and more experiences. These experiences will then be filed and filled in according to standardized criteria, allowing for further links to be consistently established, kept and transmitted. Strong connections between and among cases, recursive similarities and strong analogies that can be derived and made available are the most relevant topics.

As a learning facility in itself, a medical knowledge management system will also provide researchers with accurate models for effective reasoning about cases, which have been found relevant and have been consequently labelled and stored. If it is true that some specific categories coming from a specialized knowledge domain may be chosen as particularly significant to be inputted, it is a fact that they must be the result of accurate decision-making and consistent modelling on the expert team's side.

A medical knowledge management system is also meant to facilitate understanding of new concepts and to support redefinition of old categories and reasoning about new possible links. These links can be established productively between and among apparently disconnected events and cases, which were not available for analysis before. If reasoning by analogy is primarily based upon regressive thinking and by linking "new" to well-known and well-established criteria and points of view, then a medical knowledge management system, increasing synthetic capabilities, is meant to check and verify still unknown and unexplored connections between and among phenomena that have been only partially categorized and therefore have been labelled as "unexplained" or "exceptional."

Reasoning by analogy may result in a very significant support system for filing, indexing and labelling cases. It can trigger cases to come back once they have been appropriately analysed and found to be consistent examples by the researchers, physicians and health advisors community. Reasoning in a specific medical knowledge domain is only possible if complemented by a process of in-depth search for those relevant cases. The cases first are interpreted in their context and then appropriately recognized in all their subsequently relevant features, which may then be linked back to previously examined and filed cases or create evidence for a new case under examination.

This is why capitalizing on medical interpretation turns out to be a precious and highly articulated process, which may require a set of specific procedures to provide accurate explanation.

Specific attention should be paid to the way analogies are produced in the first place: description, explanation and narration provide qualitatively different knowledge mapping paths. Specific categories of questions need to be identified, and experts in the various knowledge domains will have to become actively involved in order to create a realistic model for relevant questions.

According to this comprehensively designed model for knowledge storing, teams of experts will be able to undergo a whole rethinking process meant to help them redefine what they have done, researched and observed. They will also be encouraged to pursue an accurate process of rethinking their own criteria and conditions for observation as well as their objects of observation. A medical knowledge management system will facilitate analogy recognition, ranking different kinds and degrees of analogy, and will also support consistent evaluation parameters by providing a whole framework of different conceptual tools for accurate analysis of highly complex settings and situations.

Experts in medical knowledge domains, supported with a whole variety of cognitive tools, will be able to see the practical advantages deriving from collaboration versus competition, and they will be able to proceed and decide for an appropriate therapy, solution, and method of further monitoring. Experts will also find precise motivation for contributing with their own experience to the progressive growth and maintenance of the overall system.

Decisions will have to be made about which cases, packaged as stories, should become part of permanent memory, as opposed to just becoming part of episodic memory. Qualitative reasoning about cases constitutes a tremendous support for accurate decision making as well as for establishing consistent links and connections. Visual schemes create a facilitated communication environment for consistent packaging and dissemination of examples. Analogous cases, which may provide further explanation and interpretation, may be added afterwards, therefore constituting a harmoniously growing body of consolidated knowledge. Qualitative reasoning about different causes and effects, symptoms and therapies, found to be analogous in some ways, may be consistently linked.

Different levels of access to medical knowledge will be based on higher vs. lower information density and will be provided to different users. Based on the user's degree of knowledge or interest, different degrees of technicality in the language used will be differentiated. Availability of information is the result of a very precise process of decision-making, selection, focusing and consistent packaging.

5. The Knowledge Grinding and Dripping Model

The Knowledge Grinding and Dripping Model (KGDM) is meant to describe the process of medical knowledge distribution within a specific area, and is addressed to different individuals involved with the process of medical knowledge access at various levels [9]. Guidelines will be made available for the appropriate solution of specific access problems that may occur most frequently.

In order to explain how such a model may be productively applied, let us first illustrate the process of specific knowledge categories definition, which has been assigned as one of the major tasks to teams of researchers and experts working within a certain medical domain. What final users are expecting is basically an accurate definition of a set of special knowledge domain categories filed according to a very precise technical terminology and complemented with specific information processed through a consistent selection procedure. This process has occurred as the result of cooperative interaction by the experts in each specific knowledge domain.

Teams of experts have, in fact, been in charge of monitoring accurately the definition process of each case as well as the corresponding category assignment. They have therefore proceeded toward building a very precise set of categories complemented by a corresponding set of respective contexts for understanding and further use. Teams have also been in charge of the selection and decision-making about "what may be relevant to whom" and "what should be maintained" and "how it should be appropriately named" [7].

If we were to create a parallel metaphor to better describe the process teams have gone through, we may add that they have been mostly in charge of "information harvesting and relevant data crop collection" [7]. No doubt they have been playing a most important role in controlling and monitoring information both quantitatively and qualitatively. Teams of experts have therefore filled in the expertise after having provided interpretation required to each given case under examination. According to different kinds of needs and demands, knowledge users have to proceed toward definition of their own information needs both quantitatively and qualitatively and case by case. They will therefore have to get access to specific knowledge after having previously expressed their own needs.

After the process of expert knowledge acquisition has been completed, it will become much easier for users to share and exchange knowledge. Dissemination and distribution of newly acquired knowledge at this level will, of course, entail adequate understanding of a commonly shared code. It will also require a very active role in the organization, sharing and dissemination of expert knowledge by the medical community of researchers, physicians and health advisors.

The "envelope language," CTML and HTML [8], will in this case provide a strong support for packaging knowledge, which is undergoing major reformulation passing throughout a whole set of transitional states. An envelope language, designed to operate between and among different states of information, will help transfer knowledge coming from one specialized knowledge domain and make it available to a wider community.

Accurate decision-making will be supported throughout the use of those conceptual tools, which are absolutely relevant to insure success for any knowledge conversion operation that is based on monitoring and control capabilities in the overall process. Individuals cooperating in the process will also be able to accurately monitor it, and this will only be possible based on a unifying system of reference and consistent task assignment. Knowledge packages based on personalized needs and demands will be carefully analysed.

Health advice information will have to undergo a process of reconfiguration according to the demand coming from those individuals who are not experts in the field and are therefore in need of precise directions and of easy access and use of basic knowledge and information. Knowledge growing as a result of the observation of new cases, found to serve as productive examples, will produce an incredible amount of new data, information and reference material to be filed consistently for proper reuse.

Some new cases will in fact serve as reinforcement for previous cases examination. Of these cases, some will constitute an important platform for further expansion of the range of applications of an already well-tested and carefully verified procedure. Some others will provide evidence for newly discovered aspects to be explored or to open up possibilities for new inferences to be drawn. New knowledge coming in and new cases supporting evidence will create a significantly wider repository for further research, based upon incoming and subsequently consolidated information.

Extra space for new experiences, found to be still significant as outside information supporting evidence seen as inside knowledge, which has already been stabilized in the form of a three-layered building structure, will have to be foreseen and provided. In order to ensure full continuity to both information spaces, the same process of selection and data organization will have to be adopted and consistently used.

6. An Annotation System With Many Possible Applications

CTML stands for Context Transport Mark up Language [6,7,8] and is a derivative language of CPP-TRS, which stands for Communicative Positioning Program-Text Representation Systems [9], a visual language based upon a set of dynamic schemes and icons to be used in combinations to indicate the kind of information contained paragraph by paragraph. CTML is a simplified and highly reliable system of visuals, more precisely textual signs and textual symbols, meant for use in specific applications, such as for controlled languages. It may also be turned into a more specialized sub-language used to meet the specific requirements of a highly characterized community of users, like that of health advice providers.

A subset of CTML annotation tags may easily allow health advice information experts and providers to map their own text as to facilitate reading and interpretation by the patient. CTML mapping devices will prevent the author from using obscure terminology, which may cause content opacity to occur as a consequence of missing explanation by the knowledge provider. This may also be the consequence of inadvertent omissions of consistent interpretive clues on the knowledge provider's side about what he or she was in fact intending to do while packaging and making available a certain piece of information for the patient. Knowledge experts and health advice providers will be supported with categories and skills, based upon qualitative reasoning on information, which will significantly enhance their abilities to organize and display tailored information and to declare their purpose in a deliverable way to the patients.

Qualitative reasoning on the nature of information health advice providers need to choose from to encapsulate some information into an effectively tailored document is made possible. That same knowledge may also be incorporated into further texts after some reformulation and repackaging of the content has occurred. This way new readers are facilitated significantly in any further redacting process.

Specific features being displayed by CTML are the following:
a) communicative function or type of a text or paragraph, conveyed by a set of ten annotation signs;
b) communicative intention or style of a text or paragraph, conveyed by a set of eleven annotation symbols;
c) communicative turn taking indicating further action to be taken upon a text or paragraph, conveyed by a set of four annotation turn taking symbols .

Conceptual mapping made available to readers prior to accessing each health advice text will not obviously incorporate the sign and symbols, which would be perceived as alien by the reader, who is already undergoing a pretty stressful experience as a patient acquiring knowledge about his or her disease or that of a relative of a patient.

Readers will therefore be provided with the verbal indication of what they are likely to find in each health advice text they are exploring, whereas CTML icons and technical terminology will have to be transparent. They will be a kind of blueprint to provide a foundation for the text that only the knowledge experts and providers will see. Health advice text reading clues ensure that correct background assumptions about the readers' needs are visible and clearly understood by the expert knowledge providers. A further viable step may be foreseen in developing an interface such that icons may be incorporated into the self-publishing software so that authors and tailored information creators can mark up their content easily according to the CTML standard.

If CTML icons and technical terminology are to be used by health advice knowledge providers as blueprints allowing more individuals to work collaboratively on the same task and to alternate, capitalize on, and consistently reuse what has been already packaged, then the same concepts conveyed by the categories CTML is based upon need to be somehow translated into viable and most understandable words. This is precisely the meaning for a both comprehensive and highly specialized HTML (Health Text Mark up Language), which translates those interpretive clues provided by CTML into a set of progressively evolving conversational sequences aimed directly at encouraging the reader to access the provided material in an easy and friendly ways in the field of health advice.

HTML marked up texts, designed to enhance content and context visibility, may provide significant help for health advice information classification and represent important items in a repository for knowledge providers that can be reused and updated at any time.

In addition, HTML may be extended easily to serve as a most effective information retrieval system. It is based upon an intelligent query system for patients and relatives of patients needing to identify the most recent, specialized, reliable, and readable information; for information-tailoring professionals needing to confront, update and upgrade information all the time to ensure its reliability; for medical knowledge workers needing to cope with enormous quantities of data coming in diverse forms and formats; and healthcare professionals needing to be updated on most recent and solid findings coming from the research field.

Actual keyword-based search engines in health advice documentation, current classifications and categories, even if increasingly sophisticated, are still not sufficient to meet all the needs previously mentioned. A set of specifically targeted searches based upon additional indications about the nature of information sought in the form of pragmatic categories may significantly reduce the quantity of hits required. For a patient or relative of a patient, searching is not a pleasurable experience, but rather a needed one, and minimizing the effort is a guarantee for successful seeking, which requires being able to go right to the target.

7. The CTML Mark Up Language [6,7] And Its Conversion Into HTML Based Discourse Sequences For Meeting The Patient's Needs.

CTML annotation signs represent the various communicative functions a text may convey, paragraph by paragraph, to the health advice information provider and document author. HTML consistently converts them into easy-to-follow and easy-to-apprehend discourse sequences for the readers, that is, the patients. They are the following:

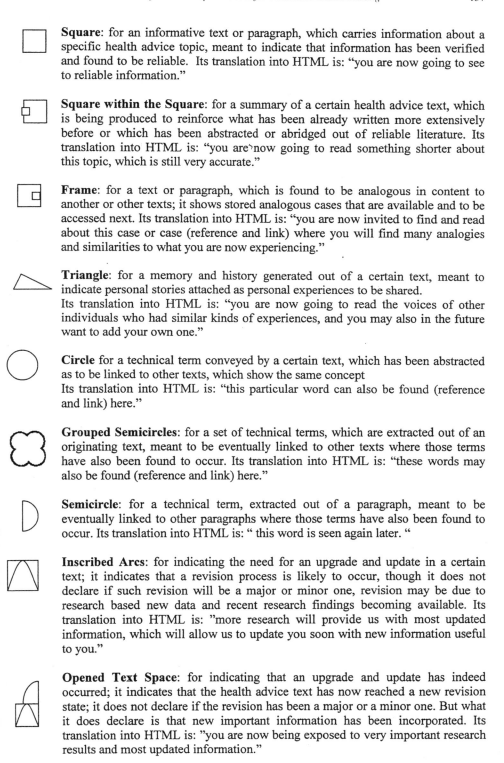

Square: for an informative text or paragraph, which carries information about a specific health advice topic, meant to indicate that information has been verified and found to be reliable. Its translation into HTML is: "you are now going to see to reliable information."

Square within the Square: for a summary of a certain health advice text, which is being produced to reinforce what has been already written more extensively before or which has been abstracted or abridged out of reliable literature. Its translation into HTML is: "you are now going to read something shorter about this topic, which is still very accurate."

Frame: for a text or paragraph, which is found to be analogous in content to another or other texts; it shows stored analogous cases that are available and to be accessed next. Its translation into HTML is: "you are now invited to find and read about this case or case (reference and link) where you will find many analogies and similarities to what you are now experiencing."

Triangle: for a memory and history generated out of a certain text, meant to indicate personal stories attached as personal experiences to be shared.
Its translation into HTML is: "you are now going to read the voices of other individuals who had similar kinds of experiences, and you may also in the future want to add your own one."

Circle for a technical term conveyed by a certain text, which has been abstracted as to be linked to other texts, which show the same concept
Its translation into HTML is: "this particular word can also be found (reference and link) here."

Grouped Semicircles: for a set of technical terms, which are extracted out of an originating text, meant to be eventually linked to other texts where those terms have also been found to occur. Its translation into HTML is: "these words may also be found (reference and link) here."

Semicircle: for a technical term, extracted out of a paragraph, meant to be eventually linked to other paragraphs where those terms have also been found to occur. Its translation into HTML is: " this word is seen again later. "

Inscribed Arcs: for indicating the need for an upgrade and update in a certain text; it indicates that a revision process is likely to occur, though it does not declare if such revision will be a major or minor one, revision may be due to research based new data and recent research findings becoming available. Its translation into HTML is: "more research will provide us with most updated information, which will allow us to update you soon with new information useful to you."

Opened Text Space: for indicating that an upgrade and update has indeed occurred; it indicates that the health advice text has now reached a new revision state; it does not declare if the revision has been a major or a minor one. But what it does declare is that new important information has been incorporated. Its translation into HTML is: "you are now being exposed to very important research results and most updated information."

Right Triangle: for a comment made about a text or paragraph, which may also contain information derived from other external sources that had to be reformulated because they had not easily available. Its translation into HTML is:" you may also want to know that ...... or that according to other authoritative sources...."

CTML annotation symbols are meant to indicate communicative intentions and styles, locally within a certain health advice text either sentence-by-sentence, or paragraph-by-paragraph.

They are particularly useful in indicating to different knowledge providers involved in the production of health advice material the contributions and choices made by each, both synchronously and asynchronously. CTML symbols support them in reshuffling or converting information many different times according to the different readers to be addressed.

Document annotation symbols, representing different modes of information conversion coming from a discourse and being packaged consistently with the originating context, may be activated at different times and may be combined and used dynamically for further information conversion purposes, such as further upgrade and update.

They may also effectively indicate transitional stages of the same text forming and evolving progressively with time. They are the following:

Describe: from the Latin *describo:* write around.

It means that the sentence identified will be complemented with as much information coming from other sources as may be found relevant to add without any specific constraints. It may also indicate the need for further information to be added to the actual text. It is represented by a spiral, which starts from the middle point, indicating the originating topical word, and proceeds toward expanding the topic at various degrees, linking it with other information coming in from different sources. Its translation into HTML is: "we will now describe your, ex: 'symptoms' etc. . . . ."

Define: from the Latin *definio:* put limits.

It means the text will be complemented with limited information about a technical word, which has been previously selected and identified as not being an obviously understood one. It is represented by the middle point of the square, and it indicates that there is a specific need to incorporate specific information about a relevant term. The term is made available and implies accurate and most selective focusing on a very limited amount of highly specialized information. Its translation into HTML is: "we are now going to define the word ex: 'mammograph.'"

Narrate: from the Latin *narro:* tell the story.

It means that the health advice text will be complemented with the narration of relevant facts and events by following a logical and chronological order. It indicates a set of major points or facts representing different diachronic   stages, which are strictly linked together. Its translation into HTML is: "I am now going to tell you my healing story . . ."

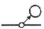

Point out: take a single point out of a story chain.
It means isolating a specific event or fact among those reported in the narration, focusing on just one event or fact and adding more detailed information, by expanding it significantly. Its translation into HTML is: " Out of this all healing story what is most important is..."

Explain: from the Latin *explano*: unwrap, open up.

It means that causes and reasons are given for certain effects, and consequences support interpretation of a certain event within a certain discourse or document.
Explanation may start by indicating the originating cause and proceed toward showing the effects. It may also start with effects and go back to the cause, decided according to what is found to be most significant. Its translation into HTML is: "We will now explain what were the causes of your health problem."

Regress: from the Latin *regredior*: go back.

It means that more information about a certain topic presented in a health advice text is absolutely needed to allow understanding to occur.
It represents a specific topic-focusing process and an in-depth information expansion,
which is activated only for that precise topic. Its translation into HTML is: "Not necessarily should you know what this, ex: cancer, is, so let me add something you may need to know now."

Inform: from the Latin *informo*: put into shape, shape up.

It means that any text is the result of some information packaging and that the kind of health advice text now provided is organized in the most unconstrained way. This lack of constraint is the result of many information conversion operations, some of which may be triggered back, if needed, out of the previous versions.
It is very rarely used by itself, and it instead leads toward two different kinds of further specification, which are respectively conveyed by the "inform synthetically" and the "inform analytically" indication:

"Inform synthetically"

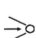

means that the information departs from a larger health advice text and proceeds toward a summary related to a specific topic identified as being the most relevant one emerging from the originating text .
Its translation into HTML is: "Let's now be very short..."

"Inform analytically" means that the information provided departs from a limited health advice text as to expand toward further information sources or to add more information, which needs to be then converted into the final form of a new text . Its translation into HTML is: "Let's now add some more about it. . . ."

Reformulate: from the Latin reformo/reformulo: change shape and shape again. It means that the kind of style will change from that adopted earlier in the same text and substituting a certain form of information packaging to a different one still related to the same health advice text. It may turn into a more or less radical transformation of the originating text according to a precisely defined request or set of requests. Its translation into HTML is: " Let me now say it in a different way . . ."

Express: from Latin exprimo: push out and press out.
It means that personal opinions will be added and individual feelings will be disclosed if related to a certain topic within a health advice text.

It indicates the most subjective mode of information organization, which is openly seen as bound to very personal evaluations, judgements and emotional states. Its translation into HTML is:" Let me tell you how much I hated to know. . . ."

CTML annotation turn-taking symbols are meant to define the mode of interpretation of a certain health advice text and to indicate if some kind of action is requested on the reader's side. They are the following ones:

Major Scale: it shows that literal interpretation is sufficient and that those sequences of text indicated and marked off have been extracted and quoted literally from a certain source that is verified and referenced or acknowledged. Its translation into HTML is: " Now let me quote what Dr. Helm, a specialist, has written about it in his article . . ."

Minor Scale: it shows that further interpretation clues need to be given and further knowledge is needed in order to really understand marked off sequences of text due to highly specialized knowledge to be provided or having been provided in abstracted or abridged parts of the text. Its translation into HTML is: "According to what Dr. Helm, a real specialist in this field, thinks . . ."

Open or Unsaturated Rhythm: it shows that accessing health advice text at its present stage may lead toward specific need for further questions to the experts. It is meant to suggest that the patient should now decide whether or not to consult with an expert. Its translation into HTML is: " We really have provided you enough information to think thoroughly if you should at this point consult with a doctor...."

Tight or Saturated Rhythm: it shows that accessing the document will lead the reader to further seek specialized knowledge once the expert has been consulted. Its translation into HTML is: " After your conversation with the doctor more elements out of this text will be more clear to you; let's therefore continue our conversation. "

The CTML annotation system here illustrated together with its HTML specialized version may apply to large bodies of health advice documentation. It can indicate specific operations, which have been performed upon text or are to be performed to connect new findings and further writings coming in different forms that have also been previously screened, encoded and accurately stored.

The whole annotation system here illustrated in its various components may, in fact, be applied at various levels of complexity with different kinds of referents and for a whole variety of possible applications. According to such a perspective, qualitative reasoning about information and quality-enhancement through accuracy-checking provide a very productive way to monitor the inherent complexity of any communicative intercourse and reduce possible distortion, which may very easily occur without constant verification of accuracy.

CTML in general may productively enhance the search of special documentation and literature, which may be easily organized under various headings after having undergone various kinds of classification processes. These processes ultimately result in compilations that can be consistently stored and then retrieved for the use of researchers and knowledge providers. HTML is more specifically aimed at providing physicians with those communicative tools and skills that are most relevant to them in order to monitor and keep track of the conversations with patients.

HTML ultimately provides the patients with gentle, effective support for searching and learning themselves. By displaying various levels of processing within the same document and by grouping them according to the various categories provided, information may be systematically arranged and consistently classified according to various layers of complexity. Health advice documents, which may have been subject to major conversion throughout HTML, coaching will still carry the essential core of their content. These documents will be accompanied by their respectively consistent context, which is specialized literature in the field or authoritative verified opinions.

Enhanced synopsis may also be easily produced in the form of skeletal displays of information provided in various ways and meant to facilitate the apprehension process by providing a quick overview of such a complex matter. Further information coming in the form of group discussions, which may be found to be of relevance, may be easily incorporated with the support of HTML tutorials and HTML guidelines.

8. Conclusions

In medical knowledge management here productively linked with health advice documentation, recognition and visualization of communicative patterns is very useful, both at a global level, which means by paragraph, and at a local level, which means by sentence. Visual encoding based upon information tailored for health advice documentation means complementing each piece of information provided with all those instructions, which are meant to enhance access and readability at various layers. Though it would seem that enhanced encoding would be an expensive process in terms of money and time, it would, in fact, turn out to be time and cost effective. Each encoded instruction will provide an enormous number of examples, which will effectively support any knowledge acquisition process.

Acknowledgments

The author wants to thank Dr. Pete Daniel, Curator in the Division of the History of Technology at the National Museum of American History, Smithsonian Institution, in Washington, D.C., for accurate reading of the present paper.

References

[1] Rimer B.K., Conaway M., Lyna P., Glassman B., Yarnall K.S.H., Lipkus I., Barber L.T., 1999, The impact of tailored interventions on a community health center population, in "Patient Education and Counseling", n.37, Elsevier Science, Ireland Ltd., pp.125-140.
[2] Lakoff, G. - Johnson, M., 1980, "Metaphors we live by", The University of Chicago Press, Chicago.

[3] Gentner, D., 1983, "Structure Mapping: a Theoretical Framework for Analogy", in Cognitive Science, vol. 7, n.2, pp. 155-170.

[4] Hofstadter, D., 1995, "Fluid Concepts and Creative Analogies", Basic Books, New York.

[5] Bushko, R.G., 1991, "Knowledge-Rich Analogy: Adaptive Estimation with Common Sense", Thesis, Massachusetts Institute of Technology, Cambridge, Massachusetts.

[6] Tonfoni,G.; 1999, "On augmenting documentation reliability through communicative context transport", in "The Proceedings of the 1999 Symposium on Document Image Understanding Technology",pp.283-286,Annapolis,Maryland.

[7] Tonfoni, G., 1998i, "Information Design: The Knowledge Architect's Toolkit", Scarecrow Press, Lanham, Maryland.

[8] Tonfoni,G., 1998ii, "Intelligent control and monitoring of strategic documentation: a complex system for knowledge miniaturization and text iconization", in "The Proceedings of the ISIC/CIRA/ISAS 98 Conference",pp.869-874, National Institute for Standards and Technology, U.S. Dept .of Commerce, Gaithersburg, Maryland.

[9] Tonfoni, G., 1996, "Communication Patterns and Textual Forms", Intellect, Exeter.

Future of Health Technology
R.G. Bushko (Ed.)
IOS Press, 2002

The Future of
Highly Personalized Health Care

Barry Robson, Ph.D.

*Strategic Advisor/IBM Distinguished Engineer, Computational Biology Center,
Exploratory Server Systems IBM Thomas J. Watson Research Center*

Jean Garnier, Ph.D.

Charge de mission for Bioinformatics, *Institut National de la Recherche Agronomique,
France and Visiting Professor, National Institutes of Health, US*

Abstract

We can surely lean well towards the optimistic in envisioning health care. In the world 10-25 years ahead of us. This optimism is based on rapid developments in genomics, the essential basis of molecular medicine, and on advances in computer power. At the time of writing this paper, the Human Genome Project was planned to have a working draft by 2000 and indeed completion was announced on June 26th from Washington. This paper describes the situation and vision at that time. Though there has been much subsequent more thought about the influence of genomics on healthcare, the aspirations and visions have not fundamentally changed from those of 2000, except for the greater attention to practical details that comes from increased confidence in the practicality of the vision.

1. Molecular Medical Science: The Acceleration Of Pace

We can surely lean well towards the optimistic in envisioning health care in the world 10-25 years ahead of us. This optimism is based on rapid developments in genomics, the essential basis of molecular medicine, and on advances in computer power. Indeed, the Human Genome Project is now planned to have a working draft by about the time of writing this Chapter, at the end of year 2000 and at the 50th anniversary of Watson-Crick Discovery. This will almost certainly be met, as progress has been exponential.

Optimism for completion is easy to understand: the first billion bp (base-pairs, nucleotides) were sequenced in 4 years in November 1999 and the second billion bp just in 4 months in March 2000. The first Chromosome, 22, was published in December1999. Some 16 international centers participated. The technique used was essentially mapping, shotgun with ten-fold coverage, assembly and finishing. According to Jill Mesirov at the Whitehead Institute, a major center in the project, the present working draft at the time of writing is estimated to have 99,9% accuracy with 97% assembled mapped clones and 85% assembled DNA sequences, a total of 2.6 billion b.p sequenced. About 90% of known genes were found in the draft. The G.C. Content was   about 41%, the known repeat elements and 38% (actual expectation circa 42%). Full completion should be in 2003 with repeated coverage done 5 to 7 times, yielding 99.99% accuracy. According to Ed Uberbacher at the Department of Energy, we had as of June 2000 some 5805 clones, 2649 contigs, 596.88 Megabases, 20792 STS hits, 3414 genes in the major data bank Genbank, 24773 genes suspected by the neural network software GRAIL. In addition to chromosome 22, human chromosomes 21,19,16,5 are already extensively completed. Some 90% of genes discovered will hopefully be publicly released.

Advances in computation have already contributed to our status in the genome projects, and some have described it as the major factor in the above-mentioned remarkable burst in efficiency in reading the genome. Certainly, much thanks is due to the fully automatic capillary sequencers, micro-electrophoresis chips, and their flat-out efforts, sequencing 24h a day, 7 days a week. However, a great deal is due to improvements in down-stream processing power, real-time process control, databases with 6 terabytes storage, as well as, in the laboratory, automated Q/C with data driven process control.

Another acceleration in progress arises in the area of the identification of genes and involves a lucky break in the relationship between human and mouse genomes. A problem so far has been that spotting a gene is not trivial. We recall that the general approach is: 1) Identify genes(s) of interest, 2) characterize genes and the SNPs and 3) test the spread of polymorphisms. One has to define the genomic organization: exons/introns (from cDNA), the regulatory elements or motifs. A major computational step once the genes are found is to discover to the function (the activity known as functional genomics). Approaches for gene recognition can be done by sequence homology (BLASTX, TBLASTX, FLASH, FASTA, SAM-T99,...) , and by statistical analysis of the nucleotide sequences (GRAIL, FGENEH, GenLang ...). However it is now likely that this essential groundwork for personalized health care will be accelerated by comparison of human and mouse genomes, since, while the genes are similar, the surrounding DNA differs quite extensively, highlighting the difference between gene and none-gene nucleotides.

Roughly half the diseases which we present our doctors are due to pathogens; the rest are genetic. How do our genes relate to our diseases? Typically, a loss of gene function is responsible. In any event, in molecular-disease studies the general approach used is: 1) identify the gene or genes of interest, 2) correlate with a disease, and 3) study it in a population. The candidate genes can be found from gene expression analysis, linkage, model systems. Linkage analysis, that gives positional candidates for genes, involves the building of a genetic tree, and it is greatly facilitated when two individuals in family share disease. The procedure is relatively straightforward for monogenetic traits, but for polygenetic traits, it becomes ambiguous. The follow-up to genome-wide linkage scan, i.e. finding variant in genes in candidate regions and interdependencies between them, is considered difficult though ultimately tractable.

Technologies using the DNA data directly most often fall into the class of diagnostics and although this is very beneficial, it is the next layer on top of genomics which is laying the groundwork for the most sophisticated medicine of the future.

This layer includes proteomics, comprising protein expression research and the understanding of protein interactions (though based of course on genomics). With microarrays chipsets one can monitor expression levels for thousands of different genes, and their correlated expression can lead to their function and their pathways of interrelationships. In studying biochemical pathway and disease, it is noted that there are many genes in each pathway and many pathways for each disease (e.g. the biological hypotheses for diabetes). In this, surprising benefits for humans come from the use of model (non-human) systems, drosphophila/yeast, C. elegans, is already beginning to lead to understanding of human function, for example by identifying genes based on homology in the insulin signaling pathway in C. Elegans. One important tool in all this involves a device which will, in future forms, doubtless also play an important role in doctors office scenarios described below: with micro-array chip-sets one can monitor expression levels for thousands of different genes, and their correlated expression can lead to discovery of their function.

By current definition, proteome, means simply the internal protein-world of the organism (as the genome represents its internal DNA world). This definition also includes the all-important issue of protein three dimensional structure, which is in turn the basis of the rational design of drugs. It also includes many other aspects, such as protein-protein and protein-drug interactions, discussed below. Within such broad definition, many companies are now active in areas which can reasonably be described as proteomics. A list is given in Appendix 1. Add to that the activity of every significant science University in the world, and this like the original Human Genome Project, is also clearly a major world effort, perhaps much more so.

There is considerable impact on both current medicine and future personalized medicine of the simple fact that it is much harder to get a proteins three dimensional structure than it is to get its sequence (i.e. essentially its chemical formula). The latter, after all, can be simply be deduced from the sequence of DNA, which is the major *raison d'être* of the Human Genome Project. The most important protein structure data bank (the Protein Data Bank, PDB) was established in October 1971 at Brookhaven following a community discussion about how to establish an archive of protein structures following the Cold Spring Harbor meeting in protein crystallography. The PDB had an exponential growth for many years. The present state of the PDB is one of continued dramatic growth, combined with transition of owners (to the Research Collaboratory for Structural Bioinformatics), curatorship, structure and format. According to Director Helen Berman, over 3951 structures were processed by RCSB since Jan 1999 (3037 primary, 458 BNL backlog, 456 Layer 1). There is less than 10day turnaround for new entries. Some 12514 structures in PDB are archived in detail. Important for drug design is the fact that the associated Ligand (HET) dictionary is now cleaned up (circa 3000 files tidied). From July 1999-July 2000 the depositions were 90% protein (82% from X ray data, 15% from NMR data), 5% nucleic acids and 5% nucleic acid/protein complexes, 56% from USA, 31% from Europe and 10 from Asia.

By this activity, most folding patterns for proteins may have been discovered, and much of the world of protein structure may be known. There may of course be many out-fliers, and data on those membrane proteins, including many drug receptors, is as yet extremely sparse. In any event, the new folds represent only 10 % of Total PDB depositions in 1999, a remarkable achievement.

To truly enable the highest fast response personalized medicine discussed below, however, requires a deep and also essentially holistic understanding of how interactions of therapeutics with one or few proteins of the patient will affect the overall patient and his/her disease state. We must obtain very highly detailed unified views of all data relating to each gene and pathway: interactions, pathway biology and gene expression, linked through to an understanding of consequences not only at the proteomic level but also the cytomic, and physiomic level, and a picture of how drugs will affect all these levels. Achievement of anything remotely like a complete picture would clearly demand a formidable undertaking, and it will be enormously computationally intensive. Nonetheless, through extensive collaborations the first steps are being made, including complete Virtual Human, effectively *homo in-silico*, projects.

In any and all events, the fact remains that the current ongoing Genome Project will continue to be a wonderful and highly productive tool for cross-comparison between model systems, for exploring function, expression, linkage, sequence data, lab data, individual variations and all the interrelations.

2. Our Molecular Individuality

A major consequence of the genome projects, giving a story significantly more refined than we ever learned from the school biology of the present generation of researchers, is a qualitative and quantitative understanding of the basis of our individuality. Approximately one in a thousand nucleotides distinguishes you and I; this corresponds to very roughly one amino acid residue difference per protein. Differences due to one base pair (or few) constitute Single Nucelotide Polymorphisms (SNP, or occasionally Simple nucleotide Polymorphisms). About 300,000 SNP's are presently known in first considering this article in summer 2000, and expect circa 1M end of 2000 and 2M end of next summer were expected.

This seems a limited sequence diversity in the human population, when compared to the difference between Chimpanzee and human 1 in just 100 nucleotides, but the roughly 1:1 correspondence of polymorphism and protein has highly significant consequences. Incidentally, there is a further coincidence in this number. The present technology is of course not error-free and produces an error of 1 in 1000 nucleotides. In other words it is, irritatingly, about the same frequency as the polymorphisms. Hence a major goal, before the achievements below are possible, is the objective is to achieve 1 error in 10,000.

What are these consequences, or having roughly one amino acid difference per protein? There is no such thing as a fraction of an amino acid coded for by a base-pair triplet. Thus, this is the minimal quantum of variation that we can expect to have to allow two otherwise identical proteins to express or function differently, or interact differently with other proteins and molecules, including therapeutic drugs. Of course, some effects will be quite neutral, others lethal. Also, of course, it is not uniformly one-to-one between polymorphism and protein: many of our proteins will be identical, and some will vary by two or even more residues. Yet we might still reasonably speculate that this quantum of variation representing the minimal possible effective individual variation within the species which is significant per protein product, is remarkable, and no mere coincidence but of important evolutionary benefit. Be that as it may, we can be sure that within the individual human lifetime it poses powerful challenges, since it effectively demands that health care must be tackled on a personal basis cognizant of the differences in our genomes and the proteins structures for which they code.

There is an assumption or two here that should be dealt with; in particular, can we expect changes with effects on health, and in responses to drugs, with just one amino acid within the human species? Certainly examples, of loss of function due to one amino acid change, are widespread: this is the most common interpretation of what happens when one inherits a recessive gene. Considering proteins which have survived the natural selection process, however, nature often seems to resist changes in the relevant functional regions despite considerable other variation. That is, the binding and catalytic sites are frequently the most conserved part of the structure. Even for distantly related proteins they can have very similar geometries. Examples considered by Arthur Lesk (he is American by origin working in England!) include YabJ (Bac) and YigF (E. coli); both are trimetric complexes with similar active sites. In another example case, Nobuhiro Go's group in Japan examined a data set of 491 phosphate binding sites with a common functional step, the binding of a phosphate group. They first compared the atomic configuration of surrounding atoms, they should satisfy: root mean square deviation <= 1.0, distance D 0<1.5 Å when the same atom type are aligned as much as possible. They found that one local atomic configuration is retained throughout each super-family, which otherwise showed considerable internal variation. Hence, we might conclude from such examples that it is hard to qualitatively affect the role of a protein, providing that the function is retained at all.

But equally well, we can sooner or later expect to find many examples of variations in function, qualitative as well as quantitative, when an amino acid residue changes and the gross function is retained. A long known example is sickle cell anaemia where the differential response to oxygen might be described as a little more significant than a quantitative difference, since, in the original homeland of the population, it confers resistant to blood parasites. Further, there are examples of functional changes even with changes in conditions around the protein which is otherwise chemically identical (so one might reasonably expect that something as drastic as a change to the chemical constitution can be very important). For example, E.coli HtrA (DegP) is a chaperone at low temperature and a protease at high temperature. Last but by no means least, we have examples in comparing proteins where the differential action of a potential drug is quite different dues to a change in one or few amino acid residues. For example, inhibitors of blood clotting bind quite differently to human and bovine thrombin due to a change in a charged residue in the protein.

In short, in the effects of single amino acid changes we may expect to see the whole spectrum, from lethal, to qualitative change in effect, to quantitative change to neutral.

These molecular individuality issues are already of contemporary concern. On the one hand medical treatment is itself is a significant killer in the United States due to the classical approach to catch all rather than personalized treatment. On the other hand, a breast cancer medication specific to an individual genetic variation is already becoming available. It is particularly interesting that, with roughly only one third of the population carrying this gene, previous classical trials and analyses, unmindful of genomic differences, would almost certainly missed this agent, classifying it as not significantly effective.

Currently, the Genome-wide SNP map is currently approached through the SNP Consortium; its goal is to get 500,000 SNPs by end of 2000, all placed in public domain in an integrated SNP map. Yet we still don't know what proportion of the SNPs alter function, understand how best can we distinguish between what is genetic disease and what is genetic individuality. We don't know what are the causes or reasons for the 10 major diseases in the US, a significant dearth of knowledge.

Nonetheless, this path ahead is not without significant cost. With conventional technologies:

2000 individiuals/500k SNPs => 1000 millions genotypes

Cost $1.0 per genotype	$1000 million Time	27 years
0.1 per genotype	$100 million	3 years
.01 per genotpye	$10 million	3 months

There is thus a current active search for cheaper, non-conventional technologies capable of achieving 100,000 allotypes per day, a considerably reduced time. For example, mass spectra high-throughput technology has been developed for determining SNPs accomplished with fully automated SNPs assay design. The technology has unlimited assay development capability using inexpensive reagents. Ultra high throughput can be obtained by pooling and multiplexing.

3. The Future Doctor's Office Scenario

Speculating on the future of health care and particularly its relation to bioinformatics, has been a considerable preoccupation of the authors for some time: Health Care will more heavily become one with protein structure science. It will interpret patient polymorphisms in terms of structural and functional effect. It will be computationally intensive, and pervasive from the doctors office to the jungle (1).

These considerations lead to an attractive scenario: It is possible to envision a time when you will be able to walk into a doctor's office and leave with pills personally tailored to suit you down to the finest molecular detail..." (2). With the above crucial role of computers in mind, Paul Horn, IBMs head of scientific research, has echoed this vision "One day you're going to be able to walk into a doctor's office and have a computer analyze a tissue sample, identify the pathogen that ails you, and then instantly prescribe a treatment best suited to your specific illness and individual genetic makeup." (3).

Strictly speaking, there are two kinds of inter-entangled vision which others, and we have considered (4).

The first form of the vision essentially uses experimental laboratory methods engineered into convenient, and highly miniaturized, desktop format. The patient walks into the doctors office, and submits a tissue sample for DNA analysis. Taking advantage of new developments in protein synthetic chemistry (5), minute quantities of protein product specific to that patient DNA might be synthesized and folded on microfluidic arrays, and used to screen potentially appropriate drugs by extensions of the methodology available in current microfluidic screening arrays, or even to direct drug development by refinements of current widely practiced combinatorial chemistry (ComChem) techniques. Tissue samples from the patient cheeks might then also be used for expression analysis using technology not far from that available today, to ensure the correct and trouble-free application of the final drug to the patient tissue (that is, including toxicity considerations).

The second form of the vision is purely computational, i.e. by simulation. Overall, the approach is the purely computational virtual reality counterpart of the above. It starts when the patient walks into the doctor's office and removes a medallion from around his neck which contains his genome. As a matter of storrage, this is already feasible. The whole DNA sequence of the human genome can readily fit on a CD (though our cells are a far more powerful storage device). Within that code Some 100,000 genes are similar to program files and almost all code for proteins, making up just 5-10% of the DNA sequence. Though the surrounding DNA once called junk DNA may well have function, and at least one defect causing cancer is known to occur there, the remaining and key information for most purposes is relatively little material by modern information standards.

In an important early step based on the genomic information for specific proteins, the relevant proteins are modeled by the computer, taking advantage of templates for standard polymorphic forms. That is to say, the challenge will, if the information is available, consist of modeling a protein from a very similar standard one of typically just one amino acid difference. As it happens, this technology is being progressively developed for modeling of proteins that are believed to be similar in three dimensional structure but have far more drastic differences than that, because experimental information on structure is far more sparse than information for protein sequences (the essential output of the genome projects). At present computational determination of protein function from structure is based on the observations between species that homologous proteins often share a function, sometimes they share only a mechanism, and sometimes homologous proteins have completely different functions (e.g. eye lens proteins: in duck: the protein is an ADH enolase that has lost its catalytic residues).

In passing we may note that there are two basic step in modeling a new or modified protein from existing data when the sequences look rather different. These are 1) identification of related proteins of known structure (i.e. The family to which the protein of interest belongs, and 2) alignment. Alignment is determination of residue-residue correspondences by pair-wise sequence alignment, multiple sequence alignment, or pairwise structure alignment, or multiple structure alignment. These underline the importance of correct alignment, based on the correct identification of conserved residues. As noted by John Moult, a founder of the internationally renowned CASP protein structure prediction experiment, predictions based on weak relationships can be as good 1.5 Å root mean square agreement between backbones, but other entries are certainly bad due to poor alignment. If one gets the alignment wrong, one gets the result wrong. The general problem with structural alignment is that the answer is not unique. As stated by Arthur Lesk: would one rather find 100 residues with rmsd =1.0 Å or 150 residues with rmsd =1.5 Å or 200 residues with rmsd =2.3 Å? Also, the solution is not unique, several substructures work equally well. The percent residue identity in the core increases indirectly/exponentially with root means square deviation in atom positions. (Chothia & Lesk showed in 1986 that protein comparisons fell on a single curve). In addition to these difficulties, even 1.5 A agreement of the backbone may not place side-chains accurately enough for drug design, in at least some cases.

Fortunately, these deep difficulties will not most generally arise in the human case in the longer term, since we mostly are interested in proteins that differ by typically one amino acid residue only. While the effect of such a small change can cause overall shifts in shape and function, these challenges do not seem intractable to the kind of computational technology that we can expect in 10-25 years.

However, the fact remains that there will be a substantial period of time in which we do not have many of the requisite templates, and the templates themselves will have to be reliably modeled by such means, for which these difficulties above are issues. A sound template library is needed. As an experimental approach to overcome such difficulties and to generate as many templates as soon possible, the structural genomics challenge is to obtain 10,000 representative structures in a 5 year period. These representative structures will demand less drastic modeling, and alleviate in particular much of the alignment problem, allowing automated modeling systems fill in what the Department of Energy workers call the white spaces between, using computer modeling. As seen by Ed Uberbacher of the DOE, the technique of threading provides a route as more and more representative structures becomes available. Protein threading is essentially just the matter of alignment again, but involves aligning each query protein sequence onto template structure in an "optimal" way with a score or threading energy function, to see which shoe fits (which is the right protein shape for the sequence). We need a threading algorithm to find sequence-structure comparison with a divide and conquer algorithm which can be done efficiently in polynomial time. One has to plan the protein structure prediction across the Entire Human Genome. (an SP3 implementation of Prospect has been bench-marked, and 100000 proteins could be threaded in approx 1 month) One could also combine NMR (Nuclear Magnetic Resonance spectroscopy) with threading to improving threading accuracy (this likely requires likely 20-25 NOE distances per protein). Of course, all the above is currently of interest to medicine right now. Even prior to the personalized medicine issues here, there is the lure that pharmaceutical companies can proceed on as a basis for truly rational drug design in which the molecular locks (proteins such as receptors and enzymes) can be seen as for design of the molecular keys (drugs).

At present, there are already several examples of automated systems which can, in the right circumstances, do a plausible job of protein modeling, especially of proteins with very similar sequences. SWISS-MODEL is a widely known Automated Protein Modelling

Server running at the GlaxoWellcome Experimental Research in Geneva, Switzerland. The purpose of this server is to make Protein Modeling accessible to all biochemists and molecular biologists World Wide. It was used in a celebrated Crunch study with Silicon Graphics, predicting as many protein structures from sequence as possible. For further details, the web site is: http://www.expasy.ch/swissmod/

After protein modeling, the computational counterparts of screening or combinatorial assembly then takes place against the protein in virtual reality (5). Related to this, there is the (admittedly tougher) aspect of simulating interaction of the patient metabolism including other extraneous protein sites at which the drug may bind. Though far from trivial, it is perhaps surprising to some to find that the screening of drugs in virtual reality is unlikely to be the hardest part, as significant advances have been made. An account of the Protherics Prometheus technology in terms of their successful public drug crunch with SGI is given on http://www.sgi.com/global/uk/news/2000/p000204.html

This was performed publicly as a crunch simulation with SGI, following, appropriately, the above protein modeling crunch. It helps that the problem of docking a relatively rigid drug to a protein is clearly a problem in far fewer variables than, say, modeling a protein from first principles (as would be necessary if there were scant information). So even in the pharmaceutical company of today, it seems that virtual screening offers the potential of rapidly and cost-effectively generating novel leads from protein structures. For example, the Protherics virtual screening technology was used to predict the binding geometry and binding affinity of a set of compounds consisting of diverse known inhibitors mixed with randomly chosen molecules (~10,000s to 1,000,000) from chemical libraries used. This method gives very good discrimination between the two sets of molecules when judged by energetic factors contributing to the binding.

But is this kind of approach quite ready for the industry yet? The above-mentioned recent Protherics-SGI blind crunch study involved computational analysis of well over 1,000,000 available chemical compounds against estrogen receptor structures. Known estrogen receptor ligands seeded in the one million randomly selected compounds were readily identifiable in the top scoring set. The project highlighted the technical feasibility of very large scale virtual screening, and its potential application in lead discovery. Using high performance computer systems available today, it is entirely practical to implement a virtual screening system capable of processing one to ten millions compounds per week. One such system could be based on the use of a large number of industry standards CPUs running the Linux operating system. This emerging technology clearly will have considerable utility in exploiting much increased number of therapeutic targets resulting from genomics. It will also create considerable informatics challenges because a large amount of data will be produced. It found important to develop a well thought out infrastructure for data storage and management, and the associated analysis and visualization tools for exploring the valuable data generated. Nonetheless, with these advances taking place already, it is not hard to imagine that the difficulties will be overcome, aided and abetted by substantial development in hardware and software over the next 20 years, giving a very high likelihood that there will be an efficient and routine doctors office version.

These possibilities are enriched by the steady progress in computing and specifically by the advent of petaflop computing (1000 teraflops), that is, a computer with the power to perform of order 10^{15} floating point operations per second. IBMs Blue Gene supercomputer with biomedical applications specifically in mind is a replicated single chip architecture with 32 Gflop processors, memory, and communications subsystems on a single chip; with 32000 chips 1 petaflop is achieved. As it happens, however, this is just a clever engineering glitch in the natural curve of computer power development over the years: we need to consider that far great computer power is likely to be available in 10-25 years, when personalized medicine really begins to bite. Almost certainly, we should be into the exaflop (1000 petaflop) range at some not too distant time, and sooner or later, beyond that, though such development will probably first demand dramatic advances in nanotechnology, quantum computing and smart computer software.

In both cases (miniature laboratory versus computational, virtual reality) one might consider, at least in the version of the scenario earlier years, that the patient must wait for his drug to be prepared in approved form, in quantity. In following years, one might imagine that the patient goes to a molecular ATM, i.e. A automated teller machine than dispenses pharmaceuticals, not money. Later still, such drugs might be dispensed much more immediately.

It is not clear which of the above (miniature laboratory versus computational, virtual reality) routes is likely to come first, though the bias of opinion seems to be towards the computational route, since there are still some tricky steps to iron out in the engineering required for the miniature laboratory approach. One might of course also conceive all combinations at any time in the evolution of the doctors office scenario. For example, the patient DNA sequence might be obtained directly, at least for relevant genes, and then sequencing of that DNA is followed by purely computational drug design. It is fashionable, and probably also reasonable, to assume that the tendency will be to move from real world to simulation as the simulations methods progressively better emulate reality. Notably, then, real world toxicity testing via something like expression array analysis might well be the last real world method to survive, but this is not unequivocal, since considerable computational progress is being made in this research area too.

4. Convergence Of Miniature Laboratory And Virtual Reality Methods

Despite the above considerations, it is likely that the methods will not be seen as mutually exclusive, although there may initially be market competition between different components of the two approaches. Indeed the present authors have considered that the protocol would be more intimately entangled, i.e. that it will be molecular-bionic, mixing real chemistry and computation technology on chips (1). Not least, in some sense, real chemistry practiced in a micro- miniaturized laboratory based on computer chip technology is just a form of analog computation using molecules (though with a more credible treatment of the forces governing intramolecular and intermolecular behavior!). Hence such a chip might play a role as a special processor within, for example, a more standard digital computer frame without jarring on the sensibilities of our future computer scientist who might be versed in such matters. Indeed, above and beyond the current interest in DNA computing which uses the copying and combining of real DNA molecules to solve problems, there is reason to suppose that lessons learned from protein structure and folding, might well lead to nanotechnological revolutions in smart materials for computation. In these the molecular scaffold carrying electrons and enabling digital processing might be adapted to include an additional analog component. Already we see that, in the matter of the original storage and presentation of the patient genomic data, the molecular biologist even of today is already in inclined to see his sample and libraries as forms of molecular-scale memory storage as real as any on a computer storage device. The extension of such dual thinking to processing operations as well as storage might well fundamentally challenge our abilities to make the miniature laboratory vs. virtual reality distinction.

Estimates for the advent the above kind of scenario have varied from 2010 to 2030. However, there are routes toward this vision which imply a more continuous, and perhaps earlier, development. On the computational side, one factor is that petaflop computing appears to be coming somewhat ahead of schedule (see above). On the experimental side as described here below, another factor is that the extension of the current use of antibodies on a chip, and imminent biosensor technology, could move us more smoothly, and sooner, through intermediate forms of practice.

5. Impact Of Pathogen Studies

Recalling that some half of disease sates are due to pathogens, and noting that the pathogen genome is generally considerably simpler, some of the first impacts might be in the area of infectious disease.

Development of such technologies may also have a catalytic effect on the technologies required for the Doctors office scenario. Notably, it is possible that a fear not just over natural epidemics but in regard to bio-warfare will be a catalytic factor for bringing forward some of the technologies. There is in fact little doubt that such research is underway in military laboratories, and would be readily adaptable. Indeed, the aims are one: we are at war with the microbes.

As noted by Colin Howard, a WHO researcher at the Royal Veterinary College, the problem for the human race is that the same holds true for pathogens as it does for human proteins: one amino acid can make a difference. Presumably, this simple fact (though undoubtedly there are other considerations) underlies the roughly comparable levels of innate and pathogen-induced disease. This also means that one amino acid is all it takes to make an otherwise innocuous organism pathogenic, or by escape from restriction to breakaway from its original host to the human population. Typically, this means escape from an animal to human populations, or at least crossing of genetic material with pathogens from animal populations. Examples include AIDS, influenza, Ebola, prion diseases. These considerations are significant even on a planetary scale. Much of mankind, especially right now in the Third World, has been devastated by such considerations.

In the laboratory approach (which may be the first routine step to routine use of human proteins on a chip in the doctors office), pathogen enzymes and receptors, are already being used with chip technology (microfluidic laboratories) for screening appropriate antibiotics. Also, because the raising of antibodies is an important step both in diagnostic and vaccine development, such diagnostic-biosesnsor arrays form a potential first step for the rapid development of cartridge vaccines, i.e. vaccines with synthetic peptide components representing B-epitopes, T-epitopes and Cytotxoic T-cell components, immunostimulatory components and so on, which are rapidly switched to cope with new epidemics.

In early studies in this direction, there are examples where that single amino acid change is again seen as important. Specifically, it can be directly important for design of vaccines and other anti-pathogenic agents. As also noted by Colin Howard, it has become a significant consideration in the war against Hepatitis B, one of the major pathogens. For example, in considering protein sequence region 139-147 (S), one of the more important of several regions of protein which might form the basis of a vaccine, the replacement of amino acid residue lysine to glutamic acid makes a vaccine only, a glycine to arginine replacement makes a vaccine and an anti-HBs agent.

In future, one may imagine pathogen data bases held upon the Internet, with input from diagnsotic-biosensor arrays. Such systems might constantly monitor for changes in the pattern of drug resistance or antibody binding which reflect epitopic changes in the pathogen, and the above-mentioned phenomena of escape from restriction which gives rise to transfer of pathogens from an old to new host group, and thereby cause epidemics.

6. Decentralization Of The Pharmaceutical Sector And The FDA

Does this mean the end of the drug industry? Almost certainly not, although realization of the above scenario would demand very profound changes. Not least, it would mean decentralization of the industry in terms of a centrifugal movement outward to real-time interaction with the patient. Specifically, one would imagine that the devices local to the doctors desk would be linked to powerful servers in the pharmaceutical companies, and the expertise of the pharmaceutical company scientists and of the Food and Drug administration would come together in directing and monitoring the final interactive drug development process for the individual patient, and the testing of safety and efficacy.

7. Decentralization of Patient Management

A common response to all the above is Why the doctors office, that is, Why not the patients home? Such a vision may be, rather brutally, considered as cutting out the doctor as middleman, and delivering health diagnosis and drug response directly into the hands of the patient. This would seem natural for two reasons, beyond just logistic convenience. First, the doctor as we know him or her now is not conversant with the management of equipment for the above kind of fast response personalized medicine in any event: indeed the whole scenario above is as alien to the current average doctor as it is to the current average patient. Second, if we extend the health care into constant monitoring both of the sick person and the everyday health monitoring preventative medicine, this naturally begs a home scenario.

Doubtless as with the pharmaceutical company the role will not be abolished, but redefined. However, there are two directions in which a current young person, aspiring to be a doctor, might go. In one direction, he could go to the home; the doctor might take on some of the role comparable to a cable TV repairman and be concerned with installation and maintenance of the requisite devices, but combined with a fine tuning to the patients needs, plus counseling general vigilance of the patient and his interaction health care devices, which demands a fairly astute level of medical, and indeed a sophisticated molecular-science, skill. Such a role might more naturally restore the role of the doctor to one of home visits and personal interaction that was reminiscent of European countries and the heyday of social medicine, when doctors, nurses and social workers house calls were the norm. Conversely, the aspiring medical worker might be driven more toward the server end of the health care business, interacting closely with the pharmaceutical and FDA scientists. Marvin Minski, the father of Artificial Intelligence, and the Future of Health Technology Institute, foresee that Caring Agents, i.e. artificially intelligent interactors and counselors, might adequately fulfill the more routine roles of the human doctor and medical counselor. Be that as it may, we may come upon some of the finer principles of the socialist idea that mechanization liberates man from his labor, in that a high degree of computer interaction will increase the amount of genuinely human face-to-face interaction.

8. ...And Why The Home Anyway?

Carrying the above trend to the extreme, it is easy to reach the concept that personalized health care should be wherever the patient is, not just at his home property. Early on, this means that pervasive computing, i.e. the wrapping of small computer, mobile phones etc.

into hand-held devices, will also embrace health matters including perhaps diagnostic kits attached to, or rolled into, those devices. But it also leads naturally to the vision of benignly invasive technology, in which diagnostic kits, biosensors and associated chips are carried within us, constantly monitoring and repairing our health. This is by no means an original vision of the future: not least it has long been considered by health care visionaries as a basis of intensive long term medicine, and by the military to monitor and unjust the status of soldiers in the field. Nonetheless, it is important to give some attention to the administrative changes that this will effect. We might suggest that they are not a great quantum leap beyond the home phase, and may even re-consolidate the more fundamentally medical role of the cable TV repairman since the safe seating and interaction of such devices with our tissues, and associated counseling, will be an issue. However, the Caring Agents may then need to transform to Guardian Angels almost literally at our shoulders, and ultimately more deeply embedded, perhaps even in direct neurological communication with our brains.

In the limit the notion of health care becomes one with an extension of the notion of augmented homeostasis, a bionic extension of the natural physiological mechanism which regulate our equilibrium of well-being, our avoidance of dis-ease. In some cases, we might consider them comparably as augmentations of our immune system, enhancing our self-defensive capability at the microscopic level.

9. Hierarchic Issues Of Well-Being

In our opinion, these visions raise in turn issues about the hierarchic level at which disease should be resolved, and particularly so in the case of genetic disorders. In effect, they enrich the number of ethical considerations, though it is not necessarily reasonable to say that they always add to the ethical burden. Rather, they might add extra opportunities, to enable resolution. For example, one might ask whether a fault be genetically resolved before conception, before birth, at somatic gene level by gene therapy, or by corrective homeostatic mechanisms which repair or edit the effects of undesirable genes. Whatever the complaint against genetically pre-selecting desirable human beings, few would argue that an individual should have to live with the pain of the consequences of not pre-selecting, if he does not have to do so. In such a case we might escape the dilemma of the early sponsoring and censoring or human worthiness, and intercept it later, at a corrective level which retains the genetic merits and existential rights of individuals.

The extra opportunities created by scientific research and technological development may help alleviate many moral dilemmas we face today. At very least, we may say that they offer us greater choices.

References

[1] B. Robson and J. Garnier , Foils to "Healthcare of the future... in the footsteps of half a century of protein structure research and computational molecular science", IUPAB Congress, India, 1999.
[2] Internet http://www.zurich.ibm.com/dcevent/compbiology.html
[3] Internet http://www.salon.com/health/log/1999/12/09/protein_folding/
[4] J. Li and B. Robson, Bioinformatics and Computational Chemistry in molecular Design. Recent Advances and their Application pp 285-307, *Peptide and Protein Drug Analysis,* Marcel Dekker NY, 2000.
[5] B. Robson (1999) Beyond Proteins Trends Biotechnology,17:311-315

Future of Health Technology
R.G. Bushko (Ed.)
IOS Press, 2002

Developing E-commerce and
Improving Resource Management

Barbara B. Friedman, MA, MPA, FAHRMM

Assistant Vice President, Support Services,
Saint Peter's University Hospital, New Brunswick, NJ, US

Albert Sunseri, Ph.D.

Executive Director, American Society for Healthcare Engineering, Chicago, IL, US

Abstract

The pressure on Materials Managers, Information Technology Managers and Chief Executive Officer's has never been greater to re-imagine, re-invent, and re-architect their operations. The need for speed and for emerging Internet skills and sensibilities has led many operations to look to E-business service providers for assistance. The United States market for E-business services, including consulting, IT outsourcing, software development, and system integration has grown from $7.01 billion in 1998 to approximately $10.3 million in 2000 according to Dataquest [1]. With the growth in E-business accelerating, the market is expected to mushroom to $59 billion by 2003. Material Managers know they must introduce E-commerce to their business strategy, but many are not sure how, which is driving them to consulting and services companies. There is confusion in the ranks on whether they need to change their business model and systems structure in order to do this, and the organization is reevaluating how to move forward in the dot.com world.

1. I-Commerce

The definition of electronic commerce infomediaries, is an Internet-based business-to-business electronic commerce marketplace for buyers and suppliers of healthcare products and services. Today what has really evolved is Intranet commerce and the definition of I-commerce is really as follows: An Internet-based electronic platform that allows for online procurement of products that also provides the vehicle to support the front-end integration of the supply chain. This element is absolutely essential to what will work in hospitals today.

Business-to-business E-commerce will only work if the integration with the legacy systems in the hospital exists. No matter which material management systems are used Matkon, PeopleSoft, Lawson, etc., if this integration does not occur, E-commerce will not work. At the end of the day, an invoice has to be paid in accounts payable and if the process of integration wasn't complete, E-commerce is worthless.

2. Current Purchasing Issues

Some of the current problems in the purchasing/material management arena today are as follows: (A) It is a totally inefficient process. There are too many cooks essentially trying to get involved with purchasing and a lot of it is just not centralized appropriately. (B) There is limited access to sellers as well. (C) There is limited product information, (D) Some of the things are just not accessible the way that they need to be, and (E) There is limited transaction data, and just a totally uncoordinated purchasing process throughout the institution, and it's offsite locations such as ambulatory care centers or physician practices, etc.

Typically, the controlling of the supply chain costs is predicated on being sequential. There are frequent disconnects throughout the organization. It is usually built around functions rather than processes, and that's one of the biggest problems in the hospitals today. Certainly a lot of people are taking a reactive approach rather than being proactive. It is historical that crisis management in hospitals, exists at most levels, and particularly in the support services. There is always a crisis from the material end, particularly at the end of the day on Friday or right before holiday weekends and there is always scrambling around trying to get that supply in.

There is a potpourri of methods, utilized including phone, EDI, e-mail, fax, etc. Essentially, there are just too many methods to choose from and people are not centralizing on one process, so that there is definitely a very high degree of uncertainty. There are lots of technology issues centering around inoperablility, data visibility, reliability, and costs.

The common state of the supply chain is as follows: What hospitals really thrive to do today is to try to have transportation cost reduction, Internet distribution processes and more inventory consignment in place many individuals still think electronic-data interprise (EDI) is still the best methodology. People think it works well, so why should they go to the worldwide Web? The utilization of group purchasing contracts is still very controversial. It is not clear whether GPOs own some of the infomediaries such as Neoforma and Medibuy or vice versa. But as the IPOs are being withdrawn and the stocks plummet, it seems that GPO's are using these infomediaries as a platform to advocate E-commerce capabilities.

3. E-Commerce Benefits

Some of the supply chain benefits with E-commerce are as follows: (A) Reducing overall product cycle time and reducing the inventories as much as possible within the organization, (B) improving product quality and reliability. (C) Providing significant source flexibility in metrics. (D) Developing key source partnerships. (E) Improvement of cash flow, improving the productivity, speed and accuracy of purchasing and payable transactions.

The E-commerce benefits to buyers and purchasing are as follows: It is an improved sourcing process. The idea is that you really go shopping on the Web worldwide. There are no new sources of supply, but still it has to be integrated in some administrative processes that allows for overseas purchasing. It gives great ability to compare and shop, whether it's with local suppliers, national suppliers, or international suppliers and certainly it gives the ability to free people up to work on more strategic, value-added tasks. It should lower the overall operation costs. In fact, it only costs a few cents to process a purchase order on the Web, as opposed to about $75.00 to $125.00 to process a purchase order. So, E-commerce enables greater control on spending, inventory levels should substantially decrease, and ultimately lower prices are paid.

4. Barriers to Success

The barriers to success are as follows: The reality is that the computer literacy of purchasing staff and other support staff in the hospital still is not up to snuff. For examples, many local supplies within the metro New York area don't even have a Web site. They clearly don't even understand what E-commerce is and they say, "Oh yeah, I think my daughter uses it for homework." It is an eye-opener to realize the amount of businesses that are still not connected to the Web and really have not developed an E-commerce strategy for their business.

In terms of what really goes on in hospitals, there are lot of hospitals even in the metro New York area that still preclude employees from being on the Internet. Some administrators that it's going to detract from employees work and decrease productivity. There really has to be greater education to CEO's in hospitals to allow the Internet to really become more pervasive in everyday use and in all of the departments within the hospital.

In effective purchasing processes, a lack of vision and strategic planning is common. When E-commerce becomes fully operable with the legacy system it is going to be tremendous. However, it is going to take time, perhaps another one to two years. Ineffective marketing by suppliers is also a big problem today. A lot of suppliers are feeling there web sites are not getting a lot of transactions on the Web, so it is not a primary motive of selling today.

5. E-Commerce Roadmap

An E-commerce roadmap, would consider the following bullet points: (A) Try to align the business goals of your organization with your E-commerce initiatives and it is very important to assemble a cross-functional E-commerce team. This will assure that in a hospital setting, everyone is basically on the same page, and that is there is one E-commerce strategy for the organization. (B) Try to determine processes that are best suited for E-commerce and try to develop a technology plan that meets the overall business needs and the strategic mission of the hospital (C) Most importantly, train staff and suppliers, and then adhere to what the three Rs: review, revise and revisit.

6. E-Commerce Summit Issues

The Association for Healthcare Resource Material Management decided to work on this checklist of deliverables to the five dot.coms companies, and ensure that they were thinking about what was really needed in hospitals, not what will give them the most profits. So number one was working together to create universal transactions standards.

Productivity enhancements such as cost saving was a primary focus. Another one, of course, was application benefits, such as the ability to interface with the legacy system. Again, this is really the crux of the matter. If the legacy systems don't integrate with the Web, this doesn't work properly.

Order fulfillment has to be at least 99 percent capacity no matter. By placing an order on the Web, if you don't get what you need the next day or when you need it, it is useless. Order fulfillment is very critical, as well as appropriate security issues. Cost-reduction benefits, use of reverse auctions, and payment terms, had to be very specifically stated companies E-commerce platforms.

The E-commerce business models and multiple delivery locations prove very interesting. Most hospitals today have many off-site campuses. Hospitals have ambulatory surgery centers, physician practices, etc., and there must be an integrated approach to accommodate all locations. Standards transaction processes including how you actually place an order, how you actually get that order confirmed, verifying the price, advance shipping notices, etc., down to the invoice process all have to be mapped down accurately so staff could understand the benefits that these infomediaries could provide.

Another set of issues cencerns the customer's perception and expectations. The first question asked was what priorities does your IDN have for the next two years? The number one reason was to improve the supply-chain model. All companies were looking for optimal productivity. The next most important reason was focusing on resource allocation and then, business partnerships.

Another key issue was what will be the primary focus for the next two years. Approximately, 76 percent said integrate the supply chain for the first reason, and grow in size as the secondary reason. Another key issue was, what is your most significant investment at this time? The answer was "IT Solutions." It is important to remember most of the hospitals are still recovering from the Y2K expenditures, so E-commerce is the priority for the year 2000. The replacement of existing equipment was a secondary reason.

Integration with hospital systems is critical and it must be a key-area focus for E-commerce companies that expect to succeed in the marketplace. Most people agree that this is absolutely essential for the dot.coms to be successful. By the year 2001, it will be difficult to find a hospital of IDN that isn't using the Internet for their materials management effort.

Most respondents were in agreement that a critical mass of successful integration within a hospital or IDN is essential   It is going to take about two years from now really for this to work out well. Most respondents stated not getting so tied into GPO's was essentially the GPO's owning the dot.com company platform.

Another issue was how should E-commerce be paid for? This was very interesting because at the April summit it was primarily material management people, who felt that the supplier transaction fees should be number one. The August response went up significantly for buyer and supplier transaction fees. The difference is that there are two more players besides the original five dot.com companies who presented in April. One of them is "Global Exchange" and there are companies today such as Johnson & Johnson and Baxter, which actually banded together and said, "Wait a minute, why should we pay these infomediaries a 12 percent transaction fee? They are working on forming their own platform. Concurrently, the distributors such as Allegiance and Bergen Brunswick banded together and as distribution companies they said the same thing. Why should we pay these transaction fees? They formulated a new platform called "New Exchange". The future success of these platforms and who actually survives will be interesting one year from now.

Most of the respondents stated the most important goal an organization expects to achieve through E-commerce was cost saving. It is critical to cut costs from the supply chain. Other goals were improving productivity, basically in the purchasing process, and an increased level of strategic versus clerical purchasing. It is now becoming clearer that more time must be devoted to more strategic ways of cutting costs in the hospitals rather than just ordering supplies and placing orders on the Web.

In order to meet management objectives, an organization will need to identify and implement an enhanced E-commerce solution. More and more people felt that by the year 2002 and primarily by the end of it, there would be a tremendous move towards people placing orders on the Web.

In terms of what is preventing an institution from using a dot.com company, other is the answer. What is other? Other is: the bureaucracy and administration in hospital-politics versus money. Many of these administrators are tied in with the GPOs and are shareholders attempting to recoup some return on their investment, and not really looking at clearly what is good the for the organization. There are a lot of issues here and material managers find themselves in a major quandry because they don't want to be the ones to say, "Well, maybe we shouldn't use that dot.com company over another." So it's still a wait and see game.

Of the five E-commerce companies present, how many will still be in business in two years? These figures are changing. The two companies that have been the major infomediaries in the past year have had tremendous layoffs. There will probably be one or two.

The questions of how much influence will a GPO have on selecting an E-commerce partner. Is very interesting. It appears that GPOs are really in the driver's seat of these dot.com companies. It remains to be seen how their platforms will continue to evolve.

7. Future Vision

The future of I-commerce will be increasing globalization and access to new markets as they integrate those legacy systems. Completed supply grids and networks will continually evolve, as hospitals will find there are more plentiful systems to get involved with. New and redefined supply channels from the manufacturing community, as well as the distributor community. Will evolve in a year from now or maybe two Dot.com infomediaries that are still thriving will probably be a handful, at most.

There will be many aggregated purchasing opportunities, as individuals understand the power of the Internet. It is clear that the Internet is a useful information tool. Everybody wants to use it, but it is not a perfect world right now and everybody needs to get involved for improvements to be made. There will be a lot more customization, particularly, in large hospitals or IDNs to really make this work properly.

For right now, there is a lot of confusion and uncertainty. Michael Dell once stated, "Ideas are a commodity, execution of them is not." E-commerce and Internet commerce is definitely wonderful and on the road to really changing the way we do healthcare in the hospital arena, but it is not quite there yet.

References

[1] WWW.DATAQUEST.COM
[2] AHRMM E-Commerce Summit, April 2000, San Antonio, Texas
[3] AHRMM Annual Conference, E-Commerce Session, August 2000, Tampa, Florida

Appendix:

E-Commerce Summit

Within this context, Association for Healthcare Resource Material Management, affiliated with the American Hospital Association had the opportunity to fulfill its mission in providing educational experiences to clarify the existing situation and to prescribe models for the future. AHRMM offered five E-commerce companies an opportunity to participate in an education summit to discuss their approaches to E-commerce within the framework of outcomes outlined below.

Specifically, AHRMM invited sixty of its chapter leaders including its Board of Directors, Past President's Council, Chapter Presidents, and Committee chairs to attend a two-day program in San Antonio, Texas in April. The Summit included five two-hour sessions with five selected firms who addressed the E-commerce outcomes and any other issues they deem appropriate.

This format provided the five sponsoring companies an opportunity to share the strengths of their approach to E-commerce and to have open dialogue with Materials Managers. The final session was an open forum for leaders in which all approaches were shared and compared. This session alone can provide valuable information on the current thinking of Materials Managers and provides information not found in the industry.

E-Commerce Summit Deliverables
1. Identify productivity enhancements through E-commerce ventures.
2. Determine measurement tools that enhance efficiencies.
3. Specify order fulfillment procedures and contingencies.
4. Specify application benefits associated with individual E-commerce firms with examples of approaches that make them unique.
5. Define standardized transaction processes and their interface with end users and E-commerce companies.
6. Develop a set of characteristics that define E-commerce companies.
7. Identify future applications and their benefits for end users.
8. Establish an enhancement concept list that can be shown to provide cost reduction synergies.
9. Establish the criteria for security and protection of information
10. (11-12)Three deliverables defined by sponsoring companies.

Future of Health Technology
R.G. Bushko (Ed.)
IOS Press, 2002

The Future of Information Technology for Health in Developing Countries

Scott C. Ratzan, MD, MPA, MA

*Senior Technical Advisor, Global Bureau at the U.S. Agency for International Development
& Editor, Journal of Health Communication, International Perspectives*

Maria I. Busquets, MA

*Chief of the Communication, Management and Training Division in the Population, Health
and Nutrition Center at the U.S. Agency for International Development*

Abstract

What is the future of communication technology for health in developing countries? This chapter sets out to answer this question by first considering the background and potential of information technology, identifying some of the issues and trends in communication, and finally following with some challenges and opportunities of how communication technologies can make a difference in health in developing countries. Past research has shown that communication can contribute to all aspects of population, health, and nutrition programs and is relevant in a number of contexts. Some of the trends in using information technology can be classified in the following categories: competition, cognitive-based presentations, comprehensive translation, convergence, and culture. Challenges include finding a way to include the South in the exchange of ideas and information. In addition, reaching a consensus on worldwide quality standards will not be easy. Yet, beyond these challenges, there are many opportunities being created for international development agencies to increase their capacity for impact.

1. Introduction

During a visit to India in March 2000, President Clinton watched a woman enter a village health center, call up a web page on the computer, and get information on how to care for her baby. This baby will live a longer life than her mother, mostly because of 20th Century public health advances and the new technological potential of the 21st Century.

Unfortunately, it is a rare occurrence for a woman in a developing country to have access to the Internet. The hopes for progress in technologies present ongoing challenges in access, quality, and equity. In fact, over half of the women in the world have never made a phone call. In Africa, which has a population of 700 million, fewer than one million people had access to the Internet in 1998, and of this number 80 percent were in South Africa. Among the other 20 percent the ratio of people who have access to the Internet to those who do not is 1 to 5000, in the United States or Europe the ratio is 1 to 6.5.

The woman in India in the example above is an anomaly as many villages still lack a working telephone. The new information technologies potentials is concomitant with the divide in the access to learning opportunities: 885 million people in the world are illiterate, and two-thirds of them are women. More than half of these adults lives in India and China, another one quarter in seven other nations in Sub-Saharan Africa and South Asia. Yet, information and communication technologies are often the hopeful solution to end these inequities, particularly among those who are poor and isolated in developing countries. [1]

A search of PubMed in December 2000 yielded 6,692 citations containing "Internet." The number is growing by at least eight per day. But of course, this is disproportionate with developing countries. Fewer than 0.1 percent of these articles are related to developing countries, despite the fact that developing countries represent over 25 percent of the scientists in the world. Similarly, a study of Medline looking back at 1992-96 showed the British Medical Journal (BMJ) had only 0.4 percent of the publications mentioning developing countries, the Lancet 0.6 percent, and the New England Journal of Medicine 0.05 percent. When you look at content and language on the Internet, the statistics are sobering—for example, only .02 percent of the Internet content comes from Sub-Saharan Africa, and while content in several languages has risen in recent years, English is still the predominant language used on the Internet.

With such a daunting challenge, we ought to answer the important question: What is the future of communication technology for health in developing countries?

To answer this question, we will first describe the background and potential of information technology (IT), some of the issues and trends in communication, and follow with some ideas of challenges as well as opportunities of how communication technologies can make a difference in health in developing countries.

While we read each day about HIV/AIDS, cancer, and emerging diseases, there has still been great progress in public health globally. Last century in both developed and developing countries, there has been a 25-year increase in life expectancy, the most rapid improvement in history. Much of the success is not due to better drugs, surgery, and diagnosis. Almost all the improvement has been the result of public health: surveillance, sanitation, nutrition, changing lifestyles, etc.

Public health actually is a field that principally focuses on the transfer and exchange of information: data collection, surveillance, information transmission, and communication. The new communication technologies have great application in public health practice.

2. Background

Recent advances in information and communication technology provide an unprecedented means of overcoming two of the root causes of extreme poverty—ignorance and isolation. The opportunity to communicate public health information and expand the flow of ideas and data coming from the South will allow for a horizontal two-way dialogue that will contribute to new opportunities to communicate public health information not available before.

Effective use of communication technology can benefit personal and public health. Past research has shown that communication can contribute to all aspects of population, health, and nutrition programs and is relevant in a number of contexts, including (1) individual's exposure to, search for, and use of health information; (2) the collection, dissemination, and utilization of individual and population health risk information (often termed risk communication); (3) individual's adherence to clinical recommendations and regimens; (4) the construction of public health policies, messages, and campaigns; (5) health provider-patient relations; (6) creation of "health as we know it" through popular culture and mass media transmission; and (7) the agenda-setting phenomenon of prioritizing public health and health care system developments. Most of the usage of communication technology has focussed on the first few areas.

Most people today think of IT as electronic mail, Internet World Wide Web sites, and interactive CD-ROMs. These are just a few of the many new communication media that provide unprecedented global access to people and information.

The landmark ideals of Marshall McLuhan represent a challenge for those of us using IT: McLuhan accurately predicted that "the new electronic interdependence recreates the world in an image of a global village."[2] Already, we have evolved communication from broadcast to multicatch, but IT is more than just the web. IT now includes the ideas of demassification—narrowcasting information to the end user, interactivity, a true exchange of information, asynchonicity, the ability to communicate whenever with our "real time" interaction, and mechanomorphism of multimedia to include all the senses (except smell at this juncture) into the communication experience.

Despite the potential of communication technology, we must be mindful. While globalization has the potential to bring people together and to provide them with tools to advance their social and economic well being and their health, it poses great risks. There is a dark side to IT: the fact that some can use it to create a "digital divide." We must be particularly concerned about Internet access for under-served populations and opportunities for girl's and women's participation in the digital information.

3. Trends

We have five basic C's that help us describe the future trends in using information technology in development:

- Competition
- Cognitive-based presentations
- Comprehensive translation
- Convergence
- Culture

These areas are creating uncharted territory as the new media evolves.

Competition—The answer to the question who's knowledge and whose information will become more complex. While there are media conglomerates and publishers that have a monopoly on communication of "knowledge" in our scientific and medical journals, this will change. Researchers and scientists have begun to bypass print journals and put research directly on the web.

Cognitive-based presentations—Powerful new cognitive formats will evolve; as this happens, the traditional format of Abstract, Introduction, Methods, Discussion, and Results could become extinct. One new format may create a new language not just for computer programmers, but consumers. A "Hypertext Comic Book" to teach children how to spot landmines in Mozambique or a Nursing School Midwifery Curriculum in Kenya that enhances by iconic "cognitive" paradigms can allow a user to point and click to icons for medical knowledge. For information or medical knowledge, the Uniform Medical Language System may evolve into cognitively based formats that maximize interactivity, hyperlinks, and memory.

Comprehension translation—Most books appear in only print format; one size fits all. The IT future allows people to indicate their backgrounds, education level, language preference, and interest with software to individually tailor a translation to maximize comprehension. These Intelligent Agents will create a digital document for an epidemiologist that will be different for a physician in Canada or traditional healer in Haiti. Translation software will evolve that can adapt for dialects, aphorisms, and other specific linguistic markers.

Convergence—The convergence of media (computers, telephones, television, radio, video, print, and audio) and the emergence of the Internet create a nearly ubiquitous networked communication infrastructure. The potential of this cannot be underestimated. Networking can be used for many purposes in public health, from creating support groups of persons trying to quit smoking to "action alert" networks for advocacy purposes. We are already seeing the creation of online communities amongst scientists, teachers, and Ministers of Health. A group of mid-level health professionals in Francophone Africa is, for the first time ever, able to share information, compare experiences, and "speak" with other professionals with similar problems.

Electronic communication can also be used for public health interventions to persuade the general public or policy makers, such as through health education, social marketing, or advocacy. Because of the capacity to segment audiences, electronic communication can be used to develop health education and behavioral change materials for specific populations (e.g., smokers, non-English speakers).

Convergence will also bring scientists to "push" new information into the world via Internet delivery. Convergence will also take place as the distinctions between the latest scientific findings, lectures, journals, and books become blurred. Schools, books, and lessons will have information days old, rather than years or decades old.

Culture—There is a problem of acculturating individuals to new technologies. Repetition has induced attitudinal change by familiarizing people with, in this case, technology through repeated exposure. Yet, the use of IT can in fact develop an information generation. This generation can change governance and policymaking. One way processes and vertical organizations will be vestiges of the 20th Century. On the Internet, interactivity will prevail; policies and research may benefit from early feedback from users. A culture of passivity on the part of the users also may ensue. People may merely access and download information, treating the Internet as an online health library. But as they spend more time on the Internet, gain access to different sites, and notice consistencies and contradictions, critical thinking ought to emerge as people pose their own questions and apply their own knowledge. Health policymakers and researchers should exploit such opportunities for interaction with users.

The health impact of interactivity, customization, cultural diversity, and enhanced multimedia is just beginning to be explored. Yet, already, interactive health communication technologies are being used to exchange information, facilitate informed decision-making, promote healthy behaviors, enhance peer and emotional support, promote self-care, manage demand for health services, and support clinical care.

4. Current Initiatives

Through a U.S. Inter-Agency Agreement launched by President Clinton in late 1998, the Internet for Economic Development (IED) Initiative seeks to empower developing countries to develop and use the Internet to boost their economies, gain access to knowledge and foster the free flow of ideas. Through this initiative, USAID Missions have supported the development of community telecenters in Ghana, Guatemala, and Haiti; and the use of the Internet for Mayan-language education.

Efforts are underway throughout the world to develop integrated national and global health information infrastructures to support health improvements. In the United States, the National Committee on Vital and Health Statistics (NCVHS) seeks to develop a system that links surveillance systems, information sources, and establishes communication linkages (on emerging and reemerging diseases).

The infrastructure makes it possible for people not only to use health information designed by others, but also to create resources to manage their own health and to influence the health of their communities. For example, community groups could use computers to gain access to survey information, health indicators, disease surveillance, and access about the quality of life in their neighborhoods and apply this information to create an action plan to present to local elected and public health officials. Information is a critical element of informed participation and decision-making, and appropriate, quality information and support services for all are empowering and democratic.

At the Millennium Assembly of the United Nations in September 2000, the right of universal access to information and communication services was discussed as a new component of the UN's principles and conventions on human rights and development. When John Chambers of Cisco and Carly Fiorina of HP joined sixty-five other CEOs in June 2000, they discussed how to make IT more accessible to the world's poor. When the G8 held their meeting in Tokyo last July, they focused on the crossroads of development and IT, and in an unprecedented move, invited developing country and civil society representatives to join the Dot Force. When they meet again in 2001 in Genoa, progress towards eliminating the digital divide will again be discussed. President Bill Clinton recently held a panel discussion on the Digital Divide in Health, Education, and Technology. The common theme was the "the global divide giving way to a global connection."

Rhetoric has given way to action. For example, the United Nations has begun ``Health InterNetwork,'' which is designed to improve public health around the globe by providing health information using Internet technologies. It links scientists in over 30 countries to the leading scientific journals, databases and discussion groups.

Under the Leland Initiative, USAID is implementing agreements with more than 20 Sub-Saharan African nations to enhance Internet connectivity and use in a competitive policy environment. Now that through the efforts of many, African countries are connected to the Internet, the Leland Initiative is supporting broadband connectivity to secondary cities and towns in select countries such as Guinea and Uganda. In addition, private and public activities are beginning to provide access to the Internet, especially through community access points, for the world's population presently without such access by the end of 2004.

In Africa, there are hundreds of initiatives developed by donor agencies—some intended to increase access to these technologies in remote areas by establishing "waystations" (resource centers that provide access to health information on CD Roms and online) and others dedicated to increasing the use of these technologies in specific areas like health and agriculture.

5. Challenges

Widespread availability and use of interactive health communication and telehealth applications create several serious challenges. One is related to the debate on whose information and knowledge appears on the Internet or on a CD-ROM. Knowledge from the "North" will need to make space for the ideas, experiences, and information stemming from other cultures and experiences. Anyone that has tried to cull through the clutter of the web will understand the challenge of creating usable content, especially content applicable to the health needs in the developing world. There are also risks associated with consumers use of poor quality health information to make decisions.

Concerns are growing about the Web making available large amounts of information that may be misleading, inaccurate, or inappropriate, which may put consumers at unnecessary risk. Although many health professionals agree that the Internet is a boon for consumers because they have easier access to much more information than before, these professionals are concerned that poor quality of a lot of information on the Web will undermine informed decision-making. These concerns are driving the development of a quality standards agenda to help health professionals and consumers find reliable Web sites and health information on the Internet.

Reaching a consensus on worldwide quality standards will not be easy. The process will most certainly move us away from the more academic and traditional quality standards that were created by the North for the North. Finally, even if we were all connected with affordable access and quality information, illiteracy and lack of computer skills remain a considerable hurdle.

6. Opportunities

The vision of new technologies cannot be underestimated. The power of technology has been described as revolutionary, and the Organization for Economic Cooperation and Development has written of a new, knowledge-based economy.

Opportunities are many—the Internet is a one trillion dollar technical infrastructure and, in theory, available to anyone; it's global and borderless with new business and development applications and models coming in from all directions; open when needed—24 hours a day—which means time zones are no longer a barrier; it's changed the way we conduct work, recreation, and even love!; and keeping it all together is *information*—it's the glue, the value-added—that keeps us coming back for more.

The information revolution can be an equalizer. Chat rooms around the world have recently been furiously debating what is a false dichotomy of computers and technology on the one hand, and health, food, and basic services on the other. It's not an either/or debate but a two-track approach to revolutionizing the way we do business.

Recognizing the challenges we face (outlined earlier), IT can still be harnessed to empower individuals and reinvent governments, promote electronic commerce, and expand access to information. In the development arena, IT has numerous applications.

International Development Agencies can use the new technologies to reinforce and modify present forms of technical assistance. Interactive multimedia training courses are being used to provide opportunities for individual and group interactions. CD-ROMs accommodate a wide range of learning styles, and their use seems to be increasing user's overall level of learning including improved engagement and retention of information.

Electronic training is becoming a reality—and big business. Hybrid CD-ROM/Web solutions are used when connectivity is a challenge. Start-up costs often appear to make electronic delivery of training appear costly in comparison to face-to-face training. However, given the large number of healthcare providers requiring training, electronic training could be very cost effective.

Virtual consultancy, where no one travels, is highly possible. Several pilot studies are already underway.

Collaborative research can take place online, as can data analysis. It is possible to do online team planning with members of the team at different points of the compass. Even real-time epidemiology is possible online.

Isolated communities can have access to online, accurate, up-to-date, quality health care information from local sources or the world's largest medical library, the National Library of Medicine at the National Institutes of Health. The MedlinePlus service provides access to extensive information about specific diseases and conditions, and has links to consumer health information, dictionaries, lists of hospitals and physicians, health information in other languages, and clinical trials.

CD-ROMs and desktop publishing offer university libraries advantages, and even African University libraries are increasingly connected to the Internet. Digital libraries are changing the work and, indeed, the idea of the library. Increasingly, it appears that scientific publishing will be available online.

Additional applications include virtual "toolkits" including communication strategic planning software, international drug price indicator guides, web courses on infection prevention, Instant Messenger for real-time training, Cyber Cafés, community forum message boards, multi-media idea bank on condoms, Technology Assisted Learning Centers, and a database of free photos.

There are numerous possibilities, almost all of which are presently 'under-exploited' in international health and development. And these possibilities will be much more attractive and valuable with the acceleration of online interactive video technology. What has become clear to the authors is that waiting for technology stability is a losing tactic.

An equally important concept to consider is the indirect impact of ICT. Many of the populations that international development agencies work with do not have access to the Internet and most likely never will. These populations receive the benefits of ICT, but it is especially hard for the public to perceive. The Famine Early Warning System[4] (FEWS) in Africa was designed to utilize high technology means to provide advance warning of the development of famine conditions. It was designed to allow acquisition and stockpiling of food in advance of market shortages. Thus the success of FEWS is marked by lower costs of food and fewer food shortages. Yet not only do most of the beneficiaries of FEWS not have direct personal access to its technology or any ICT technology, but they are not aware of the ICT benefits they receive.[5]

The new technologies provide many potential ways through the above and many others to expand the opportunities of international development agencies to maximize their impact on health concerns.

   a. The technologies are built on interaction;

   b. They are inclusive—allowing the quick identification of a range of information on an issue and the choice of the information most relevant to the setting;

   c. The information and knowledge can come from a range of perspectives and countries;

   d. They are flexible—when the information changes it can be updated very quickly; and

   e. The new technologies operate at scale.[6]

Recent discussion of the future with technology leaders in Silicon Valley and Virginia's 270 Corridor found that no one can predict which of the new technologies (or the infinite number of upcoming developments) will go mainstream. Just as Napster [recently] and the world-wide web [5 years ago] were hugely surprising in their rapid growth and use, the future is also very difficult to foresee. Some of the possible areas mentioned by the experts were:

   ❑ Wireless—continued rapid expansion of wireless access and technology (e.g., Palm Pilot, RIM, information pager networks, cell phones and WAP) with the implication of being able to access information and interact from potentially anywhere, at good speed, and not restricted by land-line capacity.

   ❑ Personalization—automated processes so that you 'pull' down the information that you want to see, not the information that the web sites are pushing at you, which provides rapid information on the most recent trends, data, and experience relevant to your work and restricts the necessity for long searches on many sites. Essentially, you take control.

❑   Video—will move ahead in leaps and bounds. VBIC already offers a guaranteed lip-synch online video facility—training, conferences, one-to-one calls, etc.—at U.S. $0.05 per minute. Virtual meetings could replace some travel because quality and cost are getting that good.

❑   Voice recognition—no typing: train your computer to recognize your voice. This software is developing very quickly and could result in better efficiencies.

❑   Data mining—the ability to sift through and manipulate (i.e., try to connect different variables and cross-reference topics) large quantities of information in a vary short time. This would really help information overload issues and lead to better, more targeted analysis.

Finally, in the midst of this technology revolution, we must:
- ensure women have equitable access to the benefits of telecommunications and are not disadvantaged by sector reform and industry changes;

- design and provide telecommunications technologies and services which take into account women's needs and requirements; and

- increase women's participation in all levels of the telecommunications sector. [7]

7. Conclusions

Even if the woman in the village at the beginning of this chapter gets access to the Internet, she will not necessarily be able to use the information to improve her child's health because as it is often said, trying to get information from the Internet is like drinking from a firehose, you don't even know what the source of water is.

The future will have more quality information provided by web sites but, realistically, only a few branded, highly credible sites will emerge (competition and convergence). Despite retrieving accurate information, the woman in the village still has to decide if the information is relevant to her situation. This hopefully will become unnecessary as more data would be generated and shared in a decentralized network linking knowledge in the developing countries, creating a so-called South to South dialogue.

Hopefully the future Medline will reference and share a number of journals from developing countries. The Internet can converge with gateways to become a Global HealthLine. The problem is complex, and possible explanations range from the difficulties encountered by researchers in developing countries in gaining funding for research)only 10 percent of funding is spent studying problems relevant to developing countries) to the existence of "ethnocentrism at its worst" in biomedical publishing circles. But now, with the availability of publishing software that can be coupled with powerful Internet search engines, it is possible for authors or local scientific societies to bypass traditional avenues of scientific publishing. They can post their research directly on their own web sites or, for example, on web sites that focus on international health or on general health and clinical research web sites like Pubmed Central or other electronic servers operated by biomedical journals.

Wireless is likely to be the principal means to access the Internet. The second billion people on the planet who access the Internet will not access it through a personal computer, but rather through wireless devices. This is facilitated by the development of less expensive technology and ease of usage coupled with a rising sense among people all over the world that they are entitled to participate openly in their government and society. Greater mobility in using the technology will be made possible through the use of pocket sized wireless devices such as Internet enabled mobile phones. Extensive tailoring of the volume and style of presentation of information can already be done using hypertext and multimedia links. This can convert any material to accessible formats that cater for different audiences.

To ensure that the envisioned future does not remain merely commercial hype, a systematic effort should be made to exploit the advances of information and communication technologies for use in developing countries. As has been described, many efforts are already being made to bring these technologies to developing countries. The long list of initiatives is impressive but how successful have their efforts been to work synergistically?

In terms of health, attention would be best directed to improving access to accurate and relevant information. Credible agencies or organizations that provide evidence based health information can increase the speed with which users are able to download information by constructing mirror or replica sites in different geographical areas. For example, the European Union funds the web site of Scientists for Health and Research for Development (www.shared.de/sharedhome.html). This web site lists potential donors, ongoing projects, and resources available to researchers in developing countries or their partners in the developed world. Medical journals that have their own web sites can follow the lead of the BMJ and provide free access to their articles.

The relevance of information can be improved partly by increasing the visibility of health research from developing countries. Technical assistance in designing web sites could be provided, preferably through the creation of templates to be easily adapted by different users. Alternatively, some agencies might offer to host other organizations on their web sites, absorbing the costs of developing and maintaining the sites. For example, Kabissa (www.kabissa.org/index.html) provides low cost domain hosting for non-profit, non-governmental organizations in Africa, including the Network on Equity in Health in Southern Africa (www.equinet.org.zw), a network of research, non-governmental, and health sector organizations seeking to influence health policy in southern Africa.

The development community is going through the same struggle as many small private sector businesses. Many tend to take small steps, especially senior management. But major shifts are warranted. It is absolutely critical to move from viewing IT as a tool to viewing it as a transformer. From the gigabytes and megahertz discussions of high end computing to low end computing such as the $10 hand held device recently developed by computer science students at MIT. From the Western perspective of desktop computers in every household to wireless and satellites. The creation and use of Web Sites should also embrace change. It is critical to move from "talking at" to "listening to" and from "brochure ware" to assessing and serving customer needs. Finally, the most often overlooked shift—the movement towards changing what's behind the web sites—the people, the processes, and the corporate cultures.

As the disparities between the information have and have-nots increase (not only between countries, but also within countries), so too do inequities in health status. Consequently, there is a great urgency to act. The new global disease threats must be addressed not only with medical means, they must be complemented by efforts to enhance literacy, economic development, and the like—what Nobel Laureate Amartya Sen has called "support led strategies". Such strategies can include communication technologies to focus on lengthening the factors that make economic development possible, of which education, health, and the empowerment of women are central components.

There are many success stories combining community effort and social mobilization to build on. Among the most promising are programs for community-based literacy education, complemented by significant social mobilization efforts using role models with high credibility from the local and national arenas, such as figures from the media and the entertainment industry.

Ideally, education could evolve just like this edited volume on the future of health so that "virtual centers," or collaboratories, where the expertise is drawn from many locations can be integrated. These do not need to be from the North or developed countries. Special consideration with new media technologies should address access issues for underserved, minority, and disabled populations. Opportunities with new communication technologies can integrate new research methodologies and approaches to respond to the swift pace of change inherent in the communication revolution. Ideally, a new connectivity can foster relationships with other public health agencies, advocacy groups, non-governmental and support organizations to the private sector.

Finally, there is an opportunity to advance a leadership position not only in publications and media channels along with the hospital, health care facility, and academic health center, but also in using communication technology for health in the private and public sector. Systematic agenda setting in keeping appropriate health issues on the political agenda in general could be of great value. This is where highly credible organizations, such as the World Health Organization, or professional organizations and governmental agencies could be most powerful by providing accurate, trustworthy data for public consumption. Developing health leadership could be the most important communication advance.

Could there be a future when people throughout the world can elicit accurate, up-to-date interpretation of study results that translates "health as we know it" into real-life daily activities? Could we communicate well enough to individuals so that we develop health "news you can use"? There are no longer technological barriers to such ideas.

While many are optimistic that we will do the right thing and create a new health as is "ought to be," health as "we know it" today might prevail—a world with disparities of income, health, and human rights, and environmental justice. Humankind often advances with market forces suggesting we have the right to just do it, rather than just doing the right thing. While we have identified the latest frontier as cyberspace, our ability to reach people for profit supercedes promulgation as a species. Perhaps, we are now at a crossroads in the third millennium.

Nearly fifty years ago, there was a different warning: "Science, which now offers us a golden age with one hand, offers at the same time with the other the doom we have built up inch by inch since the Stone Age and the dawn of any human annals. My faith is in the high progressive destiny of man."

While Winston Churchill warned of the nuclear age, I also suggest a warning of the communication age. We must empower the individual to access information with appropriate interactive health communication to enhance his/her decision-making.

References

[1] Tessa Tan-Torres Edejer, Disseminating health information in developing countries: the role of the Internet BMJ 2000;321:797-800 (30 September).

[2] McLuhan, Marshall

[3] LaPorte 1997.

[4] http://www.usaid.gov/fews/

[5] (John Daly paper for USAID) How development agencies are using information and communication technologies: examples from agriculture education, environment, and micro and small business. John Daly, InfoDev, World Bank.

[6] (Warren Feek paper for USAID) Real and Virtual - Technical Assistance - New technology opportunities for improved technical assistance by USAID Population Health Nutrition, January 2001.

[7] Engendering ICT Policy: Guidelines for Action. The Africa Information Society-Gender Working Group: Johannesburg, South Africa, 1999.

[8] Renata G. Bushko, Poland: Socio-technological Transformation – its Impact on Organizational, Process, Clinical and Service Quality of Health Care. In: W. Wieners (ed.), Global Healthcare Markets. Jossey-Bass Publishers, John Wiley & Sons, Inc. 2000, pp. 194-201.

Advancing Intellectual Leadership

Future of Health Technology
R.G. Bushko (Ed.)
IOS Press, 2002

What is Digital Medicine?

David Williamson Shaffer, M.S., Ph.D.

Lecturer, Harvard Medical School, Harvard University Graduate School of Education, Massachusetts General Hospital Department of Dermatology, Boston, MA, US

Colleen M. Kigin, M.S., M.P.A., P.T.

CIMIT (Center for Innovative Minimally Invasive Therapy), Massachusetts General Hospital Institute for Health Professionals, Boston, MA, US

James J. Kaput, Ph.D.

University of Massachusetts

G. Scott Gazelle, M.D., Ph.D.

CIMIT, Harvard Medical School, Harvard School of Public Health, Massachusetts General Hospital Department of Radiology, Boston, MA, US

Abstract

Changes in health care are a fundamental part of social and intellectual evolution. The modern practice of scientific medicine depends on the existence of the written and printed word to store medical information. Because computers can transform information as well as store it, new digital tools cannot only record clinical data, they can also generate medical knowledge. In doing so, they make it possible to develop "digital medicine" that is potentially more precise, more effective, more experimental, more widely distributed, and more egalitarian than current medical practice. Critical steps in the creation of digital medicine are careful analysis of the impact of new technologies and coordinated efforts to direct technological development towards creating a new paradigm of medical care.

1. Introduction

The last two decades have seen the beginning of a digital revolution that is creating a new information economy, and with it new paradigms for business, politics, and culture. Not surprisingly, the field of medicine is undergoing dramatic change as well.

Public conversation about health care in this time of change has tended to address questions of policy and technology. Politicians, practitioners, patients, and the health care industry more generally are concerned with access to care, reimbursement policy, improvements in quality of life, and the role that technology plays in raising or lowering the cost and efficacy of medical care. [1] [2] Much of this discussion has focused on local changes, looking at the current state of health care in comparison with the practice of medicine in the past 40 or 50 years. Policy makers ask, for example, whether Health Maintenance Organizations (HMOs) provide care that is more or less expensive — and more or less effective — than the employer-based fee-for-service insurance system that developed in the United States after the Second World War [2] [3] [4].

If we step back not 30-50 years but 3000-5000 years, we can see that the nature of medicine itself is changing. Technologies of the digital revolution do not just alter the cost of health care, the range of diseases that can be treated, or overall quality of life for patients. These technologies are fundamentally transforming the practice of medicine.

2. Background - From Healing Art to Medical Science

Disease and healing have been a part of the human condition as far back as the science of archaeology can take us. Skeletal remains of early hominids show evidence of disorders such as hypervitaminosis A and yaws, and excavations have uncovered bodies with evidence of wounds successfully treated, dislocations successfully replaced, and broken bones successfully set. [5] [6]

The development of scientific medicine is a relatively recent phenomenon, however. It is only in the last few thousand years (a blip in the span of human evolution) that early medical texts begin to define medicine "as something over and beyond mere healing, as the possession of a specific body of learning, theoretical and practical, that might be used to treat the sick." [6] It is no coincidence that the distinction of medicine as something "beyond mere healing" emerges around the same time as the development of writing. The development of medicine as a body of learning was intimately connected with the ability of physicians to record observations about specific patients and specific diseases, to share these observations, and to theorize about how the human body functions. Hippocrates and Galen, the giants of early Western medicine, made their marks by collecting, extending, and codifying medical knowledge in extensive writings.

By today's standards, the medicine of Hippocrates, Galen, and their successors appears systematic, but not yet scientific. A fifteenth century physician's admonition to "let not the sun go down behind the hill without your having gone out, or if you can not, take before meals a little exercise" [6] is good advice for general health. But these words were offered as a method for avoiding bubonic plague, against which regular exercise is little defense. Prescriptions such as this for controlling the interactions of miasmic vapors and bodily fluids were based on the notion of humoral balance — medical care based on the importance of balancing emotional states. [7] This was a theory of disease, to be sure, but not yet scientific medicine.

The development of scientific medicine as we know it today was made possible by the invention of the printing press. In 1543, just over ninety years after Guttenberg produced the first printed bibles, Vesalius published his seminal text on human anatomy. In the centuries following Vesalius, modern medicine was developed through collaborations between investigators and theorists over time and across space. While printing was not the only factor involved in the creation of scientific medicine, these collaborations were made possible in large part by the publication and distribution of medical texts. [8] [9] Scientific medicine depends on the recording, collecting, and comparing of observations, the formation of theories, and the building of new understanding on the foundation of prior work — all of which are possible on a large scale only with the ability to store and distribute information widely.

3. Human Cognitive Evolution

In a recent book, *Origins of the Modern Mind* [10], psychologist Merlin Donald describes the development of human cognitive abilities in a series of stages, where new cognitive abilities are built on top of — and co-exist with — older forms. These stages of cognitive development are associated with specific cultural practices, including the practice of medicine.[1]

In Donald's analysis, human cognition departed from its primate roots some 2 million years ago when early hominids began to develop a system for mental representation based on mimesis — the ability to represent events using gesture and re-enactment. Mimesis is, for example, when we follow someone else's gaze or pointing gesture because we understand that the gesture means they want us to look at something. Recognition that a gesture can refer to an event or object (rather than being the thing of interest itself) makes it possible to communicate intent, and is only possible if the person seeing the gesture and the person making the gesture have a shared understanding — that is, if each has a model of what is taking place in the mind of the other. Mimesis made it easier for early humans to coordinate group activities — and also provided the basis for the healing arts in gestures of understanding, support, and sympathy.

Donald argues that the social advantages of mimetic communication drove the evolution of language. Humans began to use ritualized or standardized gestures, and language developed as a more efficient way to communicate these standard gestures or symbols. The development of language created the next stage of cognitive development: a "mythic" culture based on the telling of stories or narratives that carry important cultural information. Here, then, some 300,000 years ago, was the cognitive origin of the incantations, magic, myth, and rituals of healing. [13]

Donald identifies the next stage of cognitive development as a "theoretic" culture based on written symbols and paradigmatic thought. Beginning 30,000-50,000 years ago, accounting and other complex record keeping drove the development of external representations. The existence of such external representations made it possible for literate humans to think analytically by looking for relationships among recorded ideas — and thus to develop a scientific culture based on external records and external notations for thinking such as writing and mathematics.

Theoretic culture requires large-scale storage of information, such as the accumulation of texts in a library. This "external memory field" acts as a medium in which analytic thinking

---

[1] Donald's thesis has been the foundation of much scholarly discussion, including a range of responses in a special issue of Behavioral and Brain Sciences [11]. However, despite significant controversy, the substance of Donald's argument remains intact [12].

can take place. Literate people access the cultural record (books and other written materials), use and transform that information to take appropriate actions, and make new contributions to the external corpus of human knowledge.

It is hardly surprising, then, that the development of a science of medicine depended on writing and the dissemination of medical information made possible by the printing press. It is not just that the scientific method requires accurate record-keeping. The development of scientific thinking itself is intimately linked to external recording of information. Anatomy texts and patient charts are not just symbols of modern medicine — they are essential tools in the development of scientific medicine in a theoretic culture.

Donald's picture of a theoretic culture based on the external storage of information has been extended into the digital age by authors such as Shaffer and Kaput [14], who suggest that new digital tools are creating a fifth stage of cognitive evolution where computers and other new media not only *store* information for us, but *process* information as well. This has profound implications for the practice of medicine.

4. A new stage of development

Donald's theoretic culture depends on the externalization of memory. Cognitive theorists whose information-processing perspective matches Donald's analysis [15] explain cognition as an interaction among long-term memory, short term (or working) memory, and the process of transforming information internally. There is some doubt as to whether mental activity can be as cleanly segmented as such a model suggests; [16] however, it is clear from Donald's analysis that theoretic culture depends on external *storage* of information and internal *processing* of information.

What happens when information can be transformed externally as well? To take an example from Shaffer and Kaput, computers make it possible for a researcher to perform a statistical analysis without making a single computation by hand. Software does the necessary calculations and produces a results table or visual representation of data that the researcher can use to understand the phenomena in question. The computer is processing the information so the researcher can focus on the more interesting problem of interpreting the results of the analysis. In the same way, a clinician who orders a CT or MRI relies on a computer to gather and process a vast amount of information and render it into a useful model of internal anatomy. In both cases, the computer is not just storing information; it is taking information in one form and returning it in a fundamentally altered form without additional action by the researcher or clinician.

We are thus on the verge of a new cognitive culture, dependent on the externalization of symbolic processing as well as on externalization of symbolic representation.[2] As humans developed gestural communication, language, and writing, they created mimetic, narrative, and analytic ways of thinking that interact and compliment each other. Mimetic, mythic and theoretic cultures, in turn, developed the art of healing into the science of medicine, where the experimental method and the other tools of modern medicine augment — but do not replace — compassion in the delivery of health care. The development of computational media makes possible a digital culture, and with it, we argue, a new era of digital medicine.

---

[2] We are not suggesting here that information-processing is the only important aspect of mental activity. We argue here that a new digital culture is being created as we develop new ways to execute well-specified algorithms, which are a limited by important subset of thinking.

5. Information and Knowledge

In order to understand how computers will create an era of digital medicine, we need to understand what it means to "process medical information." If processing medical information means only keeping more detailed medical records, or making sure that a medication delivered matches the medication ordered, then digital medicine will be a useful adjunct to clinical practice, but hardly a transformation of medicine as we know it.

It is true, of course, that computers can not imbue data with meaning. But this does not prevent them from transforming information and thus making it more available and more useful. As Wendell Berry writes: "Knowledge refers to the ability to do or say the right thing at the right time." [17] Knowledge in this sense requires the selection of (and ultimately action upon) information appropriate to a particular context: knowledge is what remains after the irrelevant and distracting pieces of information are removed and only the useful information remains.[3]

By transforming information, computers generate knowledge any time they sort through, discard, and simplify information and raise its utility. The table of results from the regression is easier to use and more meaningful to a researcher than listing of the raw data. A CT scan is more useful to a clinician than a collection of individual x-ray images. Both are examples of how a computer can generate knowledge.

Of course, generating knowledge is not the final step in most activities — clinical or otherwise. There is a long way to go between completing and interpreting a statistical analysis and answering a research question, just as conducting a CT scan is only one step in the process of diagnosis and treatment.

Knowledge is context-appropriate information: a window into a particular system. We turn knowledge into understanding as we view the same situation from enough perspectives to develop a robust mental model of the underlying system. The goal of a clinician in assembling medical knowledge — whether general knowledge about physiology and pathology, or specific information about an individual patient — is to come up with an understanding of what is happening in the body and why. Finally, understanding leads to action. This produces new information, which can be turned again into knowledge, and then used to refine understanding. Wisdom is built up from this accumulated experience of creating understanding, taking action, and evaluating the outcome in clinical (and other) venues.

Computers can be good at generating knowledge, but computers are notoriously bad at generating understanding and wisdom [16]. So-called expert systems have a terrible track record in medical diagnosis [19]— and in many other complex domains to which they have been applied. The first chess playing program to beat a human chess master (the famous

---

[3] Theorists of information make distinctions between data, information, and knowledge.[18] Information, they argue, is data combined with "meaning" — with some framework for interpretation. Knowledge is internalized information and the ability to apply that information in action. In this scheme, data is what can be stored on a computer disk. Information is the meaning of that data in "the collective mind of a society." Knowledge exists in an individual person's mind. In a theoretic culture, these distinctions are sensible: data is the external memory field which forms the medium of culture and thought. What matters is how people acquire the data (turn it into information) and how they put it to use internally (act knowledgeably). In this view, however, a computer *by definition* can do nothing more than store data. Data transformed remains data, and only human beings can add value to data by giving it meaning and turning it into knowledge. But in transforming data, computation augments "thinking" as well as "memory." Instead of data, information, and knowledge, we suggest in the following paragraphs that in digital culture the critical progression is from information, to knowledge, to understanding, and finally to wisdom. These two frameworks can be summarized in the following table:

Digital Culture	Information		Knowledge *selection of context-appropriate information*	Understanding *creation of a mental model of situation based on multiple contexts*	Wisdom *choice of appropriate actions based on understanding of situation*
Theoretic Culture	Data	Information *data + meaning*	Knowledge *information that is internalized and used*		

Deep Blue) was able to match human performance in a relatively simple domain (chess is far less complex than even a relatively trivial task like doing the dishes after dinner). In the foreseeable future, human beings may come to rely on machines to help generate knowledge about the world. But we will almost certainly rely ultimately on ourselves and on other people to develop understanding and act with wisdom.

6. So, What Is Digital Medicine?

Put simply: digital medicine is the transformation of health care that is coming about as computer technology is used in the creation and application of medical knowledge.

The traditional role of the clinician is as the intellectual agent of patient care. The clinician examines a patient. From the examination comes a diagnosis, and from diagnosis a plan for treatment, which is also carried out by a clinician. At each stage in the process (examination, diagnosis, planning, treatment), the clinician turns information into knowledge by deciding what data are relevant, what the data mean for the health of the patient, when and how to use instruments or administer medication.

In digital medicine, technology helps in the process of turning clinical information into medical knowledge. CT and MRI scans are digital examinations because they collect raw data and produce segmented images of the underlying anatomy. Implantable cardiac defibrillators are digital treatments because they collect information about cardiac function and determine, based on parameters set by the clinician, whether at a given moment the heart needs artificial stimulus. Modern health care policy is digital because computer simulations and statistical tools are used to evaluate cost-effectiveness and quality of life impacts of data too complex to be analyzed using pencil and paper. [20] [21] [22] Tissue engineering, genetic sequencing, and telemedicine are digital medicine because none are possible without the power of modern computers to transform complex information into medical knowledge. [23] [24] [25]

Although digital medicine is made possible by advances in information processing, the changes brought about by digital medicine will be more than just diagnostic and analytic; digital medicine will impact therapeutic interventions as well. Minimally invasive techniques such as MR-guided therapy and radiation therapy are digital procedures because they make it possible to destroy or excise tissue using computer-augmented images of patient anatomy more precisely and with less damage to healthy tissue than is possible with traditional instruments alone [26] [27] [28]. As digital medicine improves our ability to generate and act upon medical knowledge using technology, robotically-augmented tools will be able to use sophisticated sensors to deliver drugs or carry out procedures beyond the limits of human performance, such as guiding a micro-catheter through a tortuous distal vessel, or delivering extremely precise bursts of energy to destroy cells along a tumor margin. [29] [30]

Digital medicine, in other words, is the augmentation of human abilities through the external generation and application of medical knowledge that will make health care safer and more effective by enhancing our ability to diagnose and treat disease.

7. The Ten-thousand Foot View

It is impossible at this early stage in the development of digital medicine to predict what specific diagnostic and therapeutic techniques will be developed as digital technology transforms medicine. It is possible, however, to identify some of the ways in which digital medicine will differ from the practice of scientific medicine overall.

7.1 Digital Medicine Will Be More Precise

Digital tools will make it possible to create knowledge about the human body at a level of detail previously unimaginable. Computers can collect information that is difficult to obtain or hidden in signals too noisy to interpret, and then render that information into medically-useful knowledge. [31] Mappings of the human genome have already provided a new class of treatments (gene therapies) [32]. Minimally-invasive tools make it possible to deliver drugs, energy therapies, and devices to more parts of the body with less disruption to surrounding tissue [33] [34]. New imaging techniques make it possible to diagnose complex conditions quickly and accurately: where today we can use CT to characterize tumors and response to therapy, tomorrow we may be able to target specific neurons for pain or as the cause of seizures [35] [36]. As computational technology advances, we will be able to gather more precise diagnostic information and intervene with computer-guided and computer-assisted therapies that are less invasive and more effective at treating specific conditions.

7.2 Digital Medicine Will Be More Effective

Digital tools will make it possible to target therapies more precisely to specific diagnoses. External generation of medical knowledge is a critical component in the emerging sciences of modeling and decision analysis. [20] [21] [22] As patient data becomes more standardized and more portable,[4] and as more sophisticated tools are developed for monitoring the course of treatments, it will be possible to assess the impact of interventions — and thus to manage conditions — more effectively.

7.3 Digital Medicine Will Be More Experimental

One of the most important effects of digital tools is to make it possible to simulate anatomy, physiology, pathology, and therapeutic interventions. Computational chemistry has made it possible to generate and perform preliminary tests on candidate formulations for new drugs [37] [38], and first-generation simulation systems are currently available to help train clinicians with new devices and procedures [39] [40] [41]. As computing power advances, simulations will become more realistic and more robust. Data from real patients will make it possible to plan procedures and tailor treatment regimes to individual idiosyncrasies. High-fidelity simulations will increase the rate at which new devices and therapies can be developed, as prototypes can be rapidly created, tested, and adapted in the simulated environment, and safety and efficacy can be tested in a virtual patient before clinical trials are conducted. Digital tools will make it possible to experiment and explore *in silico* more rapidly and far more safely than is possible *in vitro* or *in vivo*.

---

[4] We recognize, of course, the central importance of protecting patient confidentiality as new tools are developed to help clinicians evaluate the impact of treatments.

7.4 Digital Medicine Will Be More Distributed

As more procedures can be done less invasively, conditions that once required inpatient hospital stays can be done in a doctors office, with the patient returning home the same day. Telemedicine is already making it easy to get expert consultations from remote locations [42] [43], and the ability of digital tools to transform information by altering its location makes it easy to create and access knowledge and expertise across wide areas. As digital technology produces new sensors and new communications tools, inexpensive monitors will able to gather data about patients during the course of their everyday lives and transmit it the physician. [44] Telecommunications will make it possible for examinations to be carried out from a patient's home [45], and digital networks will make it possible for patients to get high-quality information and medical advice from virtually anywhere at virtually any time. [46]

7.5 Digital Medicine Will Be More Egalitarian

New tools are making it easier for patients to make informed decisions about their health care options: from pre-packaged medical decision support systems [47] to internet forums where patients can "ask the experts", chat with people who share their conditions, or look up the latest medical information on a wide range of topics. Home testing kits are available for ovulation, pregnancy, insulin level, and other assays that previously required access to a sophisticated laboratory. In each case, the delivery of context-appropriate information — that is, the generation of medical knowledge — is made more accessible by new technology. As digital technology makes it easier for patients to access medical information — both general medical information, and information about their own health — the doctor/patient relationship will have the potential to become more of an equal partnership. The clinician will continue to have specialized knowledge and skills. But patients will increasingly have the opportunity to use the doctor as expert advisor, to help them weigh alternatives and make a wise and well-informed decision, rather than relying on the clinician as sole source of medical knowledge.

Taken together, these transformations will potentially change the role of the clinician in the health care system. As medical knowledge is generated in partnership with digital tools, clinicians will be able to focus their attention on their higher calling: the role of the physician will be to manage a wide range of clinical resources for the good of the patient, with the emphasis on complex problems of ethics, on the wise application of the power new technology brings, and ultimately on making sure that the vast medical knowledge of digital tools is grounded in human compassion.

8. Looking ahead

What medicine will become in the digital age is impossible for anyone at this point to say with certainty — just as Vesalius himself would not have been able to predict the transformation of medicine made possible by the development of the printing press. In the field of health care, it is clear that computers and other computational media will have a tremendous impact on the practice of medicine. Computers make it possible not just to store medical knowledge, but to create it. In doing so, they make it possible to develop digital medicine that is potentially more precise, more effective, more experimental, more distributed, and more egalitarian than modern scientific medicine.

Of course, this process is neither inevitable or deterministic. The development of scientific medicine was made possible by the invention of the printing press, but it would be ridiculous to suggest that the invention of the printing press alone created modern medical practice. Digital tools have already had an impact on health care, and fortunately the effects have been, for the most part, for the better. But there is thus much to be gained by taking a proactive approach to the development of digital medicine.

In an era of rapid and fundamental change, we can stand by passively and allow events to unfold, or we can take an active role as agents of change, trying to understand the impact of new technologies and directing them to the best possible ends. Critical steps in any such effort will be a careful analysis of the impact of new technologies and coordinated efforts to direct technological development towards creating a new paradigm of medical care. We hope that the ideas presented above will begin a larger discussion about the potentially deep and lasting effects of new technology on the practice of medicine.

References

[1] Halperin, J., *Setting health standards for the 21st century*. J Am Pharm Assoc, 1998. **38**(6): p. 762-6.
[2] Bryce, C. and K. Cline, *The supply and use of selected medical technologies*. Health Aff, 1998. **17**(1): p. 213-24.
[3] Zimmerman, R., T. Mieczkowski, and M. Raymund, *Relationship between primary payer and use of proactive immunization practices: a national survey*. Am J Manag Care, 1999. **5**(5): p. 574-82.
[4] Lyles, A. and F. Palumbo, *The effect of managed care on prescription drug costs and benefits*. Pharmacoeconomics, 1999. **15**(2): p. 129-40.
[5] Kiple, K., *The History of Disease in The Cambridge Illustrated History of Medicine*, ed. R. Porter. 1996, New York: Cambridge University Press.
[6] Nutton, V., *The rise of medicine in The Cambridge Illustrated History of Medicine*, ed. R. Porter. 1996, New York: Cambridge University Press.
[7] Maher, B. and W. Maher, *Personality and psychopathology: a historical perspective*. J Abnorm Psychol, 1994. **103**(1): p. 72-7.
[8] Palmero, J., *Nephrology from the middle ages to humanism: the Italian influence in Spain (12th-16th centuries)*. Am J Nephrol, 1994. **14**(4-6): p. 290-4.
[9] Fye, W., *The literature of American internal medicine: a historical view*. Ann Intern Med, 1987. **106**(3): p. 451-60.
[10] Donald, M., *Origins of the modern mind: three stages in the evolution of culture and cognition*. 1991, Cambridge, MA: Harvard University Press.
[11] Donald, M., *Precis of Origins of the Modern Mind: Three Stages in the Evolution of Culture and Cognition*. Behavioral and Brain Sciences, 1993. **16**: p. 737-791.
[12] Gardner, H., *Thinking About Thinking*, in *New York Review of Books*. 1997. p. 23-27.
[13] Abrahamsen, V., *The goddess and healing. Nursing's heritage from antiquity*. J Holist Nurs., 1997. **15**(1): p. 9-24.
[14] Shaffer, D. and J. Kaput, *Mathematics and virtual culture: an evolutionary perspective on technology and mathematics*. Educational Studies in Mathematics, 1999. **37**: p. 97-119.
[15] Simon, H., *The Sciences of the Artificial*. 1996, Cambridge, MA: MIT Press.
[16] Dreyfus, H. and S. Dreyfus, *Mind over machine: the power of human intuition and expertise in the era of the computer*. 1986, New York: Free Press.
[17] Berry, W., *"On Choosing Health"*, in *The Plain Reader*, S. Savage, Editor. 1998, Ballantine Pub. Group: New York.
[18] Devlin, K.J., *Logic and information*. 1991, Cambridge: Cambridge University Press.
[19] Engle, R., Jr., *Attempts to use computers as diagnostic aids in medical decision making: a thirty-year experience*. Perspect Biol Med, 1992. **35**(2): p. 207-19.
[20] Kucey, D., *Decision analysis for the surgeon*. World J Surg, 1999. **23**(12): p. 1227-31.
[21] Chalfin, D., *Decision analysis in critical care medicine*. Crit Care Clin, 1999. **15**(3): p. 647-61.
[22] Gelman, A. and D.B. Rubin, *Markov chain Monte Carlo methods in biostatistics*. Stat Methods Med Res,

1996. 5(4): p. 339-55.

[23] Fray, T., et al., Quantification of single human dermal fibroblast contraction. Tissue Eng, 1998. 4(3): p. 281-91.

[24] Mahairas, G., et al., Sequence-tagged connectors: a sequence approach to mapping and scanning the human genome. Proc Natl Acad Sci USA, 1999. 96(17): p. 9739-44.

[25] N/A, Telemedicine: an overview. Health Devices, 1999. 28(3): p. 88-103.

[26] Kettenbach, J., et al., Computer-based imaging and interventional MRI: applications for neurosurgery. Comput Med Imaging Graph, 1999. 23(5): p. 245-58.

[27] Gould, S., et al., Interventional MR-guided excisional biopsy of breast lesions. J Magn Reson Imaging, 1998. 8(1): p. 26-30.

[28] Mageras, G., et al., Computerized design of target margins for treatment uncertainties in conformal radiotherapy. Int J Radiat Oncol Biol Phys, 1999. 43(2): p. 437-45.

[29] Davies, B., A review of robotics in surgery. Proc Inst Mech Eng, 2000. 214(1): p. 129-40.

[30] Mohr, F., et al., The evolution of minimally invasive valve surgery--2 year experience. Eur J Cardiothorac Surg, 1999. 15(3): p. 233-8; discussion 238-9.

[31] Giele, E., et al., Reduction of noise in medullary renograms from dynamic MR images. J Magn Reson Imaging, 2000. 11(2): p. 149-55.

[32] Davidson, S., The monster code: biology and the computer sciences. Healthc Forum J, 1997. 40(6): p. 48-51.

[33] March, K.L., Methods of local gene delivery to vascular tissues. Semin Interv Cardiol, 1996. 1(3): p. 215-23.

[34] Keane, D., et al., Catheter ablation for atrial fibrillation. Semin Interv Cardiol, 1997. 2(4): p. 251-65.

[35] Davis, K.D., The neural circuitry of pain as explored with functional MRI. Neurol Res, 2000. 22(3): p. 313-17.

[36] Krings, T., et al., Hemodynamic changes in simple partial epilepsy: a functional MRI study. Neurology, 2000. 54(2): p. 524-7.

[37] Kirkpatrick, D., et al., Structure-based drug design: combinatorial chemistry and molecular modeling. Comb Chem High Throughput Screen, 1999. 2(4): p. 211-21.

[38] Hall, A.H., Computer modeling and computational toxicology in new chemical and pharmaceutical product development. Toxicol Lett, 1998. 102-103: p. 623-6.

[39] Torkington, J., et al., The role of simulation in surgical training. Ann R Coll Surg Engl, 2000. 82(2): p. 88-94.

[40] Chaudhry, A., et al., Learning rate for laparoscopic surgical skills on MIST VR, a virtual reality simulator: quality of human-computer interface. Ann R Coll Surg Engl, 1999. 81(4): p. 281-6.

[41] Bro-Nielsen, M., et al., PreOp endoscopic simulator: a PC-based immersive training system for bronchoscopy. Stud Health Technol Inform, 1999. 62: p. 76-82.

[42] Schulmeyer, F.J, A. Brawanski, Telemedicine in neurosurgical daily practice. Stud Health Technol Inform, 1999. 64: p. 115-18.

[43] Kangarloo, H., et al., Improving the quality of care through routine teleradiology consultation. Acad Radiol, 2000. 7(3): p. 149-55.

[44] Vering, T., et al., Wearable microdialysis system for continuous in vivo monitoring of glucose. Analyst, 1998. 123(7): p. 1605-9.

[45] Kinsella, A., Becoming a virtual caregiver. Caring, 2000. 19(1): p. 36-7.

[46] Coile, R.C., Jr., The digital transformation of health care. Physician Exec, 2000. 26(1): p. 8-15.

[47] Frosch, D. and R. Kaplan, Shared decision making in clinical medicine: past research and future directions. Am J Prev Med, 1999. 17(4): p. 285-94.

Future of Health Technology
R.G. Bushko (Ed.)
IOS Press, 2002

Evaluating New Health Information Technologies: Expanding the Frontiers of Health Care Delivery and Health Promotion

Gary L. Kreps, Ph.D.

Chief, Health Communication and Informatics Research Branch, National Cancer Institute Behavioral Research Program, Division of Cancer Control and Population Sciences

Abstract

The modern health care system is being irrevocably changed by the development and introduction of new health information technologies (such as health information systems, decision-support tools, specialized websites, and innovative communication devices). While many of these new technologies hold the promise of revolutionizing the modern health system and facilitating improvements in health care delivery, health education, and health promotion, it is imperative to carefully examine and assess the effectiveness of these technological tools to determine which products are most useful to apply in specific contexts, as well as to learn how to best utilize these products and processes. Without good evaluative information about new technologies, we are unlikely to reap the greatest benefits from these powerful new tools. This chapter examines the demand for evaluating health information technologies and suggests several strategies for conducting rigorous and relevant evaluation research.

1. Evaluation Research and Health Technology

New health information technologies (such as specialized websites, innovative new communication devices, and powerful health data analysis tools) are being developed and introduced at a rapid rate into the modern health system to facilitate improved health care delivery, health education, and health promotion [1; 2]. While these new technologies are likely to revolutionize the modern health system, it is imperative to carefully examine and assess the effectiveness of these technological tools to determine which products are most useful to apply in different contexts, as well as to learn how to best utilize these products and processes. Without good evaluative information about new technologies, we are unlikely to reap the greatest benefits from these powerful new tools [3; 4].

Evaluation research is an essential process in developing and implementing health information technologies [2; 5]. Failure to engage in careful and concerted evaluation research is pure hubris (a fatal miscalculation) that is likely to doom the success of new health information technologies. It is unlikely that new technical products will work well for users without the use of relevant evaluation data. Effective development and institutionalization of new technological products involves a series of product adaptations. Good evaluation data provides needed direction for product refinement.

Every new health technology should have both **formative** and **summative** evaluation strategies built right in to the development process from the very beginning [6]. (Formative and summative evaluation will be discussed in more depth later in this chapter). Evaluation data provides technology developers with a broad range of critically important information about:

- level of demand for new health information technologies,
- environmental constraints and specifications for the implementation of new products,
- specific design flaws and limitations of new products,
- assessments of the relative efficiency and effectiveness of new products,
- the appropriate fit of these products for specific audiences and contexts, and
- strategies for adapting new health information technologies to fit the idiosyncratic demands of different users and unique social situations.

2. Research and Reinvention; What Do We Already Know?

Technological innovation is a process of invention and **reinvention**, however it appears that reinvention is the process that is most often utilized in health technology development and implementation [7]. It is usually unnecessary to develop radically new products or processes to effectively address current health care/promotion needs. In fact, the more radical the technical innovation is, the more difficult it will often be to integrate within the health care system. The technical interventions that typically work best within the health care system are developed incrementally through a process of reinvention, reinventing current processes and products to better meet health care/promotion needs.

Prior to the development of new health information technologies, comprehensive reviews of relevant literature should be conducted to identify key findings from literature in the scientific and professional fields most closely related to the technological product. It is foolish to reinvent the wheel, when good information about product demand and practices is already available. Key established research and practice findings should guide product development and implementation.

3. Formative and Summative Evaluation Research

Formative evaluation is an essential process in the development and refinement of new health information technologies. Formative research is used to test the adequacy of technological interventions, providing relevant data for improving the technologies. By examining key components of new technologies, the ways the technologies are used, and identifying constraints to system performance, formative research data can provide clear directions for the development of improvements to these technologies.

Summative evaluation research is used to measure overall new technology impact and outcomes. Summative research is used to document the positive and negative influences and impacts of new health technologies. These data provide important measures of the utility of health information technologies for health care and promotion. Summative data should examine the costs and benefits of the technology and help health care systems determine the effectiveness and long-term utility of employing specific technological products and processes.

Formative and summative evaluation research should not be viewed as separate and unrelated research processes. Rather, formative and summative evaluation can be viewed as different ends of an evaluation research continuum. Formative research looks at the small pieces of the technology, providing a microscopic analysis of the individual components of the product or process. Conversely, summative evaluation looks at the big picture, providing a macroscopic global evaluation of the way these different components work together to accomplish relevant health care/promotion goals. Formative and summative research should work together in the evaluation of new health information technologies. Ideally, formative data informs summative research, providing pieces of the data needed to evaluate overall system impact and outcomes. Results from formative evaluation should be mined and combined in compiling summative evaluations.

4. Audience Analysis Research: Targeting the New Health Technology

Successful technological innovations depend on data gathered through audience analysis research to design programs to fit audience needs. *Needs analyses* are initial applications of audience analysis evaluation research that gather data from potential product users to establish levels of audience demand and opportunities for new health information technology products and processes [6]. Are there significant performance gaps (differences between the intended and actual outcomes) in current health system products and processes that necessitate technological innovation and intervention? It is essential to begin the process of health technology innovation and product development by examining the perceptions of potential users (audience members) about current technologies in the health care system, identifying limitations to these products, and developing strategies for extension and innovation to increase the effectiveness of products that are not delivering satisfactory service. Careful evaluation of current products and processes in health care/promotion is essential for guiding technological reinvention.

All technological interventions should be based upon clear evidence of what works. There is a wealth of important data often lying dormant in every health care/promotion setting that indicates what has and what has not worked in the past to achieve health care/promotion goals. Needs analysis data should reveal whether there is sufficient demand for new technological products and processes for achieving health care/promotion goals to initiate development of new health technologies. Furthermore, audience analysis research will help identify many important user expectations and predispositions that will undoubtedly influence product acceptance and utilization [8].

It is also important to get to know the orientations, attitudes, beliefs, and expectations of audiences for new health information technologies so user interfaces can be designed to meet consumer communication orientations [8; 9]. The more revealing data health information technology developers have gathered about the intended audiences for their products, the better they can target development of products to fit user characteristics and skills [10]. Usability testing will help technology developers to assess the extent to which they have targeted technologies to match the technical skills and needs of users [11]. (The importance of usability testing as a particularly rich evaluation research strategy for determining the extent to which health information technology programs match individual user skills and abilities will be discussed in more depth later in this chapter.)

5. Evidence Based Technological Intervention Efforts

The best technological interventions are based upon strong evidence. Evaluation data should provide evidence about what has and has not worked in the past within the health care/promotion system. It should help demonstrate the need for change and intervention within the system. It should help identify the kinds of technologies that best fit the needs of users and the demands of the social context for interventions. It should demonstrate the utility of proposed interventions, identify the most promising implementation strategies, and test the effectiveness of new health information technologies in action.

There are rich **natural data sources** that should be identified during audience analysis research efforts that can help provide evidence for directing technological intervention and provide data about the relative success of new technological interventions. For example, the evaluation researcher can identify "natural" (normally collected) records of key events (such as product performance, employee attendance, quality control, error rates, usage levels, and sales records) that can provide the researcher with interesting trend data to track system performance before and after the implementation of new health information technologies [6; 12]. Natural data collected before new technology implementation can help provide a clear **baseline measure** from which to track system changes that, at least in part, can be tied to the influences of the new health information technologies. (Care must be taken to recognize multiple influences on system performance due to uncontrolled events and extraneous variance, and not to overstate (or understate) the influences of new technologies. Control measures in similar contexts that have not implemented the new technologies can provide important points of comparison for clarifying the impact of new technologies.)

It is a good idea for health information technology evaluation researchers to implement **user response mechanisms** that are built right into the new technological products [13]. These response mechanisms can be both **passive** (provide invisible data collected automatically by tracking and recording characteristics of technology use) and **active** (requesting feedback, comments, and suggestions from users). Passive usage data is relatively easy to collect, but can often be misleading if analyzed in isolation of other data. For example, high time of use data may seem to indicate a successful new technology, but it might just as easily indicate that the technology is time-consuming and cumbersome to use. Active response data can suffer from validity issues concerning self-report data (discussed in more depth later in this chapter). Passive user response and active user response data should be analyzed together to clarify user reactions and ideas about the new technologies.

Prior to implementation of new technologies, as well as after technologies have been implemented, it is important to conduct **usability tests** of new health technologies. Usability tests are hands-on evaluations of users' perceptions about and abilities to operate new health information technologies [11]. Usability tests assess technology users' evaluations of their experience with products, including the ease, comfort, efficiency, speed, and effectiveness of use, as well as track these users' actual abilities to navigate the technological products and achieve health care/promotion goals [6]. Can users accomplish the goals the new technology was designed to help them accomplish? How readily can a new user learn how to use this system? Are there ways to improve the usability of this system? Usabilty data will help answer these questions and suggest strategies for refining health information technologies.

6. Methodological Issues and Constraints in Conducting Evaluation Research

A major limitation in the way that evaluation research is often conducted is the **over-use of single point of data collection** evaluation studies, based on the false assumption that one cross-sectional data set will suffice in evaluating new health information technologies. One point in time cross-sectional data will not provide the depth of information needed for most evaluations. It is important to see how new technologies are accepted and utilized over time. There are peaks and valleys in technology use. Users have to learn about new technology products, get used to them, learn how to use them, experiment with them, and figure out how to adapt the technologies to different applications and situational demands. This learning process takes time. Gathering cross-sectional data (one point in time) is likely to miss the key moments in evolutionary trends of technology implementation and usage, missing both potential strengths and weaknesses of the technology.

A common problem experienced in evaluation efforts is **over-reliance on the use of self-report data**. Self-report data is information requested from respondents through the use of survey research tools (typically with questionnaires and interviews). In many cases self-report data has become the default measurement approach used in evaluation studies. While surveys often provide interesting information, there are serious questions about the veracity of survey responses leading to threats to the validity of survey data, especially in organizational contexts where socio-political pressures can influence responses. It is all too common for respondents to praise new technologies because they fear organizational reprisals from management for providing negative information (the mum effect threat to validity) [7]. Respondents also often try to provide the "right" answers to surveys to please researchers and management (the Hawthorne effect threat to validity) [6]. Sometimes survey respondents just give the same, most expedient answers to survey questions to get through with the survey quickly (the response-set threat to validity) [6]. Due to these threats to validity, caution must be taken in interpreting survey data in evaluation studies.

Evaluation researchers often focus on **tangential variables** (variables that are not directly relevant to research goals), especially with the use of standardized survey instruments. These standardized scales can be attractive to use due to their established reliability, availability, and ease of use (the law of the hammer) [6]. The variables measured in many of these standardized scales (such as health beliefs, personality attributes, and attitudes) are not always relevant to the technological products and processes being evaluated. These tangential variables inevitably provide weak and equivocal evaluation data. Technological evaluation research depends on the measurement of important variables that provide data of direct relevance to the goals set for the products and processes under examination.

Another problem that often limits the effectiveness of evaluation research efforts conducted for new health information technologies is over-reliance on **shallow data**, such as the number of web hits. Such data are very equivocal and difficult to interpret due to limited information. Conclusions made based on such data are often unwarranted. For example, does increases in the number of hits (log-ons) to a new web-based health information dissemination program indicate the program has been successful at achieving health promotion goals? Not necessarily. Additional information is needed. Who is accessing the website? What is their experience with navigating and using the website? What kinds of information are users getting from the site? How are these individuals using information from the site? What impact has the information they have accessed had on their health behaviors and health conditions? Effective evaluation research of health information technologies must answer these key questions.

7. Data Reduction and Information Overload

The way that evaluation research results are presented is fundamental to making the findings from the research useful. Consumers of evaluation research need to understand the strengths, weaknesses, and overall influences of new health information technologies. All too often, evaluation data are presented in ways that do not communicate well to different audiences, increasing information overload in health care systems, rather than increasing understanding. Statistical presentations of evaluation research results are often complex and confusing for many audiences. To get the most out of evaluation research, researchers have to translate findings in clear and compelling ways. Strategic use of tables, charts, and examples can help technology managers and users interpret and apply evaluation research findings [6]. Researchers must clearly identify the implications, applications, and limitations of evaluation research.

8. Methodological Recommendations for Conducting Evaluation Research

The following suggestions are designed to help researchers increase the effectiveness of their efforts to evaluate new health information technologies:

- **Longitudinal Evaluation Research Designs**. It is important to develop longitudinal evaluation research designs that gather data at multiple points in time to capture the evolution of technological implementation and use. In fact, it is a good idea to build in strategies for continuing measures of both passive and active evaluation data over the life of the health information technology, beginning from before implementation to establish clear baseline data.
- **Multi-methodological Research Designs**. Multimethodological research designs combine different methods to offset the weaknesses of each method with the strengths of other methods [6]. It is a particularly good idea to augment the use of self-report survey research with other measures to help establish the validity of survey results. Multiple measures can provide important complementary perspectives for analyzing health information technologies.
- **Combining Quantitative and Qualitative Data**. While quantitative data can be powerfully analyzed statistically, quantitative data often fails to provide great depth of explanation. Alternatively, qualitative data (gathered from unstructured interviews, focus groups, observations, etc.) can usually provide great depth of information and can be profitably combined with more traditional quantitative research methods in evaluation efforts [6]. Triangulation of quantitative and qualitative measures can afford the evaluation researcher both precision and depth of analysis.
- **Unobtrusive Evaluation Measures**. Wherever possible, evaluation researchers should design non-reactive data gathering strategies into evaluation efforts, such as measures that do not depend upon respondents self reports (unobtrusive measures) to increase the validity of evaluation research [12]. By observing naturally occurring data, such as examination of archival records and the natural build-up (accretion) or wearing away (erosion) of observable elements in social contexts, researchers can often reach strong conclusions about social behavior that are not influenced by social and political constraints. Unobtrusive data can also be used to check the validity of self-report data, increasing confidence in conclusions reached from survey research [6].

- **Communication and Health Outcomes Variables.** By measuring relevant health outcome variables, evaluation researchers can assess the impact of new health information technologies on important health consequences, such as users' knowledge, attitudes, behaviors, and health states [14]. Measurement of important health outcomes is especially important in summative evaluation to identify the contributions of the technological programs and processes.

- **Translating Data into Practice.** A significant advanced step in the evaluation research process is interpreting data and applying them to action strategies for increasing the effectiveness of health information technologies. It is not enough to just describe evaluation data; data must be leveraged into real activities for achieving important health care/promotion goals [9]. Too often rich evaluation research data are merely reported and not applied to the development of interventions for refining and improving health information technologies. Translating data into practice is an essential culminating step in evaluation research.

- **Using Evaluation Data to Demonstrate Progress.** Evaluation research should provide clear information about the contributions of new technologies to the accomplishment of important health care/promotion goals and outcomes [15]. By tracking progress, evaluation researchers can identify the achievements and shortfalls of new technologies, helping to direct the development of future health technologies for enhancing health care and health promotion [16].

References

[1] AHCPR (Agency for Health Care Policy and Research). Consumer health informatics and patient decision making. Final report. US Department of Health and Human Services, Agency for Health Care Policy and Research. AHCPR publication 98-N001, Rockville, MD, 1997.

[2] T.R. Eng, & D.H. Gustafson. (Eds.). Wired for health and well-being: The Emergence of interactive health communication. Office of Disease Prevention and Health Promotion, US Department of Health and Human Services, Washington, DC, 1999.

[3] T.R. Eng, A. Maxfield, K. Patrick, M.J. Deering, S. Ratzan, & D.H. Gustafson. Access to health information and support: A public highway or a private road? Journal of the American Medical Association, 280 (1998), pp. 1371-1375.

[4] F.A. Sonnenberg. Health information on the Internet: Opportunities and pitfalls. Archives of Internal Medicine, 157 (1997), 151-152.

[5] M. Chamberlain. Health communication: Making the most of new media technologies. Journal of Health Communication: International Perspectives, 1: 1 (1996), 43-50.

[6] L.R. Frey, C.H. Botan, & G.L. Kreps. Investigating communication: An introduction to research methods (2nd ed.). Allyn & Bacon, Boston, MA, 2000.

[7] G.L. Kreps. Organizational communication: Theory and practice (2nd ed.). Longman, White Plains, NY, 1990.

[8] E.W. Maibach, G.L. Kreps, & E.W. Bonaguro. Developing strategic communication campaigns for HIV/AIDS prevention. In S. Ratzan (Ed.), AIDS: Effective health communication for the 90s (pp. 15-35). Taylor and Francis, Washington, D.C., 1993.

[9] I. Rootman, & L. Hershfield. Health communication research: Broadening the scope. Health Communication, 6: 1, (1994), 69-72.

[10] T. Albrecht, & C. Bryant. Advances in segmentation modeling for health communication and social marketing campaigns. Journal of Health Communication: International Perspectives, 1: 1, (1996), pp. 65-80.

[11] J. Neilsen.. Designing web usability. New Riders, Indianapolis, IN, 2000.

[12] E. Webb, D.T. Cambpell, R.D. Schwartz, & L. Sechrist. Unobtrusive measures: Non-reactive research in the social sciences. Rand McNally , Skokie, IL, 1973.

[13] V.S. Freimuth, J.A. Stein, & T.J. Kean,. Searching for health information: The Cancer Information Service model. University of Pennsylvania Press, Philadelphia, PA, 1989.

[14] G.L. Kreps, & D. O'Hair, (Eds.). Communication and health outcomes. Hampton Press, Cresskill, NJ, 1995.

[15] G.L. Kreps, L.R. Frey, & D. O'Hair. Applied communication research: Scholarship that can make a difference. Journal of Applied Communication Research, 19: 1, 1991, pp. 71-87.
[16] G.L. Kreps, S.M. Hubbard, & V.T. DeVita, The role of the Physician Data Query on-line cancer system in health information dissemination. In B.D. Ruben (Ed.), Information and Behavior 2 (pp. 362-374). Transaction Press, New Brunswick, NJ, 1988.

Future of Health Technology
R.G. Bushko (Ed.)
IOS Press, 2002

Future of Security and Privacy in Medical Information

Gio Wiederhold

Professor of Computer Science, Medicine, and Electrical Engineering,
Stanford University, Stanford, CA, US

Abstract

Today, issues of privacy and confidentiality in healthcare are dealt largely informally. Little legislation exists, and the awkwardness of accessing paper records makes violations of patients' privacy sporadic. As healthcare institutions move towards a future where all information is kept in an Electronic Medical Record (EMR), the casual attitudes that are prevalent will be in conflict with the desires and expectations of the patients. Legislation has been passed to make the holders of medical data responsible for securely protecting the patients privacy. Specific implementation guidelines are still lacking. There is much institutional resistance to the adoption of rigorous rules, but we expect that in the near future reliable procedures will have to be implemented to comply both with legal guidelines and patient's expectations. .

After introducing the issue more precisely we provide an overview over the concepts needed to understand the roles of technology of privacy and security and the people that must manage the technology. We then discuss the components of secure EMR systems and will point out where adequate technology exists and where future improvements are essential. We conclude with some advice to healthcare management facing the demands for security and privacy that the future will bring.

1. Introduction

This chapter considers that in the near future most patient information will be stored in an Electronic Medical Record (EMR) [1]. The participants in the EMR expect that required patient information will be rapidly and completely available to persons who should receive that information, and that its contents will not be revealed to anyone else. To achieve that simple objective many pieces of technology have to work correctly and reliably. We will identify most of these technological components because they are all interrelated, but not discuss many of them in depth because they are common to all computer-based information systems. We will focus on issues that are particular to the medical record domain. Unfortunately there are problems with medical records that are not handled adequately by the methods that are supplied in broad-purpose software [2]. Issues of security and privacy are not unique to medical information, but we will see that they become more complex in health care.

Protection of privacy depends greatly on having a secure system. Security first of all requires that persons accessing the system are properly identified, or authenticated. Once they are authenticated, they can be authorized to read or manipulate specific parts of the EMR. Healthcare records contain a wide variety of information, from relatively public demographic data to data that could be misused to embarrass a person or deny them employment, insurance, social, or residence opportunities. In between those categories is information of value to various organizations. Of primary concern is the delivery of information to a variety of caregivers, the physicians, consultants, nurses, pharmacists, etc. that depend on having complete and correct information to carry out their duties. External laboratories exchange crucial test information with the EMR. Hospital management has the duty to monitor the spread of infections within the hospital [3]. There are legitimate demands for certain information from public health organizations, insurance companies, and other third-party payors. There may be legal injunctions to obtain data, for instance in accident settlements. There is a need for medical treatment data and the effects of such treatments for medical research and pharmaceutical development. An important application is drug surveillance, checking if new drugs have side effects not found during the clinical trials that led to their approval. Last, but not least are the patient themselves, who have the right to know what is happening to them. However, sometimes the patient's rights are abrogated by medical practitioners in the interest of the general well-being of a particular patient. Sometimes those rights are assigned to family members, who have assumed responsibility for the care of minors or senile patients [4].

1.1 Complexity

We see that the EMR must serve a very wide variety of purposes. At the same time medical information cannot be as well structured as, say, banking or merchandising records. While the IRS has legitimate rights to survey some of our bank records, the variety of information seen in them is much simpler. The privacy of merchandising records is also a concern, and although the information in them rarely has the potential to be damaging, we expect that it will not be released with any personal identification. Unfortunately, personal identification is essential for many of the purposes in a medical record. For continuing treatment, for tracing the origin of an epidemic, for understanding a delayed effect of a drug treatment, etc., personal identification is crucial to information linkage. Even when, say for medical research, anonymous data is adequate, investigators, legitimate or not, still have means to identify individuals. For instance, in an anonymized research record the dates of visits to a clinic will be stored to understand the temporal course of a disease. A visit pattern is likely to be unique for any individual. Matching this pattern against the relatively public records of the clinic's operation is certain to identify particular patients.

1.2 Reliability

Security, and hence protection of privacy, can not be obtained unless the underlying computer systems are reliable. When failures occur, not only availability, but during repairs and downtimes the privacy of the records is easily compromised. If a large number of computer specialists have access to the computers for maintenance and repair security is easily compromised, since these wizards rarely go through the full authentication and authorization process demanded during normal operations. These issues are common to all computer systems, so will not discuss them further. We do observe that today, perhaps because of poor funding and high availability demands of computer systems in healthcare, that many systems are not run as carefully as they must be if security is to be assured. System reliability is not the focus of this chapter, but a reasonable level of reliability must be attained if security of information is to be achieved.

Whenever data are transmitted through outside of an institution there is chance that it may be misdirected or overheard. To protect again this type of loss, the contents of any transmission to a remote site should be encrypted, and decrypted upon receipt. Encryption technology for communication is routinely available, and has only modest effects on system performance and costs [5]. On the other hand, it is not effective to store medical records for the long-term in encrypted form. The variety of accessors is such that means for decryption will have to be provided at many points, adding little protection and a high costs to assure that requests can be issued when and where needed.

Another aspect of reliability pertains to the stored data themselves. Errors in data collection, data entry, filing, and data manipulation will occur even in well-managed systems. There are some differences in the management of errors between data kept on paper or handled in the EMR, but the final error rate is not drastically affected. Marking questionable entries on paper is easy, but few EMR system designers have included equally convenient provisions to mark possible errors and eventually correct them. A good EMR can distribute any corrections made automatically to all destinations that have received erroneous data. Since there is less transcription in an EMR fewer eyes have a chance of finding errors, so that errors are less likely to be caught in an EMR. Computer systems can automatically identify simple inconsistencies in patients' histories, laboratory results, and the like. Historically, physicians are well aware of the limitations of data, and will rarely commit to procedures based on a single indication. Now, and even more so in the future, economic pressures are reducing the redundancy of laboratory testing and status recording that provided a safety margin in earlier systems.

Security and privacy is indirectly affected by the presence of errors in data records. Reporting misfiled data about a patient to an external destination can be embarrassing and even costly. Data errors, data processing errors, and security failures will all be seen as failures to properly protect data.

2. System concepts

We will now summarize the system concepts that underlie the protection of healthcare information. Basic to any approach is the need to define what information is to be protected, authenticate the people that have access to the records, and manage their authorization with respect to the data. In a subsequent section we will introduce the technical means for achieving the security objectives, but first we must first address how the system must deal with people. Figure 1 illustrates the relationship among relevant concepts.

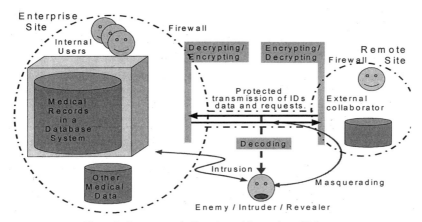

Figure 1: Components in Security and Protection of Privacy

2.1 Authentication

Authentication of individual requires that some personal identification be submitted. Today, the entering of passwords into a computer is most common way. There is tension between requiring secure passwords, that are lengthy and uncommon, versus passwords and personal identification numbers (PINs) that are easily remembered. Uncommon passwords are often written down, perhaps kept in the drawer of the terminal desk. Common passwords, as names of family members, pets, or birthdays are easily guessed. Even if only one user of a computer system chooses a poor password, the contents of an entire system may be compromised [6]..

In the near future identification cards will gain acceptance. They are combined with simple identification numbers that require little recall but still protect access in case of loss. Identification cards are less likely to be misplaced or left near the computer terminal if they are also needed to gain access to the buildings, the parking lots, etc. However, we will also have to deal with remote accessors where issuing individual cards is not feasible.

More stringent means of authentication employ biometric technologies that depend on unalterable physical characteristics of an individual. Methods that are being proposed to control authentication include automated checking of voice prints, fingerprints, facial features, iris and retinal patterns, or hand dimensions [7]. Devices for these methods are becoming routinely available, although they will not be found at every site where requests to access to medical information may be made. For acceptance in critical settings these devices must demonstrate a very high reliability in practical situations; for instance, the voice analysis must not deny access when practitioners express stress in their speech. Since identification is only one link in having secure systems a disproportionate investment in high-tech authentication is not warranted.

2.2 Domain of protection

It is equally crucial to properly define the boundary of protection. In networked computing, as is common now, the boundary of protection is not simply the physical perimeter of a computer system, it extends to all the computer systems that share a common protection system. Such a virtual perimeter is best defined by a firewall [8], software that is intended to prevent both inappropriate requests and inappropriate release of information. It is at the firewall that authentication is validated. A simple firewall may wrap one specific record system [9], several interoperating systems, or all computers within a healthcare enterprise. Sites outside of the perimeter may be accessed via the Internet, increasing the need for firewalls [10]. The complexity of providing protection depends on the scope of the system.

In a major institution here may be multiple domains, each protected by their own firewalls. For instance, financial information may be segregated from patient care data. Some applications must span the domains, for instance, to justify billings to a third party information from the medical record is required, but the release of such information should be mediated, since the insurance company has no right to obtain information not related to the current case.

Within the health care system are many types of data, but central to our concern is the medical portion of the EMR. This portion is the most problematical, since much of its is relatively unstructured text. The text will contains both highly private information as well as information that must be made available for billing and external reporting. An EMR instance can refer to multiple diseases, although the rules for release of information may differ among those diseases. For instance information about HIV infections must be dealt with more carefully than, say, cardiac problems. Pregnancies, diabetes, trauma, etc. all have differing sensitivities to release of data. Keeping the variety of information in the medical record disjoint is not practical. For proper healthcare the total picture is essential, so that a rigorous partitioning is inappropriate. We do want that a nurse who takes care of a patient can be aware of any infections that can be transmitted, even if the current task is to deal with another problem.

2.3 Authorization

Within a domain an authenticated accessor will have certain rights. Rights may pertain to certain files, or certain records. For instance, nurses on a ward should have access to all medical information for patients in the ward, while the physicians will need access to the patients under their care in various localities. The rights to append information, as entering orders, is more restricted. Authorization to actually change stored medical information is rare, since inhibits the audit trail for decisions that have been made.

For convenience, a specific type of authorization may be assigned to groups having specific roles, say the billing clerks in an institution, so that the number of entries in an authorization table remains manageable. Then there must be mapping table from individuals to such a group. It is inappropriate to assign a single identification to multiple individuals. If that is done, and one member departs, new identification cards or passwords have to be given to all. The attendant costs and risky delays are worse than the cost of authenticating every individual.

Where access requests are issued by a remote organization, say a clinic, the issuing of EMR identifications can be delegated to that site. Again, individuals should be properly identified, even when they share an identical authorization. Such a policy encourages responsible protection of information and is essential to provide an audit trail. Remote access does have additional risks. To mitigate them, additional constraints may be imposed. For instance, insurance companies may be restricted to have access to otherwise authorized information only during their working hours, to prevent unsupervised access. Emergency overrides will not be needed for such types of access.

Authorizations follow professional conventions. Physicians and nurses that are bound by a code of ethics will receive broader rights than clerical personnel [11]. Staff working within an institution and receiving guidance on privacy protection will have fewer restrictions imposed on them than external staff [12]. Where data retrieval is not urgent, say for medical research, delays due to a more careful validation are acceptable. Data for research may also be transformed to reduce the risk of inadvertent disclosure [13]. Figure 2 sketches the interaction of authorizations and health care data.

The information defining assigned authorizations should be kept so that it can be easily inspected and updated when needed. That information also must be represented in a way that computer programs which enforce access can interpret the rights and assign them to authenticated individuals or roles as needed [14]. The table containing the rights assigned to individuals and groups with respect to the types of data represent a major part of the institutional policy for security and protection.

2.4 Logging

Authorized transactions within an EMR can be easily be recorded or logged. The storage capacity of computer systems is such that transaction logs can be quite comprehensive, recording who accessed what, when, and how. When data leave the institution, the actual contents should also be recorded. For periodic audit tools can be sued to spot atypical activities, and in case of problems definite conclusions can be drawn.

Here computer systems can perform much better than humans, who have fallible and often opinionated recall. To encourage that all data access are mediated by the security services, The computer system must be able to handle any transaction that has been permitted by a responsible authority, including exceptional requests. If systems do not have the capability to allow exceptions, users will use improper means, such as copying files and removing them physically, when a legitimate need exists. The log and resulting audit trail then becomes incomplete. If problems arise, legitimate versus wrong use of improper methods are hard to distinguish.

Since the logs contain confidential data, the computer that collects the logs must be included in the protected domain, and access to it should be even more severely restricted, since conventional authorization mechanisms do not apply there. When log tapes or disks are removed from that machine they must be kept in a physically secure location. The retention requirements of security logs are not as well defined a those for medical and legal data, so typically the same retention rules are applied.

2.5 Management of protection

The decisions that define what types information to protect from what classes of individuals, and to what extent to invest in protection must be made a high institutional level. It s the management of an institution who ultimately have responsibility when access fails or when a patient's expectation of privacy is violated [15]. Once the policies are set, their execution is delegated to specialists. In our description we will assume that the execution of protection policies is delegated to an institutional security officer. Such a person maintains the communication between management and computer and communication technologists who manage the actual software. The translation of policies to enforceable rules is always problematic. Not all desirable policies can be fully implemented. For instance, automating the policy that in an emergency case all data must be available, requires that the computer can unambiguously recognize an emergency. The policy may be implemented to make all information available recognize an emergency. The policy may be partially implemented by making all information available to emergency room personnel; but not all emergencies occur in the emergency room.

Having an individual on duty who is authorized to override restriction is wise. Such overrides can also be logged, so that a complete audit trail is maintained. The security officer can establish such rules in order to best implement the institutional policies. Today, the responsibility for implementation is often assigned to technical personnel as a secondary responsibility. When, for instance, the database manager is responsible for security, very liberal rules are likely to be established, since the primary function of this person is to make data available, not to protect them from inappropriate access. Similar concerns arise when a networking manager is assigned the responsibility for security and privacy, since for that person the primary objective is to keep the system accessible, not to protect data from inappropriate access.

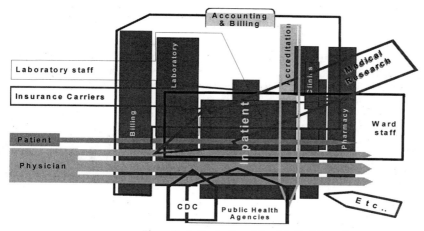

Figure 2. Authorizations into a Medical Record

3. Technologies

In order to provide security a number of technologies are in common use. We listed various means for authentication above, but also have to worry that transmissions are save from intruders, that authorizations are obeyed, and that only appropriate information is released. We assume now that management policies are in place, and that that operational responsibilities have been assigned to a security officer.

3.1 Cryptography

Transmission of information, including the passwords or identifications needed for authentication, can be protected through encryption. Encryption causes a message to be transformed according to an encryption key. The encryption key can direct shuffles, boolean transforms, reversible multiplications, and the like. Cryptography can provide an arbitrarily high level of protection by lengthening the key. The difficulty of breaking encrypted information increases proportionally to the power of the size of the encryption key. Software using 56-bit keys has been in common use since 1977 [16]. With current high-performance computers data encrypted with such a key can be decoded within a few days. Still, the information to be gained by breaking into an EMR rarely warrants even that effort. Cryptographic procedures with much longer keys are now becoming available. Existing and future capabilities of cryptographic software seem to be adequate for healthcare.

Managing the keys is still a problem. The key used for encryption has to made available to the destination, so that decryption can be performed. Loss of the key makes all of the information inaccessible, and a stealing a copy of the key makes encryption meaningless. Key losses can be dealt with be depositing copies of the keys with a responsible part, an escrow agent. Law enforcement agencies have been favoring schemes where keys would always be deposited with an escrow agent, so that encrypted files could be decoded when a legal search warrant is issued. It appears unlikely that they will get their wish, since such restrictions can easily be ignored by criminals and people suspicious of the government.

Public-key encryption use two keys to overcome the problem of key management. Data to be transmitted are encrypted with two keys, one supplied by the sender and one by the receiver. A private version of the key is retained locally and derived keys are made publicly available. Encryption uses the local private and the remote public keys. Decryption requires the remote public and the local private keys. Public-key encryption is effective for modest data volumes, for sharing keys used to encrypt larger quantities of data, and to authenticate remote requestors [17].

Although cryptography is an essential tool in protecting information from intruders, it only provides protection for well-defined tasks, and cannot distinguish among the many types of requestors that need to get to an EMR. All legitimate requestors of a record would need the same encryption key, and could not be distinguished. All others are viewed as potential enemies.

3.2 Firewalls

Firewall software is now widely available, and is effective in defining the perimeter of an enterprise. They analyze the headers of incoming information, and sometimes outgoing, information packets and can limit access to sites that have known Internet Protocol (IP) addresses. It has been hard to protect computer systems from intruders who masquerade themselves as coming from legitimate Internet sites by faking IP numbers..

Many products can also validate submitted authentication information. Mobile requestors, say physicians on travel, typically do not have a fixed IP addresses, and for those individual authentication is essential. Since these identifications are submitted over public pathways, it is important that the transmissions are protected, so that potential intruders cannot copy legitimate name-and-password combinations.

Firewalls do not check the specific authorizations or contents of requests, submitted, or retrieved. For those aspects internal software, perhaps database systems must be responsible. If a legitimate user, either inadvertently or through subterfuge obtains inappropriate information, the filtering provided by a firewall is of no help.

3.3 Partitioning of the medical record

The authorization table relates requestors, be they individuals or groups, to categories of the stored data. Implicit in this approach is that the data to be presented or retrieved are partitioned into disjoint cells, so that for every authorization types cells with the appropriate rights can be identified. The process of assigning categories to information involves every person who creates, enters, or maintains information. When there are few cells, originators of data can understand what is at stake, and can perform the categorization function adequately, although errors in filing will still occur. When there are many cells, the categorization task becomes onerous and error prone. When new applications are created, surveillance for more diseases is needed, or new collaborators must share the existing information system, the categorization task becomes impossible.

3.4 Multi-level secure systems

A technology that has been advocated mainly in the military domain is to have the a database systems, and the underlying operating system, be aware that there may be several layers of authorization that subsume each other: top secret, secret, confidential, etc. Impressive software has been demonstrated to deal with such multi-level data in a single environment [18]. However, the hierarchical approach of those systems does not deal with the overlapping access rights we find in health care. Furthermore, even where appropriate, these systems have not been put into practice because their cost. Much of their cost is due to the delays in implementing and validating multi-level secure capabilities, which causes them to lag one or two generations of commercial software. We will not consider this technology further.

4. Problems to be addressed in the near future

We have seen that we deal in the medical domain with many types of collaborators, all sharing access to information in the EMR. These collaborators are important in our complex enterprise, and cannot be viewed as enemies. The medical record cannot be partitioned into sections that are distinct for each group of authorized users. Such sections will overlap, and the number of possible combinations will be unmanageable [19].

Today, security provisions for computing focus on controlling access.
Relying on access control makes the assumption that five conditions are fulfilled
1. Authentication of all persons requesting access
2. Perimeter control by use of a firewall or its equivalent
3. Authorizations that are complete and well-maintained
4. Secure transmission wherever physical access is not controlled
5. Partitioning of the information to match the authorization pattern

Unfortunately, in health care espcially, the last condition, namely perfect a partitioning of the information into cells for disjoint access for each type of auhorization, is not realistic. We have many requestors whose needs overlap. We cannot expect that medical staff can foresee all the uses that medical information will serve, so that partitioning at the time of data collection is impossible. Delaying a partitioning of data later is not acceptable, since patient care demands that the record be accessible in a comprehensive form and up-to-date [20]. Furthermore, enforcing data partitioning to obtain security would greatly increase the cost of healthcare.

Changing patterns of outsourcing of services imposes exacerbates the problem. Reorganizing healthcare databases to deal with developing needs for external access is costly and disruptive, since it will affect existing users and their applications. The problem has been recognized, but not yet addressed in industry; for instance, security concerns were the cited as the prime reason for lack of progress in establishing *virtual enterprises* [21].

5. A Complementary Technology

A solution that addresses this dilemma, *result checking,* has been demonstrated in our Trusted Interoperation of Healthcare Information (TIHI) project [22]. Result checking is a function provided at the firewall which complements the conventional tasks of access control with a filter for outgoing information. Now the results of any information request are checked before releasing them to the external world. The system also allows checking of a large number of parameters about the release. Result checking mimics the manual function of a security officer when checking the briefcases of collaborating participants leaving a secure meeting in a protected setting. No checking of result contents is performed in current firewalls. Result checking need not depend on the sources of the result, so that it remains robust with respect to weaknesses in information categorization, software errors, and misfiling of data.

5.1 Filtering System Architecture

Since result checking requires more work than firewalls can provide the new functions are implemented in a dedicated *security mediator* workstation, to be managed by a security officer. Such a *security mediator* system interposes security checking between external requestors of information and the data resources to be protected, as shown in Fig.3. The mediator can also carry out the functions of authentication and access control to the extent that such services are not, or not reliably, provided by network and database services. It will not process requests issued by trusted internal users, so that the performance of the system, as seen internally, is not impacted.

It is a management decision, of course, where domain boundaries are to be drawn. We'd assume that clinical personnel is inside, and all others collaborators would be external to the perimeter defined by the mediated firewall. Gray areas remain: should billing clerks be inside or external to the primary protected perimeter?

To assure effective management control, the security mediator software is designed to operate on a distinct workstation, owned and operated by the enterprise security officer (S.O.). It is positioned as a pass gate within the enterprise firewall, if there is such a firewall. In our initial commercial installation the security mediator also provided traditional firewall functions, by limiting the IP addresses of requestors [23].

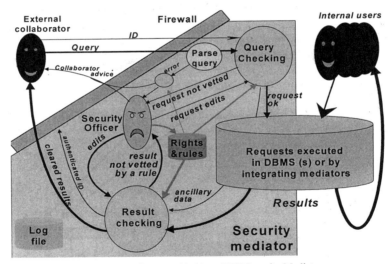

Fig.3. Functions provided by a TIHI Security Mediator.

Since all requests that arrive from the external world and their results are processed by the security mediator, the databases behind a firewall need not be secure unless there are further internal requirements. When combined with an integrating mediator, a security mediator can also serve multiple data resources behind a firewall [24]. Combining the results of a query requiring multiple sources prior to result checking improves the scope of result validation.

5.2 Operation

Within the workstation is a rule-base system which investigates queries coming in and results to be transmitted to the external world. Any request and any result which cannot be vetted by the rule system is displayed to the security officer for manual handling. The security officer decides to approve, edit, or reject the information. An associated logging subsystem provides an audit trail for all information that enters or leaves the domain. The log provides input to the security officer to aid in evolving the rule set, and increasing the effectiveness of the system.

The software of our security mediator is composed of modules that perform the following tasks

1. Optionally (if there is no firewall): Authentication of the external collaborator
2. Determination of authorization type (role) for the collaborator
3. Processing to vet the request for data (pre-processing) using the policy rules
4. If the request is in error or dubious initiate interaction with the security officer
5. Communication to internal databases (submission of vetted request)
6. Communication from internal databases (retrieval of unfiltered results)
7. Processing to vet the results (post-processing) using the policy rules
8. If the result contents are dubious: interaction with the security officer
9. Writing origin identification, query, actions, and results into a log file
10. Transmission of vetted information to the requestor

Authentication, secure communication, query parsing, integration of results from multiple sources, and many other tasks remain are carried out identically in a system using security mediation as in other secure systems. A supporting database systems can still implement its view-based protection facilities [14]. The system need not be fully trusted, but its mechanisms will add efficiency.

Item 7, the post-processing of the results obtained from the databases is the critical additional function. Processing to vet the contents of results retrieved from databases is potentially quite costly, since it has to deal thoroughly with a wide variety of data. Applying such filters selectively, specifically for the problems raised in collaborations, as well as the capabilities of modern computers and text-processing algorithms, makes use of the technology feasible. Furthermore, for many external collaborations, as disease reporting and research support speedy response is not critical.

To control the filtering a rule-based system is used in TIHI. The rules provide flexibility, allowing security policies to be set that achieve a reasonable balance of cost to benefit. It's operation will be described in the next section.

Having rules, however is optional. Without rules the mediator system will operate in fully paranoid mode. In that case, each query and each result will be submitted to the security officer. The security officer will view the contents on-line, and approved, edit, or reject the material. Adding rules enables automation. The extent of automation depends the coverage of the rule-set. A reasonable goal is the automatic processing of say, 90% of queries and 95% responses.

Unusual requests, perhaps issued because of a new collaboration, will initially not have applicable rules, but can be immediately processed through interaction with the security officer. In time, suitable rules can be entered to reduce the load on the officer.

The actions performed by security mediator software remain under the control of the enterprise since the rules are modifiable by the security officer at all times [25]. In addition, logs are accessible to the officer, who can keep track of the transactions. If some rules are found to be to liberal, policy can be tightened. If rules are too stringent, as evidenced by an excessive load on the security officer, they can be relaxed or elaborated.

5.3 The Rule System

The rule system comprises the rules themselves, an interpreter for the rules, and primitives which are invoked by the rules. The rules embody the security policy of the enterprise. They are hence not preset into the software of the security mediator.

In order to automate the process of controlling access and ensuring the security of information, the security officer enters rules into the system. These rules trigger analyses of requests, their results, and evaluate a number of associated parameters. The interpreting software uses these rules to determine the validity of every request and make the decisions pertaining to the disposition of the results. Auxiliary functions help the security officer enter appropriate rules and update them as the security needs of the organization change.

The rules are simple, short and comprehensive. They are stored in a database local to the security mediator system with all edit rights restricted to the security officer. Some rules may overlap in a given situation, in which case the most restrictive rule applies. The rules may pertain to requestors, cliques of requestors having certain roles, sessions, databases tables or any combinations of these.

Rules are selected based on the authorization rights determined for the requestor. All the applicable rules will be checked for every request issued by the requestor in every session. All rules will be enforced for every requestor and the request will be forwarded to the source databases only if it passes all tests. Any request not fully vetted is posted immediately to the log and sent the security officer. The failure message is directed to the security officer and not to the requestor, so that the requestors in such cases will not see the failure and its cause. This prevents that the requestor could interpret failure patterns and make meaningful inferences, or rephrase the request to try to bypass the filter [26].

The novel aspect of this approach is that security mediator checks outgoing results as well. This is crucial since, from the security-point-of-view, requests are inclusive, not exclusive selectors of content and may retrieve unexpected information. Furthermore, helpful, user-friendly information systems often return more information than requested. From a security point-of-view being helpful generous is risky. Thus, even when the request has been validated, it is important that the results are also subject to screening by a set of rules. If the rules cannot assure that the results can be released the cause and the information are sent to the security officer but not to the requestor.

5.4 Primitives

The rules invoke executable primitive functions which operate on requests, on submitted or retrieved data, on the log, and on other information sources. As new security functions and technologies appear, or if specialized needs arise, new primitives can be inserted in the security mediator for subsequent rule invocation. In fact, the suppliers of security mediation software should not expect to be the source of all primitives. All primitives, supplied or added, should be sufficiently simple so that their correct function can be verified. Primitives which have been demonstrated are shown in Table 1.

Table 1. Primitives to support filtering rules

- Assignment of a requestor to a role-group for authorization
- Limit access for clique to certain database table segments or columns
- Limit request to statistical (average, median, ..) information
- Augment query with data useful for result analysis
- Provide number of data instances (database rows) used in a statistical result
- Provide number of tables used (joins) in computing result for further checking
- Limit number of requests per session

- Limit number of sessions per period
- Limit requests by requestor per period
- Block requests from all but listed sites
- Block delivery of results to all but listed sites
- Block receipt of requests by local time at request site
- Block delivery of results by local time at delivery site
- Constrain request to data which is keyed to requestor's own name
- Constrain request to data which is keyed to request site name
- Filter all result terms through a clique-specific good-word dictionary
- Disallow results containing terms in a clique-specific bad-word dictionary
- Convert text by replacing identifies with non-identifying surrogates [27]
- Convert text by replacing objectionable terms with surrogates
- Randomize responses for legal protection [28]
- Extract text out of x-ray images for further filtering [29]

Not all primitives will have a role in all applications. Primitives can vary greatly in cost of application. For instance, checking for appropriate terms in results is costly in principle, but modern spell-checkers show that it can be done fairly fast. For this task we create clique-specific dictionaries, by initially processing a substantial amount of approved results. In initial use the security officer will get false failure reports, due to innocent terms that are not yet in the dictionary. Those terms will be incrementally added, so that in time the incidence of such failures will be minimal.

For example, we have in use a dictionary for ophtamology, to allow authenticated researchers in that field to have access to patient data. That dictionary does not include terms that would signal, say HIV infection or pregnancies, information which the patients would not like to see released to unknown research collaborators. Also, all proper names, places of employment, etc. are effectively filtered. Figure 4 shows a screen of the interaction when a physician name, that should not be released, appeared in a result. The action for the security officer may be edit the document by removing the name, so that it can be released.

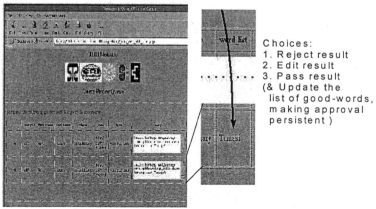

Choices:
1. Reject result
2. Edit result
3. Pass result
(& Update the list of good-words, making approval persistent)

Figure 4. Extract from a report to the Security Officer

Several of the primitives are designed to help control inference problems in statistical database queries [30]. While neither we, nor any feasible system can prevent all leaks due to inference, we believe that careful information release management can greatly reduce the probability [13]. Furthermore, providing the tools for subsequent audit, as logging all accesses will reduce the practical threat [31],. The primitive to enforce constraints on access frequencies will themselves refer to the log. Here again the principles for traditional database support and security mediation diverge, since database transaction are best isolated, where as inference control requires history maintenance.

5.5 Logging

Throughout, failures to vet queries and responses, as well as the request text, the source of the data, and any actions taken by the security officer, are logged by the system for audit purposes. Having a security log which is distinct from the database log is important since:

- A database system logs all transactions, not just external requests, and is hence confusingly voluminous
- Most database systems do not log attempted and failed requests fully, because they appear not to have affected the databases
- Reasons for failure of requests in database logs are implicit, and do not give the rules that caused them.

We provide user-friendly utilities to scan the security log by time, by requestor, by role, and by data source. Offending terms in results are marked.

No system, except one that provides complete isolation, can be 100% foolproof. The provision of security is, unfortunately, a cat-and-mouse game, where new threats and new technologies keep arising. Logging provides the feedback which converts a static approach to a dynamic and stable system, which can maintain an adequate level of protection. Logs will have to be inspected regularly to achieve stability.

Bypassing of the entire system and hence the log remains a threat. Removal of information on portable media, as floppies is easy. Only a few enterprises can afford to place controls on all personnel leaving daily for home, lunch, or external sites. However, having an effective and adaptable security filter removes the excuse that information had to be downloaded and carried out because the system was to stringent for legitimate purposes.

6. Summary and Status

We have presented security mediation as a service that can coalesce many functions needed to protect healthcare information. Such specialization allows concentration of the responsibility for security Architecturally the concept expands the role of a gateway to the external world in the firewall from a passive filter to an active pass gate. The service is best implemented on a dedicated workstation, owned by the security officer. Isolating security management from other operational demands and their changes decreases the risk of unintended breaches. Existing technologies, as constraining authorization views over databases, encryption for transmission in networks, password management in operating systems, etc., can be managed via the security mediator node.

The specific, novel service presented here, result checking, complements traditional access control. We have received a patent to cover the concept. Checking results is especially relevant in systems with many types of users, including external collaborators, and complex information structures. In such settings the requirement that systems that are limited to access-control impose, namely that all data are correctly partitioned and filed is not achievable in practice. Result checking does not address all issues of security, as protection from malicious actions, although it is likely that such attacks will be preceded by processes that extract information. A side-effect of result checking that it provides a level of intrusion detection. Assuring that the data contents is trustworthy still relies on a minimum level of reliability in the supporting systems. No security technology can compensate when information is missing or not found because of misidentification. In general, a security mediator cannot protect from inadvertent or intentional denial of information by a mismanaged database system.

The rule-based approach allows balancing of the need for preserving data security and privacy and for making data available. Data which is too tightly controlled reduces the benefits of sharable information in collaborative settings. Rules which are too liberal can violate security and expectation of privacy. Having a balanced policy will require direction from management. Having a single focus for execution of the policy in electronic transmission will improve the consistency of the application of the policy.

Traditional systems, based on access control to precisely defined cells, require a long time to before the data are set up, and when the effort is great, may never be automated. In many situation we are aware of, security mechanisms are ignored when requests for information are deemed to be important, but cannot be served by existing methods. Keeping the security officer in control allows any needed bypassing to be handled formally. This capability recognizes that in a dynamic, interactive world there will always be cases that are not foreseen or situations the rules are too stringent. Keeping the management of exceptions within the system greatly reduces confusion, errors, and liabilities.

Our initial demonstrations have been in the healthcare domain, and a commercial version of TIHI is now in use to protect records of genomic analyses in a pharmaceutical company. As the expectations for protection of the privacy of patient data are being solidified into governmental regulations we expect that the mediated approach will gain popularity [32]. Today most of the healthcare establishment still hopes that commercial encryption tools will be adequate for the protection of medical records, since the complexity of managing access requirements has not yet been faced [33]. Expenditures for security in medical enterprises are minimal [2]. Funding of adequate provisions in an industry under heavy economic pressures, populated with many individuals who do not attach much value to the privacy of others, will remain a source of stress.

7. Advice

Even when traditional security protection methods succeed in disallowing access from enemies, break-ins still occur. Most of them are initiated via legitimate access paths, since the information in our systems must be shared with customers and collaborators. Once someone is permitted into the system, protection becomes more difficult. In that case the access control technologies provide no protection, and the burden falls on the mappings and the categorization if the information.

In the near future the requirements keeping the medical record secure, be it on paper or in electronic form, will be increasing. Protection of what patients perceive to be their private information is becoming important. Legal obligations will arise as well, but limiting to protection to what appears to be legal minimum may well be inadequate. In time, case law will define more precisely public and legal obligation.

The management of healthcare institutions must be prepared to define policies and supervise their implementation. Assigning responsibilities for medical record security to database or network personnel, who have primary responsibilities of making data and communication available, will conflict with security concerns and is unwise. These people are promoted to their positions because they have a helpful attitude and know how to overcome problems of system failures and inadequacies. This attitude is inherently in conflict with corporate responsibilities for the protection of data. Outside vendors of products will not advertise the weaknesses of their approaches to security, especially in respect to the complexity of the requirements imposed on a medical record.

Acknowledgements

Research leading to security mediators was supported by an NSF HPCC challenge grant and by DARPA ITO via Arpa order E017, as a subcontract via SRI International. Shelley Qian and Steve Dawson were the PIs at SRI. The commercial transition was performed by Maggie Johnson, Chris Donahue, and Jerry Cain under contracts with SST (www.2ST.com). Work on editing and filtering graphics is due to Jahnavi Akalla and James Z. Wang. Some of this material has appeared in earlier publications [34].

References

[1] Richard S. Dick and Elaine B. Steen (eds.) *The Computer-based Medical Record:; An Essential Technology for Health Care;* Institute of Medicine, National Academy Press, 1991.

[2] Paul Clayton (chair): *For the Record; Protecting Electronic Health Information*; National Academy Press, 1997.

[3] R. Scott Evans et al.: "Computer Surveillance of Hospital-acquired Infections and Antibiotic Use"; *J. of the AMA*, Vol.256 No.8, 1986, pp.1007-1011.

[4] Molla S. Donaldson and Kathleen L. Lohr (eds): *Health Data in the Information Age: Use, Disclosure, and Privacy;* Institute of Medicine, National Academy Press, 1994.

[5] Thomas Beth: "Confidential Communication on the Internet"; *Scientific American*, December 1995, pp.88-91.

[6] S.Castano, M.G. Fugini, G.Martella, and P. Samarati: *Database Security;* Addison Wesley Publishing Company - ACM Press, 1995.

[7] J.P. Holmes, L.J. Wright, and R.L.Maxwe: A Performance Evaluation of Biometric Identification Devices; Sandia Report SAND91-0276, Sandia National Laboratories, June 1991.

[8] William R.Cheswick and Steven M. Bellovin: *Firewalls and Internet Security;* Addison-Wesley, 1994.

[9] Wietse Venema: "TCP wrapper: Network Monitoring, Access Control, and Booby Traps"; *Proc.3rd Usenix Security Symp.*, Baltimore MD, 1992.

[10] D. Brent Chapman and Elizabeth D. Zwicky: *Building Internet Firewalls;* O'Reilly and Associates, 1995.

[11] American Medical Association: "Confidentiality: Computers"; *Code of Medical Ethics*, Aamericamn Medical Assiciation, 1994.

[12].Computer-based Patient Record Institute: *Guidelines for managing Information Security Programs*; Work Group on Confidentiality, Privacy, and Security, CPRI, 1996.

[13] Latanya Sweeney: "Guaranteeing anonymity when sharing medical data, the *DATAFLY* system"; *Proceedings, Journal of the American Medical Informatics Association*, Washington DC, Hanley & Belfus, 1997.

[14] Patricia P. Griffiths and Bradford W. Wade: "An Authorization Mechanism for a Relational Database System"; *ACM Trans. on Database Systems*, Vol.1 No.3, Sept.1976, pp.242-255.

[15] Priscilla M. Regan: *Legislating Privacy, Technology, Social Values. and Public Policy;* University of North Carolina Press, 1995.

[16] A.G. Konheim, M.H.Mack, R.K. McNeil, B. Tuckerman: The IPS Cryptographic Programs"; *IBM Sys. J.*, Vol.19 No2, 1980, pp.302-307.

[17] Whitfield Diifie: "The First Ten Years of Public-Key Cryptography"; *Proc. IEEE,* Vol.76 No.5, May 1988, pp.560-577.

[18] Therea Lunt et al.: "The SeaView Security Model"; *IEEE Trans. on Software Eng.*, Vol.16 No.6, 1990, pp.593-607.

[19] A. Luniewski et al. "Information organization using Rufus" SIGMOD '93, *ACM SIGMOD Record*, June] 1993, vol.22, no.2 p. 560-561

[20] Thomas C. Rindfleisch: Privacy, Information Technology, and Health Care; *Comm. ACM;* Vol.40 No. 8 , Aug.1997, pp.92-100.

[21] M. Hardwick, D.L. Spooner, T. Rando, and KC Morris: "Sharing Manufacturing Information In Virtual Enterprises"; *Comm. ACM*, Vol.39 no.2, pp.46-54, February 1996.

[22] Gio Wiederhold, Michel Bilello, Vatsala Sarathy, and XiaoLei Qian: A Security Mediator for Health Care Information"; *Journal of the AMIA,* issue containing the Proceedings of the 1996 AMIA Conference, Oct. 1996, pp.120-124.

[23] Gio Wiederhold, Michel Bilello, and Chris Donahue: "Web Implementation of a Security Mediator for Medical Databases"; in T.Y. Lin and Shelly Qian:*Database Security XI, Status and Prospects,* IFIP / Chapman & Hall, 1998, pp.60-72.

[24] Jeffrey Ullman: Information Integration Using Logical Views; *International Conference on Database Theory (ICDT '97)* Delphi, Greece, ACM and IEEE Computer Society, 1997.

[25] Tor Didriksen: "Rule-based Database Access Control – A Practical Approach"; *Proc. 2nd ACM workshop on Rule-based Access Control*, 1997, pp.143-151.

[26] T. Keefe, B.Thuraisingham, and W.Tsai: "Secure Query Processing Strategies"; *IEEE Computer*, Vol.22 No.3, March 1989, pp.63-70.

[27] Latanya Sweeney: "Replacing personally-identifying information in medical records, the *SCRUB* system"; J.J.Cimino, ed. *Proceedings, Journal of the American Medical Informatics Association*, Washington, DC: Hanley & Belfus, 1996, Pp.333-337.

[28] E. Leiss: "Randomizing, A Practical Method for Protecting Statistical Databases Against Compromise"; *Proceedings of the Conference on Very Large Databases (VLDB)*, Morgan Kaufman pubs. (Los Altos CA) 8, 1982, McLeod and Villasenor(eds), pp 189--196

[29] James Z. Wang, Gio Wiederhold, and Jia Li: Wavelet-based Progressive Transmission and Security Filtering for Medical Image Distribution"; in Stephen Wong (ed.): *Medical Image Databases*; Kluwer publishers, 1998, pp.303- 324.

[30] N.R.Adam andJ.C. Wortmann: Security-Control Methods for Statistical Databases: a Comparative Study; *ACM Computing Surveys*, Vol. 25 No.4, Dec. 1989.

[31] T. Hinke: "Inference Aggregation Detection in Database Management Systems"; *Proc. IEEE Symposium on Security and Privacy*, Oakland CA, April 1988.

[32] Bill Braithwaite: "National health information privacy bill generates heat at SCAMC"; *Journal of the American Informatics Association*, Vol.3 no.1, 1996, pp.95-96

[33] David M. Rind, Isaac S. Kohane, Peter Szolovits, Charles Safran, Henry C. Chueh, and G. Octo Barnett: "Maintaining the Confidentiality of Medical Records Shared over the Internet and the World Wide Web"; *Annals of Internal Medicine*, 15 July 1997. pp.127-141.

[34] Gio Wiederhold: "Protecting Information when Access is Granted for Collaboration"; in B.Thuraisingham, Z.Tarri, K.Ditttrich (eds): *Proc. IFIP WG11.3 in Database Security;* IFIP-Kluwer, pp.3-11.

Future of Health Technology
R.G. Bushko (Ed.)
IOS Press, 2002

Future of Technology to
Augment Patient Support in Hospitals

Marina U. Bers, Ph.D.*

Assistant Professor, Eliot-Pearson Department of Child Development,
Tufts University, Medford, MA, US

Joseph Gonzalez-Heydrich, M.D.

Assistant Professor of Psychiatry, Harvard Medical School &
Medical Director, Outpatient Psychiatry Programs, Children's Hospital, Boston, MA, US

David Ray DeMaso, M.D.

Associate Professor of Psychiatry,
ırvard Medical School & Associate Psychiatrist-in-Chief, Children's Hospital, Boston, MA, US

Abstract

This chapter explores the potential of using computer technology to support and augment psychotherapeutic interventions in hospitals, communities and homes. We describe two applications piloted at Children's Hospital Boston. The first pilot explored how patients with pediatric heart disease used the Storytelling Agent Generation Environment (SAGE) computer program to create interactive storytellers and share their personal stories. The second involved youngsters on hemodialysis for end stage renal disease using the Zora graphical multi-user environment to create a virtual city and form a therapeutic virtual community. In this chapter we show how computer technology can be used to help patients explore their identity, cope with their illness and provide mutual support and interaction. We also present design recommendations for future interventions of this kind.

1. Introduction

Advances in medical care have greatly increased the life expectancy of children and adolescents suffering from a myriad of physical illnesses. Despite these advances, many youngsters must continue to contend with a chronic physical illness and ongoing treatment [1, 2]. It has been recognized that enhancing adaptive coping strategies improves health outcomes and resiliency in many patients. Interventions that provide information, facilitate expression of feelings, and allow mutual support are important components of psychoeducational interventions that have been found to be useful. In addition there is an emerging recognition that both emotional and physical benefit can be gained through the development, expression, and understanding of an individual's personal narrative or "story" of a physical illness [3]. Personal narratives often include how a physical illness has changed or not changed who they are, their relationships and life choices, and "what it means to them."

Parallel to these psychotherapeutic developments in the support of physically ill patients, computer technologies have evolved that facilitate mutual support networks, the exploration of the self, and the development of personal narratives. The recent increase of home pages, chat-spaces, virtual worlds, multi-user environments and Internet-based role-playing games are "real world" examples of these technologies. Turkle [4] suggests that the "Internet has become a significant social laboratory for experimenting with the constructions and re-constructions of self that characterize postmodern life." Despite these technologic advances the challenge remains of how to design environments that leverage the characteristic of the computer to purposefully support explorations about identity that can lead to therapeutic personal narratives and better mutual support.

Identity construction environments [5] can serve this purpose. They are designed following the philosophy of constructionism [6] that asserts that people learn best when engaged in creating meaningful projects that they can reflect upon and share with others. Therefore identity construction environments enable children to design their meaningful computational projects to explore their sense of self. In this chapter we present two examples of identity construction environments, SAGE and Zora. SAGE enables children to design interactive storytellers, while Zora provides them with tools to create a virtual city. This chapter describes the use of these two identity construction environments in Children's Hospital Boston.

2. SAGE: Telling Stories With An Interactive Soft Rabbit

SAGE (Storytelling Agent Generation Environment) is an identity construction environment that supports the creation of individualized "wise or sage storytellers" by children. It was developed at the MIT Media Laboratory in Cambridge, Massachusetts to help children "play out" what is happening in their lives by telling and listening to stories. In order to encourage child's emotional engagement, the wise storyteller's assistant was embodied in an interactive stuffed animal (rabbit) — a *soft interface*. With SAGE, children became the designers as well as users of their creations. Thus, SAGE supported two modes of interaction. In the first mode, children share their personal stories with a wise sage, and his rabbit assistant, who "listen" and then offer a relevant tale in response. In the second mode, children can add to the collection of wise sages by designing their own storyteller for themselves and others to interact with. They then write stories for their sage to tell [7].

In order to support children in creating their own characters, a visual programming language was developed to design and program: (1) the scripts that are used by the storyteller, (2) the conversational structure or flow of the interaction, (3) the body behaviors of the interactive toy, which behaves as the pet assistant of the storyteller, and (4) the database of tales that are offered in response by the character. SAGE also has multimedia capabilities allowing children to record their own stories and to draw their own characters. SAGE was designed to focus on creating stories and storytellers that invite reflection about the child's inner world.

SAGE seeks cognitive and emotional engagement. Hence, the decision to embed the assistant of the sage storytellers in a programmable interactive stuffed animal (see figure 1). The stuffed animal is capable of some of the types of nonverbal behaviors that humans use to indicate engagement and which are commonly found in conversational narratives between people (i.e., the rabbit moves as the children converse with it). In design mode, children are able to decide on the toy's communicative behaviors as well as the different personalities it might have.

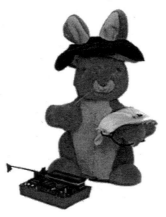

Figure 1: Interactive programmable stuffed rabbit

3. Stories From The Heart

Patients admitted on the hospital's cardiology ward (ages 7 to 16) were asked to use the SAGE to tell their stories and to create interactive characters. Informed consent was obtained from all families as part of a larger project by the authors to understand and promote family coping with cardiac illness, hospitalizations, and invasive medical procedures. The aim of this project was to explore the feasibility of physically ill children to use SAGE as well as its usefulness and safety in the hospital setting.

To engage hospitalized youngsters in the project, we created special characters for SAGE that could tell stories relevant to the medical environment. This began with "Mrs. Needle" who was a cartoon-type character that engaged children around the common child fears of "needles or pokes." This character used humor as a way to "break the ice" with these children. These characters proved quite successful as evidence by the creation of new hospital characters, e.g., "Mr. Tape", by the children themselves. Interestingly hospital professionals even created their own characters, e.g., "Mr. Squeeze".

The following are two examples of how two patients used the system to write stories of their medical experiences.

■   Lisa created a character (herself) called "Sadly Alone." The character asks the user, "Are you feeling sad?" and then told Lisa a story. In response, Lisa worked on her own story with a close family member. Lisa was gravely ill when working with SAGE wrote the following.

> *"My name is Lisa, and I have a problem. I'm 16 years old and I have a real bad heart problem and I am getting ready to have a heart transplant really soon but the hardest thing is my mother [is very sick] And I have a little brother, so it's so hard*

to leave them alone so I just stay strong and do what I have to do and if you ever have this kind of problem just stay strong for your family and think of me."

■   Samuel is a 13-year-old boy who had had a successful heart transplant. He wrote three stories about this experience and put them together into a trilogy called "The heart transplant dictionary".

"At first I felt very sick and I had to go into the Emergency room. First I had an IV which I never had before which I was pretty scared about and then I had a blood test on my arm and I never had one of those either which I was very scared about too but the IV was much scarier because I didn't know how much it was going to hurt. And another scary part was a lot of different doctors coming in all the time and that made me nervous because it made me think that there was something very wrong with me [...] but then I got better and I got to go home and I thought that everything will be OK but then I got sick again and I had to go back to the hospital and then they realized that I had to have a heart transplant.

After my heart transplant I was very sick because my body was rejecting my heart and it made me feel very sick and I had to go in for medicine and get biopsies twice a week where they go through a vein in your neck with a needle and they thread a catheter through and then they scrape a little piece of the heart tissue to see if you have any rejection. Rejection is when your white blood cells do not recognize your heart and think it is some bad virus or disease because it is not your original heart and your white blood cells try to attack your heart. So I kept having rejection [...] so they sent me to [another hospital] to go on a experimental drug [...] and felt better and the new drug is working very well and now I have no heart rejection at all [...]

The following example is from actual SAGE logs of interactions that a 16-year-old patient had with different storytellers (some already existing and others created by the patient). Interaction between the patient (*CHILD*) and SAGE happens through the keyboard (i.e., typing input and text-to-speech or recorded output).

■   This is a log of an interaction between Damian and the rabbit, best friend of "Mrs. Needle."

CHILD: I guess yes
SAGE: Well, Mrs. **SAGE**: *Hi, what is your name?*
CHILD: Damian
SAGE: *Welcome, Damian. I am Bunny, the best friend of Mrs. Needle. She hides in the computer because she is a little shy. She thinks that all the kids hate her. So she asked me to talk on her behalf. Is that OK with you?*
CHILD: yes
SAGE: *Wonderful, wonderful, Damian! Mrs. Needle is worried because kids scream when they see her. But, have you met Mrs. Needle before?*
Needle is my best friend and she hides in the computer. Tell me, Damian, how old are you?
CHILD: 16
SAGE: *Damian, you are older than me. I wonder if you are you scared of needles as I am ? I hate them, all except my friend Mrs. Needle. What about you?*
CHILD: They are all right

SAGE: *As I was telling you, Damian, I am Mrs. Needle's best friend and she asked me to find out why children hate her so much. She thinks that it is because she stings, but she is not sure. What do you think?*

CHILD: yes no kid is excited to get any needles

SAGE: *I see Damian ... what else can you tell me about this?*

CHILD: the kids are afraid of it because it hurts and they don't like it to hurt and I guess that is it

SAGE: *Well, Damian, let me see if I understand. I am sure that Mrs. Needle is very happy to hear what you have to say. Yes no kid is excited to get any needles the kids am afraid of it because it hurts and they don't like it to hurt and you guess that is it. Am I right?*

CHILD: yes

SAGE: *Guess what, Damian? Mrs. Needle has a story for you. She is shy but she loves to tell stories. She always says that they have power...Listen to her...*

Ms. Needle's Story: *They built me to sting, but that is not all I do. If you were a flower I could water you without hurting you. But you are not, and I am not a water pot. My nose is like a hose or like a straw and my belly has goodies than can help you to heal. When my belly is empty, the goodies are yours and you can feel better. But sometimes it is the other way around. My belly starts completely empty, and then it becomes full with your goodies. You can think of me as a someone that only stings, but I also do good. The problem is that this is not always immediately obvious.*

SAGE: *I loved Mrs. Needle's story, but how about you? Does it somehow relate to what you told me before, Damian?*

CHILD: yes it does

SAGE: *I see, Damian, please explain me the connection. I don't get it.*

CHILD: The children don't realize that the stuff can help them, the medicine.

SAGE: *I see, Damian, you got the power of the story. I am sure my friend Mrs. Needle will be very happy. I wish that you will always have the courage to keep telling and listening to stories. I hope to see you soon....Bye !*

- After playing with "Mrs. Needle", Damian decided to create his own character called "Mr. Tape." He created the conversational structure, the scripts that "Mr. Tape" says, and also the stories that he tells. After, he interacted with the character and invited other people in the Cardiac Unit to play with him. This is a saved log of Damian's interaction.

SAGE: *Hi my name is Mr. Tape. What is yours?*

CHILD: Damian

SAGE: *Well hello, Damian, my name is Mr. Tape. I am very sticky, as you probably may know, a lot of children don't like tape because when you have to take it off it hurts. Some kids like me to put me anywhere, like the face, hands, just for fun. Do you like tape?*

CHILD: no

SAGE: *I am sorry, why don't you like me. Does it hurt you?*

CHILD: sometimes, yes

SAGE: *Well, I am good for taping things up that are broken and I come in different kinds. I try to do the best I can with making things back to normal. So, Damian, how old are you?*

CHILD: 16

> **SAGE:** *You are lucky to be able to live that long. My life expectancy is only two to three years. Some people use me up fast and sometimes I am forgotten in the junk drawer. I get pretty lonely in there. Would you like to hear my story?*
> **CHILD:** *yes*
> **SAGE:** *When I am used as medical tape I am the number 1 user for nurses and doctors. I go on IVs and wrap things up. I am good to write on for the nurses to put on IV medication. You can use me just about everything in the hospital but I am not very sticky for heavier objects. I could be colored on and used for decorations for kids that are very bored. Some people just throw me around and drop me which hurts my feelings, I can't pick them up and drop them, but I thank them for using me as their number one choice. Well it was nice talking to you, maybe you will talk to me again and listen to my story. Bye*

As shown in these examples (as well as many others) youngsters with pediatric heart disease were able to readily use the SAGE to express significant fears and feelings. SAGE proved feasible, safe, and useful. It enabled children to adaptively express emotions through the creation of stories and narratives along with the development of innovative and interactive characters with whom they could converse. Nevertheless the SAGE did not engage children in sharing their stories with others in a community. When an individual is facing adversity it can be helpful to share one's personal narrative and becoming part of a social network that shares similar concerns. Recognition of SAGE's limitation in developing a supportive community led to the next prototype, Zora.

4. ZORA: Designing And Inhabiting A Virtual City

Zora is a 3D graphical multi-user environment designed at the MIT Media Laboratory [8]. Users build virtual rooms and populate them with objects and characters representing aspects of themselves, program them with storytelling behaviors, and converse with others in real-time through an avatar. Young patients used Zora in the hospital's dialysis unit. These patients form a community because they share a common medical condition and treatment in their end stage renal disease. Yet, at the same time there is little opportunity for social interaction with each other as they are confined to a single bedspace where they are attached to a dialysis machine for several of hours three times each week. The aim of this project was to explore the potential of the Zora identity construction environment to facilitate mutual patient support. In order to investigate this potential, the study examined the feasibility and safety of using the Zora virtual environment in a hospital setting.

Zora is a 3D graphical multi-user environment designed to support the exploration of identity through storytelling and programming. Users can create a virtual city and populate it by designing spaces, objects and interactive characters that can be programmed to engage in interactions with other users. The environment also has a story writing capacity. The name Zora was inspired by one of the cities that Italo Calvino describes in his book Invisible Cities, *"This city is like a honeycomb in whose cells each of us can place the things we want to remember...So the world's most wise people are those who know Zora."* [9].

Users are graphically represented by avatars with the owners' image. Children can visit each other's homes and can communicate in real-time through their avatars via text or gestures. Avatars can gather in the "City Hall" to decide the laws of the virtual city as well as to discuss cases related to community self-government and current controversial news. Users cannot only navigate around the 3D virtual city, but also construct the city's private and public spaces: personal homes, community centers and temples. Temples are shared public spaces that represent cultural traditions or interests. Both personal homes and temples are spatial representations of identity composed by artifacts symbolizing intangible aspects of the self.

Zora is an object-oriented environment, meaning that users can make new objects by cloning existing ones and inheriting its attributes. Objects have the following attributes: 1) presentation attributes, *graphical appearance* and *motion*; 2) administration attributes, *ownership*, which determines who owns the object and therefore can edit it, and *permissions*, which set if the object can be cloned; and 3) narrative-based attributes, *textual description, stories, values* and *conversations*. Zora is implemented using the Microsoft's Virtual Worlds platform, a development kit for building distributed multi-user environments [10].

5. A Virtual City in the Hemodialysis Unit

During a five months pilot study in the hospital's hemodialysis unit patients had access to a networked computer at their bedside and used it to create their own virtual city (see figure 2). The unit staff was also involved in participating in the study. Informed consent was obtained from all participants.

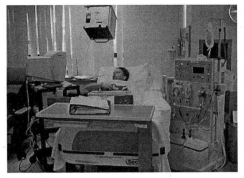

Figure 2: The Zora Computer and the Dialysis Machine

During this study, participants designed a total of 16 virtual places (see figure 3). Interestingly the hospital staff created 3 spaces including the *Nurse's Room* and the *Temple of Feeling Better* (described by the staff as a place to tell each other ways to cope with hard things). The MIT Medial Laboratory staff created 3 spaces including *the Restaurant*. Patients designed personal homes as well as several common spaces including the *Music Room* and the *Renal Rap* (described by the patients as a virtual space for dialysis patients to get together do fun things).

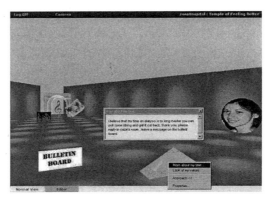

Figure 3: The Temple of Feeling Better

Participants made a total of 94 objects ranging from pictures of the hospital staff to favorite cartoon characters to video games. Overall, the patients created 14 characters generally cartoon characters that they called "heroes." The values dictionary of the city had 13 values with their definitions, e.g., *"friendship", "doing something positive to help myself or someone else"* and *"respect" with the definition "people should be aware of what they do to other people's things."*

During the study, the patients created 5 "cases" which are special types of objects representing events or circumstances to be discussed and agreed upon. They require community members to take action to resolve them. For example one case dealt with setting up the social organization of the virtual city, e.g., *"...someone changed the appearance of my door and I don't understand why...I would like to suggest as a rule that there is no tampering with other people's stuff..."* Participants posted in the bulletin boards 17 messages e.g., *"I really liked what you guys have done with the renal rap room".* They engaged in interactions with each other more on an asynchronous way than on a real-time way. This is not surprising since not all the participants were in the same dialysis shift and not all of them felt healthy to use Zora at the same time.

6. Feasibility and Safety

In order to assess the feasibility and safety of using Zora in a hospital, in the midst of the hemodialysis treatment, participants (both patients and staff) were asked to rate the application using a 7-point Likert scale anchored at one end by "1=not at all" and at the other end by "7=a great deal". Descriptive statistics were calculated for each of these rating scales. Participants were also asked several open-ended questions.

Feasibility
The patients (n=7) reported that they were very satisfied with Zora (mean = 5.3; standard deviation =1.3) and that they enjoyed very much participating in the experience (mean = 5.7; standard deviation =1.6) (see figure 4). *"It was really nice to have something fun to do at the hospital that could keep my mind off dialysis and that it was not schoolwork, but entertaining",* said a 15-year-old patient.

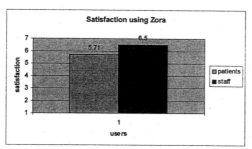

Figure 4: Satisfaction of Using Zora

When designing this pilot study there were some doubts about how patients, who are usually tired or sleep during most part of their treatment, would engage with Zora and if they would even use it at all. Zora was found not only feasible to use with patients undergoing hemodialysis treatment, but that was also an enjoyable and positive experience.

Hospital staff rated the experience very high (mean = 6.5; standard deviation =0.58) (see figure 4). For example, one staff member noted that being involved with the project helped her learn about the infinite potential of computer applications designed with a structure that might support different forms of therapy. Nurses did not find that Zora interfering with the patient's medical care. On the contrary, they enjoyed seeing their patients using Zora. One of the nurses said: *"I liked it a lot because I noticed that kids could say things in the computer that they might not say face to face and this has a lot of potential. It is a wonderful program for kids who are restricted and limited to the outside world."*

Nurses also enjoyed being involved with different logistical tasks, such as helping kids move the computers around and connect to the Internet. At a personal level, the hospital staff enjoyed the fact that Zora helped them learn new computer skills. They regretted that they could not devote more time to participate in the experience and the lack of a dedicated computer.

Safety
Overall, the seven patients reported that Zora was safe (mean = 5.93; standard deviation =1.84) and that participating in the experience was not hurtful (mean = 1.43; standard deviation =1.13). When asked about the safety of using Zora, a 17-year-old replied *"It might be unsafe if you put certain things in your room that younger kids shouldn't see. But that's the whole point with having the [virtual] city hall, where we set the rules and laws for Zora. I don't think it's not safe for kids."* Safety was a significant concern given the multi-user and open-ended nature of Zora and the fact that it runs on the Internet where children could easily find inappropriate content. This patient's response shows the importance of having in Zora as a space for community participation and democratic decision-making. In his perspective it was the patients' responsibility to make Zora a safe space, and not just a matter of obeying a code of behavior imposed by outsiders.

Hospital staff reported that using Zora was safe (mean = 5.63; standard deviation =1.49) and they all agreed that participating in the experience was not hurtful at all (mean = 1; standard deviation =0). One of the nurses said: *"Zora was a safe place and a safe way for patients to get their feelings out. It was an appropriate way to discuss their feelings. Rather than going out an punching a wall they had an opportunity to discuss things and to learn and to ask anything in Zora."* Another staff member agreed but pointed out the importance of supervising what children were doing and saying, in case that intervention from an adult was needed. In the five months that the program was running, there was no need of intervention. However, the community of users was small and they all belonged to the same institution.

7. Exploration of Personal Identity

When the study was designed it was hypothesized that patients would use **Zora** to explore their illness as a key component of their identity. We imagined kids would build virtual rooms populated by kidneys, dialysis machines and nurses. However, this did not happen. On the contrary, all of the patients consciously avoided any mentioning of hemodialysis in their virtual rooms. As a 15-year-old said: *"I am already on dialysis and I don't want to put things in my [virtual] room that remind me of dialysis; I don't want to go to other rooms that have that kind of stuff either."* It is not surprising that, when asking kids if participating in **Zora** helped them gain perspective about their illness, most of them replied that it did not (mean 2.43; standard deviation =2.30).

Children used Zora as a way to escape from the harshness of dialysis, not to think about it. Patients escaped in two different ways. First, they used their avatars to "move around" the Zora virtual city, while being "tied down" to bed and hooked up to the hemodialysis machine. Patients decided where to go and visit in the virtual city and were able to make decisions regarding how long to stay in the different places. This sense of autonomy and control was one way of escaping the frustrations of dialysis where there is no possibility to move around in a free way, neither to make many choices.

Second, patients escaped the harshness of dialysis by using their rooms to represent aspects of their identity that are usually underplayed during treatment. In general while undergoing hemodialysis, patients spend their time sleeping or watching TV. Their identity is represented by "passive" activities. However, when outside the hospital, like most people of their age, they participate in active endeavors, such as working, going to school or going out with friends. Their image of themselves is not the same inside and outside dialysis. Zora provided a way to bring back the self-image of patients as active agents. It offered a different venue of how to use their extensive time in dialysis in a creative and fun way by engaging in the creation of a personally meaningful project. When asked what she learned during the experience, a 14-year-old said: *"I learned new things about computers, like how to work with pictures and design my room, but I guess that I also learned about myself because I realized the things that I really care about and what my interests are and how to talk to others about that. In my room in Zora I could put both computers and other things I like."*

Since undergoing dialysis was a common factor for all of the participants none of them felt the need to make it explicit in their rooms. Instead they chose to represent other aspects of their identity. For example, Sharon created an Elvis Presley room with animations of the singer performing in the walls while Rina created a horse haven, with stories and pictures of her horse at home. In future studies it might be worth looking at what happens if patients create a Zora city together with kids that do not share their medical condition and treatment. Will they want to highlight the fact that dialysis is part of their identity? Or will they prefer to ignore it? Another question is what would happen if kids were using Zora at home instead of at the hospital. By being removed from the machines, would they use the opportunity to reflect about their experiences?

8. Facilitating Mutual Patient Support and Interaction

In order to facilitate mutual patient support and interaction, Zora provided both synchronous and asynchronous ways of communicating and sharing experiences. The patients talked with each other in real-time through their avatars and they also posted messages and wrote stories for their objects and characters.

Patients reported that using Zora helped them make friends or get support from other kids on dialysis in a moderate way (mean = 3.86; standard deviation =2.41). At the same time, they reported that it greatly helped them to feel more part of a group on dialysis (mean = 4.43; standard deviation =1.62). *"I think that I always was part of the dialysis group but using Zora helped me to get to know the people better because I could talk with them and see their interests, what they like and do not like by going to their virtual homes"*, said a 13 years old patient. Hospital staff perceived that using Zora helped patients a lot to make friends (mean = 4.50; standard deviation =1) and a little less in making them feel part of a group (mean = 3.75; standard deviation =0.5) (see figure 4).

Synchronous Communication: A Private Way to Talk in a Public Space

The hemodialysis unit is a public noisy space where patients are physically together for long periods of time. However, since their beds are far apart from each other, they cannot communicate with each other in a private way. Although the dialysis patients have all the characteristics to form a community, they lack the means to converse while undergoing treatment. Most of the patients particularly liked the fact that Zora provided a good way to communicate with each other in a private way, while undergoing the public event of dialysis. *"I really liked that I could use Zora to talk to other kids who were at a distance. Otherwise I would have to yell across the room. But using Zora was great because others could not eavesdrop on my conversation and I felt more comfortable discussing things. I particularly liked to talk with others about our favorite nurses, without being heard"*, said a 13-year-old patient. On-line conversations were not about dialysis per se, but about favorite video games, movies and activities done during the weekend. Most of the conversations were task-oriented such as helping each other to resolve technical problems and use some of the Zora features.

Asynchronous Communication: A Space to Voice Opinions

Patients used Zora to post messages in each other message boards and to write stories for their objects and characters. This asynchronous way of communicating their feelings was, as one of the nurses noted, *"a way to help patients that weren't on the same shift together to get an understanding of the other patients when visiting their rooms"*.

Asynchronous communication facilitated the creation of a social network by providing a space for patients to voice their opinions, without the burdens of face-to-face and real-time conversation. For example, 17-year-old Larry dropped a case in the *"Temple of Feeling Better"* in which he complained about the increase of his time on the dialysis machine: *"I believe that my time on dialysis is too long. Most of the patients are on for only three and half-hours. Maybe you can pull some string and get it cut back. Thank you. Please reply in Caza's room. Leave a message on the bulletin board"*. He attached the value "pity" to the case but did not define it. At first Larry made his case very small and hid it behind other objects in the virtual temple. Only a very skilled Zora user could find it. Meanwhile, one of the hospital staff noted that Larry was upset and could not talk about what was bothering him. When we pointed out to her the case that he created in the virtual temple, she used it as a jumping board to engage in a conversation with

Larry. Shortly after, Larry made his case big and put it in the center of the temple, thus recognizing the legitimacy of his feelings. Later, Larry engaged with Dr. Joe (a physician) in an exchange by leaving messages in each other's rooms and expressed that he was very happy to be able to voice his opinions and be heard.

9. Zora Design Recommendations

A crucial study outcome was to identify not only the positive aspects of Zora, but also problems. This is important to the design of future interventions tailored to the particular needs of this complex real-world setting.

- **Need of a broader community.** In each dialysis session only three patients were able to connect to Zora at the same time. This was due, on the one hand, to the lack of computers, and in the other hand, to the lack of motivated participants in the required age range and the difficulties of having a broad patient population feeling up to work at the same time. Therefore the Zora community logged in on real-time was very small. *"It is kind of lonely in there [Zora] because when you get on there are not many people with you and it is hard to talk with others"*, said a 15-years-old girl. Other patients pointed out that they felt embarrassed to talk with kids they see everyday about their feelings towards dialysis. They rather talked anonymously. In the future it might be important to increase the number of Zora participants such as involving other dialysis units. Another possibility would be to extend the experience to a large community by including renal transplant and/or at home dialysis patients.

- **Need of more intervention.** Another goal was to observe how patients would use Zora on their own and how they would create a participatory community. However, this patient population requires a lot of direct intervention and guidelines in order to be engaged and motivated in any activity for long periods of time. As the child life specialist noted *"after a point in time the kids get bored with anything, they want bigger and better to keep them entertained, and a lot of them just want to sleep... they don't want to do anything because they are not feeling good."* In future experiences it would be helpful to designate a project coordinator that would propose a tailored syllabus. The creation of a syllabus is a big challenge because, due to their medical treatment, not all the patients can engage in the same type of activities at the same time.

- **The question about dialysis content.** All of the patients agreed that they did not want to encounter in the Zora virtual city any content related to dialysis. They wanted Zora to be a space to escape from dialysis. However, all hospital staff had exactly the opposite opinion. They thought that Zora would be an excellent medium to teach kids about dialysis and to engage them in thinking about the process. For example, one of the social workers suggested the creation of a restaurant because food is a big issue for kids undergoing dialysis. The MIT Media Laboratory staff set up the virtual space and asked patients to create the menus. For our surprise, none of the created menus took in consideration the particular dietary restrictions of this patient population. Following is an excerpt of a conversation that happened in the virtual restaurant:

> *Vitor says 'Washu, do you have any idea about what should we have in the menu?'*
> *Washu says 'shrugs'* ||
> *Vitor says 'What drinks do you think we should have in the menu?'*
> *Washu says 'coffee, tea, ice water, etc....'*

Vitor 'Which ones do you like best?'

Washu says 'I like tea with cream and sugar'

Vitor says 'I've never tried that, what about desserts'

Washu says 'ice cream and there is a Chinese dessert that all the nurses love'

Vitor says 'What kind of food do you like?'

Washu says 'I like Chinese food and Italian foods...noodles and fried rice spaghetti and meat balls"

Marina says 'I wonder if there should be a special menu for people on dialysis...what do you think?'

Washu says 'I guess that is helpful to people but I don't like to be reminded that I need different food'

The question is how to create spaces that engage children in learning and talking about dialysis. These spaces should go beyond displaying information produced by professionals. Patients need to take an active role in their creation. For example, they could be the ones who, working together with the professionals, design the virtual rooms to teach visitors about dialysis. For this to succeed it is important that the activity be authentic, namely real visitors should be invited to walk around these rooms and engage in conversations with the patients. For example, visitors can be kids recently diagnosed with end stage renal disease, medical staff, parents of patients, elementary and high school students interested in medicine.

- **Visualizing data.** Patients reported that using Zora did not help them gain perspective or understanding about their illness (mean = 1.86; standard deviation =1.21). At the psychological level, children did not use Zora to talk about dialysis, but as an escape from it. At the physiological level, Zora did not support patients to explore what happens in their bodies while undergoing dialysis. However, Zora can support both types of interventions in future experiences. On the one hand, a mental health professional can coordinate virtual meetings in the same style than therapeutic communities. On the other hand, the Zora environment can support the collection and display of physiological data provided by the dialysis machines and other medical charts. This data indicates progress in the treatment as well as the level of compliance between visits. If patients were encouraged to pay with this data in a friendly, creative and educational way they could explore "what if" possibilities regarding their own health care. And it would allow researchers to investigate correlations between engagement with Zora and successful medical compliance.

10. Discussion

More and more hospitals are acquiring the means to connect to the Internet. However, connectivity by itself is not enough. We should ask ourselves how can we use the Internet to support therapeutic work already going on in medical facilities. Identity construction environments, such as SAGE and Zora, open up new possibilities for health care. As shown in this chapter, the use of well designed computer technologies to implement well grounded psychotherapeutic interventions is feasible, safe, and useful to patients and staff. Introducing a fun, self-exploratory and community-building computer activity can provide patients with the opportunity to be creative. It help them express themselves and explore aspects of their identity in ways that are generally underplayed and even avoided in the medical setting.

A computer based application that promotes increased coping and resiliency in the face of pediatric illness can make accessible psychotherapeutic interventions that otherwise is only available to those living geographically close to a major pediatric medical center. Identity construction environments such as SAGE and Zora can provide an important opportunity for patients and staff to participate in the process of gaining self-understanding and shared understanding, which are cornerstones to coping and resiliency [11].

Acknowledgements

We thank Seymour Papert, Mitchel Resnick and Sherry Turkle for their advising role, undergraduate research assistant Daniel Vlasic for the implementation of Zora, Darcy Raches for doing the interviews and Matt Pots for his work with patients. We are grateful to Dr. William Harmon, Kristen McGee, and Evelyn Corsini and the nurses and patients at the dialysis unit of Children's Hospital Boston. We also thank Linda Stone, Lili Cheng and the Microsoft Virtual Worlds research group.

* This work was done as part of Marina Ber's doctoral work at the MIT Media Lab.

References

[1] Brem AS, Brem FS, McGrath M, Spirito A. (1988) Psychosocial characteristics and coping skills in children maintained on chronic dialysis. Pediatric Nephrology 2:460-465.

[2] Brownbridge G, Fielding DM. (1994) Psychosocial adjustment and adherence to dialysis treatment regimes. Pediatric Nephrology 8:744-749.[3] Gonzalez-Heydrich J, Bromley D, Strohecker C, Marks J, DeMaso DR, Ackermann E, Gibson S, Shen C, Umaschi M. (1998) "Experience journals: Using computers to share personal stories about illness and medical intervention." MedInf'98, 9th World Congress on Medical Informatics. IOS Press. 1998, pp. 1323-1327.

[4] Turkle, S. (1995) *Life on the screen: Identity in the Age of the Internet.* NY: Simon & Schuster

[5] Bers, M. (forthcoming) " We Are What We Tell: Designing Narrative Environments for Children " In *Narrative Intelligence.* Edited by P.Sengers & Mateas. Amsterdam: John Benjamins.

[6] Papert S. (1980) *Mindstorms: Children, Computers and Powerful Ideas.* New York: Basic Books.

[7] Bers, M.; Ackermann, E.; Cassell, J.; Donegan, B.; Gonzalez-Heydrich, J.; DeMaso, D.; Strohecker, C.; Lualdi, S.; Bromley, D.; Karlin, J. (1998) "Interactive Storytelling Environments: Coping with Cardiac Illness at Boston's Children's Hospital" In Proceedings of Computer-Human Interaction (CHI'98) ACM,pp.603-609.

[8] Bers, M. (1999) "Zora: a Graphical Multi-user Environment to Share Stories about the Self." In Proceedings of Computer Support for Collaborative Learning (CSCL'99), pp. 33-40.

[9] Calvino, I (1972) *Invisible Cities,* NY: Harcourt Brace Jovanovich

[10] Vellon, M. Marple, K. Mitchell, D. & Drucker, S. (1995) "The Architecture of a Distributed Virtual Worlds System". Virtual Worlds Group. Microsoft Research.

[11] Focht L, & Beardslee WR (1996), "Speech after long silence": The use of narrative therapy in a preventive intervention for children of parents with affective disorder. *Family Process* 35:407-422

Future of Health Technology
R.G. Bushko (Ed.)
IOS Press, 2002

Our Wealth, Our Health –
Bellwether Industries for Decision Tools
and Symbiotic Stewardships

Jean A. Wooldridge, M.P.H.

*Strategic Advisor for Cancer Communication Technologies, National Cancer Institute,
Division of Cancer Control and Population Science, Office of the Director, Bethesda, MD,
USA (on loan from the Fred Hutchinson Cancer Research Center, Seattle WA) &
Principal, St. Cloud Communications*

Abstract

This chapter examines the tea leaves of emerging technologies for the most fruitful areas of crossover value to health decisions, by spotting bellwether industries of similar information asymmetries. It examines changing tools and roles for growing consumer-centrism in personal finance, healthcare, private aviation, and law. It seeks to understand the technologies of managing and measuring, the transformations of growing transparencies in our processes, and how an increasing sense of collective stewardship forged between people and their machines can lead beyond effectiveness to wisdom, for individuals, communities, and the world.

"The whole thing reminds me of the uncomfortable feeling I experienced when I first sought out investment advice. . . . .I concluded that I had to undertake the generalist's job myself; I had to take the high-level management of my investments into my own hands. Similarly, given the structure of the medical practice associated with prostate cancer, that's the only viable choice any patient has."
Andy Grove, Co-Founder and Chair, Intel [1]

"In the end, a symbiotic culture composed of human and digital individuals may be a more effective steward of the earth's resources than humans would be by themselves."
Donald D. Chamberlin, author and ACM Fellow [2]

1. Introduction

As ubiquitous computing becomes a reality, individuals and communities will find their bodies and their actions creating an exuberant wellspring of rich, complex data. These biological and sociological data can be ignored, used alone or shared with others for various reasons – for personal gain or for social good. Issues that will seem fractal in nature will spring from these converging technologies in genomics, proteomics, nanotechnology, biosensors, body networks, agent technologies, distributed networks and supercomputers, and smart environments. They will spur entire industries and advocacy movements, and puzzle even the most far-sighted policy makers.

So, where should our short-term strategic binoculars for health decision tools be focused?

The industries that can serve as bellwethers are those with the greatest information imbalances among stakeholders, have similar characteristics for their consumer decisions, and use new technologies in different ways and at different rates of adoption than healthcare [3]. The ones we consider here are: financial, private aviation, and personal law.

Technology most transforms industries with the greatest information asymmetries. These bellwether industries share sharp asymmetries, demographics, rising consumer demand, and some overlapping impact of economic and environmental issues. (For example, just as today's physicians will not be able to serve the aging population and their chronic diseases, today's 36,000 certified financial planners cannot serve all 100 million U.S. households.)[4]

Consumer-centrism is the future for all these industries, as seen in how people are currently using new self-help tools in finance, health, private aviation, and personal and small business law, and how they will be using them. AOL/Time Warner understands this shift wherein consumers will purchase "customized bundles of content properties across various media", on demand [5]. Tools in retail, entertainment, and education [6] are also significant because of the level of private investment and early adoption.

In finance, there is a customer self-service revolution. Celent Communications predicts that rapid growth will bring online financial users to 20 million by 2005 in the U.S. It finds that services are moving from a marketing ploy to a competitive necessity, and, at the same time, moving from simple calculators to sophisticated planners and probabilistic simulators to give people more control of their wealth [7]. Increasingly personalized tools, even "bots" (cyberspace robots), are appearing to add more natural consumer interface choices.

In healthcare, industry, government, and academic thinkers are also acknowledging a customer revolution, following the lead of pioneer self-care advocates such as Tom Ferguson, M.D., of The Ferguson Report and Harvard [8]. Dr. Ferguson proposed the transition from industrial-age medicine to information-age health care in The Millennium Whole Earth Catalogue" in 1994, with individuals managing their health, pulling in various resources, including peers, and using health professionals in well-defined roles of facilitator, partner, or authority [9]. CEO Craig Froude, of WellMed, online health management services, states, "We are often compared to the financial world and we enjoy that comparison. People are taking more and more control over their financial welfare and well being, and we can do the same with their health assets, so that in one place they can manage their entire family's well-being." [10]. Federal agencies increasingly recognize this in funded programs:

- In 1995 the Office of Disease Prevention and Health Promotion began a series of conferences around public/private partnerships for networked consumer health information, and began a science panel to explore an evidence-based approach to interactive health communications using emerging technologies, which led to the report "Wired for Health and Well-Being" and a summit for public and private technology developers [11]

- In 1995, the National Institute of Technology Standards, Advanced Technology Program began funding research with matching industry partner funds for healthcare information infrastructure, including applications to directly meet consumer needs [12]

- In 1997 the U.S. government's National Library of Medicine opened up the world's largest database of medical literature, MEDLINE, to the public on the Internet [13]

- In 1998, a Food and Drug Administration survey reported a major trend for home medical devices for prevention and disease monitoring by consumers [14]
- In 1999, the National Cancer Institute held a conference on risk communication and helping health decision-makers[15], and in 2000 launched a three-year budget initiative, "Extraordinary Opportunities in Cancer Communications" to leverage technology for all audiences [16].
- In 2001, Institute of Medicine reports, ("Informing the Future: Critical Issues in Health" and "Crossing the Quality Chasm: A New Health System for the 21st Century"), recommended revamping the entire health system over the next decade to make patient needs and preferences the centerpiece of care [17,18]. In June, 2001, the Robert Wood Johnson Foundation released "The eHealth Landscape: A Terrain Map of Emerging Information and Communication Technologies in Health and HealthCare" [19]

Alex Pentland and The Media Lab's Health Special Interest Group of the Massachusetts Institute of Technology present a reasonable view of the future:
"Nanotechnology, biosensors, body networks, and smart homes are combining to give consumers the tools to take control of their health and maintain their lifestyle. This emerging network of technologies can also help create a web of interpersonal relationships that reinforce healthy behaviors and medical compliance. The detailed, continuous and individual data from such a network is synergistic with advances in both human genome and conventional medical research, and offers the potential for creation of a data-rich, personalized, and preventative medical science." [20]

General aviation and law have smaller audiences than finance, but their tools and trends offer good lessons for healthcare and share many of the issues (high risk, incomplete knowledge, history of information asymmetries among stakeholders, shifts of power, etc.). In general aviation, for example, a multimillion-dollar program for small aircraft called, "Highway in the Sky", funded chiefly by NASA, with the aviation industry, will bring an advanced set of pictorial tools armed with intuitive menus to the cockpits of future small airplanes. An MIT researcher involved in pilot interfaces predicts, "I could take someone with no training and in five minutes have him flying a plane all the way through a landing." [21] In personal law, the article, "Online Law: Why the Legal System Will Never Be the Same Again" shares important perspectives:
"The movement to reform American's inaccessible, overpriced legal system has puttered along for years, scoring some small successes, but few significant ones. The Internet is fast changing all that. Commercial, government and nonprofit websites are making legal information and self-help law tools directly available to tens of millions of average Americans. By giving consumers so much more information and so many more choices, the Internet is fast changing how people find, hire and work with lawyers. That makes it possible for people to accomplish legal tasks -- from getting a divorce to filing a patent application -- that until just a few years ago had to be left to lawyers"[22]

2. Management

The following observations explore the usefulness of bellwether industries for helping us to wisely tend these shifts to self-management in healthcare. Of critical importance, is to ground these devices and analytic tools with a deeply personalized context of values. For as we grow in understanding of how technology is transforming our healthcare, we will also grow in understanding of how our individual health is embedded in the rich fabric of the health of our communities and of our world and how that translates to a wider stewardship of resources. This human stewardship increasingly appears to be in symbiosis (hopefully) with our technological progeny, as noted by such thinkers as Ray Kurtzweil (*The Age of Spiritual Machines*) [23], Michael D. McDonald [24,25], Bill Joy [26], Howard Bloom [27], and Leonard Kleinrock, the UCLA scientist who established the first Arpanet node three decades ago [28].

2.1 Management: You Can't Manage What You Can't Measure

Businesses know this. Individuals forget. Perhaps that is one reason why people tend to have trouble managing their wealth and managing their health.

To make good decisions in wealth and health, people need to have equal access to information, understand the critical impact of their decisions on their quality of life (particularly for decisions made early in life), be able to work with incomplete and dynamic data within time and fiscal constraints, understand risk, have various literacies (financial, economic, health, scientific, and technological), and be able to evaluate and work with a variety of professionals and resources. Real time measurements set into meaningful contexts for influencing our daily decisions and long-term planning are hard to come by. Particularly for decisions made when young, such as diet and saving.

Financial planning tools and advice, once the province of high net-worth households, are now within the reach of the average online family. Even the cheapest basic service of, for example, Netfolio, provides customized annual advice of which stocks to sell or keep to get the best tax outcome. Managing personal spending habits has been revolutionized by online banking and by software programs like Money and Quicken, but they still take continual self-discipline and attention to detail. How these habits fit into larger contexts and investment decisions along a lifetime of decision making are becoming easier to understand via analytical and graphical interface software.

Personal health management is receiving increased attention, as the burden of disease shifts to chronic care and as the role of behavioral choices in disease, such as diet, exercise, smoking, and alcohol consumption, is increasingly acknowledged. It's estimated that "lifestyle behaviors alone contribute to 50% of an individual's health status." [29] This, combined with the swelling demographics of older Americans bringing their emerging health problems to bear on overworked medical systems, has prompted the investment community and research agencies to pay attention to personal health management technology for monitoring devices and planning programs.

Behaviorally-generated health data is difficult to obtain and demands self-discipline: try tracking calories and fat grams. The current medical devices aren't uniformly tied to useful planning tools and many, like telemedicine home devices, were developed more with the health professional, than with a self-caring patient, in mind [30].

However, pieces of the puzzle are present. We don't have yet a smart tooth with a chip that discreetly chirps when we are within 10% of our desired caloric intake for the day, but we can strap on an electronic pedometer that synchs with our computer to graph our athletic progress. Online diet sites offer customized interactivity. At least one study found that weight loss tripled for people monitoring themselves interactively with the Internet versus people only using the Internet for information [31]. Monitoring will become more convenient, as interactive textiles translate lab breakthroughs to store shelves, with shirts (Sensatex) that can track heart rate and breathing, and parkas (Columbia) that can track and respond to body temperatures [32].

Consumers will gain more control as the locus of health management moves back to the home, where it was before 1900. William A. Herman, of the Food and Drug Administration's Center for Devices and Radiological Health, observes, with regard to the current demographics, economics, and technology forces: "Ironically, it's beginning to seem that this period of apparently normal centralization [*..to special facilities..]* was a temporary aberration. A century later, gains in technology are moving care back to home settings". He predicts that "...home-centered capability is expected to become a catalyst for a huge health paradigm shift from 'last-minute heroic intervention' to 'consumer-driven individualized prediction, prevention, early detection, and maintenance.'" [33,34]

2.2 Management: Sometimes You Can't Manage What You Can Measure

Good data doesn't guarantee good management. In wealth as in health, often we know what we're supposed to do or even want to do, but we don't do it. Other times, the biggest challenge is figuring out what we do want to do.

Citibank Private Bank has a full-time psychologist available for wealthy clients and estate matters. In many industries, multi-disciplinary teams, including cultural anthropologists, are forming to help us to become more self-aware. Affective computing using robots, computers and sensing devices that can mirror our emotional states by measuring physical gestures, unconscious movements, and physiological responses will help us to learn (more than we wanted) about ourselves. These sensing technologies will collect data independently and transform it into personalized learning tools, intimately responsive to our needs.

For example, a posture-monitoring chair covering that recognizes fidgeting was presented at the year 2000 International Mechanical Engineering Congress and Exposition [32]. Are you having trouble following some complex treatment choice information in a teleconference with your doctor about a recently diagnosed heart condition? A future chair, programmed with information about how you learn under pressure, could, even before you're aware of discomfort, prompt a change in camera angle, or in learning modality - from real time face-to-face to text, video, or instant messaging with another doctor – to help you stay on track in your discussion

2.3 Management: Sometimes You Shouldn't Manage What You Can Measure

Measurement tools are imperfect. Sometimes the very data they leave out are the critical ones for the best decisions. Wall Street is responding to this by moving from deterministic, linear retirement calculators to probabilistic simulations, which add in worst-case scenarios. In making decisions in wealth and health even the most sophisticated simulation will leave out the historical and loving knowledge of us that an old friend would bring.

Fortunately, there are researchers wrestling with these "ineffable" factors in our decision-making. In trying to measure intuition, compassion, empathy, and aesthetics, you can lose the ability to access them, according to Boisot's E-space theories and other recent educational models like Kolb's learning cycle, and Sch n's reflection-in-action and reflective practicums. Joseph V. Henderson, M.D., M.P.H., Director of Dartmouth Medical School's Interactive Media Lab, is ensuring that these dimensions are brought into technology, theory and applications for physician education. He is developing a model for virtual education for primary care physicians on topics such as HIV counseling that capture these important dimensions [36].

3. Transformations

Technology transforms industries with the greatest information asymmetries. As technology progresses through different societal sectors and industries, we can watch to see where there is the greatest unequal distribution of information (read "power"). That point of "pain" is where we will see the greatest changes in stakeholder roles and how people work together. The mere existence of diverse information channels implies opacities and imbalances of information and power, and affects people's bargaining power and their ability to make a sound decision. Because the financial sector and the health sector have striking imbalances, their transformations by technology will be equally impressive. Many people, besides ourselves, create the data context in which we manage our wealth and health; channels and "informational chokeholds" abound.

3.1 Transformations: Technology In Wealth And Health

Transformation watchers are alert not only to points of pain, investment dollars, and policy changes and demographics, they also watch technology convergence, early-stage venture capital fund flows, and "people flows" as industries transform.

In the wealth arena, in the late 1990's, the growth of online day traders influenced the market with their collective individual actions, and spurred regulatory bodies to curb their effect. Consumers demand more sophisticated tools. Of the top U.S. financial institutions surveyed in 2000, over 80% already offer some form of simple online planning tool (calculators), but only 20% offer sophisticated planning tools, like Monte Carlo simulations. By 2005, Celent expects this proportion to flip [37]. Some of the technologies shaping online personal finance include streaming/real-time portfolios the direct live stock quotes to PCs, direct-access trading that bypass the middleman brokerage personnel, account aggregations that work as "screen scrapers" to find all of your accounts at various websites and compile them on one screen, and in-car investing, such as the partnership between Fidelity and GM's OnStar that allows you to use voice commands to access your account or place a trade while you are stuck in traffic [38].

In the health arena, the effect of the individual is also becoming measurable, at least in process measures. Healthcare futurists advise of the coming consumer-centric healthcare world, fueled in part by the demographics of the aging boomers who have assertively transformed most institutions on their march through life's milestones, and most certainly will do so with a healthcare system ill-equipped to provide the level of personalized service they expect.

The technologies developed in other industries and appearing in other parts of our lives also will lead to expectations for health care technologies. The "worried well", are becoming the "wired well" [39]. They are seeing that other industries, such as automotive safety, are using sensors to monitor critical functions, in addition to helping customers use their products. Backup warning systems can prevent you from backing into a wall or a car or keep you from running over a tricycle, or a child [40].

In the public agenda, evidence of change is appearing in government standards for health privacy, and culturally and linguistically appropriate service in health care are making processes more transparent and including previously excluded stakeholders [41].
Scientists are reaching out through online multimedia projects, such as "Coffee Break", a collection of interactive tutorials at the National Center for Biotechnology Information at the National Library of Medicine. A recent title under "What's Brewing?" was "Honey, I shrunk the genome [42]." Consumer advocacy programs are securing heightened recognition within agencies. Trusted government sites, such as Healthfinder and CancerNet are often the first stop for savvy patients." [43] Dramatically:

"In 1997 the U.S. government's National Library of Medicine opened up the world's largest database of medical literature to the public on the Internet. Use of MEDLINE, once the near-exclusive domain of doctors and scientists, soon skyrocketed from 7 million to over 200 million searches a year. 'Consumers have powered that explosion,' says Eve-Marie Lacroix, chief of the public services division of the National Library of Medicine. 'They're starved for medical information.' " [44]

The demographics of caregivers and the approaching "juggernaut of chronic illness", also will force change and bring investment into assistive technologies. Molly Mettler of Healthwise, Inc, notes: "The blossoming of new consumer attitudes, the codification of evidence-based medicine, and the reach of the Internet are combining to turn current day practice of disease management upside down. These trends, all documented by various forecasts, point to a near-future in which the majority of chronic illness care will be custom designed for and by each individual partner. (*Chronic illness*) is huge, it's costly and it's accelerating. Consider this – by the year 2010: 120 million Americans, about 40% of the total population, will be living with a chronic illness. ...If we try to extend today's approach to chronic care, which is fragmented, system-centric, and non-empowering, the system will simply collapse. We just can't train enough providers to meet the need."[45]

The impact of the government's Human Genome Project will be felt across the entire health continuum from prevention to end-of-life issues. It will lead to profound changes in medical practice and accelerate consumer-centrism, with genetic scans for diagnoses, accelerated drug discoveries, tissue engineering, nano-machines for medical tasks, cloning for transplants, phamacogenomics for personalized drugs and targeted deliveries, and a shift in paradigm from treating acute illness to predicting and preventing diseases by managing their risks [46].

Efforts to address these demographic and scientific challenges and coming consumer-centrism, include research by the Center for Future Health at the University of Rochester, NY, where its "smart medical home" encourages academe and industry partners to focus on the individual, and affordable home-based technology.

3.2 Transformations: Transparencies and tools

Processes and information are being made more transparent by emerging tools and the expertise of "information architects", such as Richard Saul Wurman and Edward Tufte [47,48].

Bots (robots in cyberspace) are migrating from the video game world to bridge text and live chat. Pioneer Funds introduced three financial "CyberGuides" of artificially intelligent "bots" [49] and photo-avatars are helping patients and families feel more comfortable when undergoing extensive treatments far from home [50].

Collaborative filtering software and intelligent agent technologies, such as those developed by the Intelligent Agents Lab at MIT, under Patti Maes, which can give rise to "communityware", which connects like-minded large, decentralized groups of people for pursuing interactions. Applications include "personalization, user profiling, information filtering, privacy, recommender systems, electronic commerce, communityware, learning user profiles" and reputation, negotiation, and coordination mechanisms [51]. These technologies can build trust in online communities, and speed comparative healthcare analyses.

Groupware combined with visualization tools help stakeholders make better decisions. A collaborative graphical interface from IBM facilitated a Colorado land use issue discussion "by airing political, economic, emotional, and environmental concerns in a controlled, moderated setting." [52]

Distributed computing (peer-to-peer applications) involves the public in research, especially for biotechnology, by creating "distributed" supercomputers with cycle-sharing and large databases. It began with the SETI (Search for Extraterrestrial Intelligence) project in Berkeley, California in 1999. Intel's "PC Philanthropy" project, launched in 2001, wants cycle-sharing to be as common as signing up to be an organ donor when you get your driver's license. Brigham Young University is constructing a global genealogical genetic database with the help of individual volunteers who provide a pedigree chart, one tablespoon of blood, and a consent form. File-sharing a la Napster will enable cancer patients to enrich current online communities. Some commercial companies, like Porivo Technologies, are beginning to pay people rent for sharing power from their PCs [53].

Affective computing aims to create machines that can "sense, recognize and understand human emotions, together with the skills to respond in an intelligent, sensitive, and respectful manner toward the user and his/her emotions"[54] Work at the MIT Media Lab, under Roz Picard, includes expressive glasses which can learn an individual's learning patterns and graphically display their interest or confusion expressions, by measuring muscle movement in the corrugator and frontalis (eyebrow) muscles. At the Blue Eyes project at the IBM Almaden Lab, cues of users' emotional and physical state are captured on video cameras, and analyzed to provide information that can be used by machines to adjust how they interact with humans and, even more directly, devices such as the emotion mouse, are being prepared that can correlate physiological data with emotional states [55].

Visualization tools for "live" dynamic databases create transparencies of complex data, adaptable to different learning styles. The World Economic Forum uses technology from The Brain as a Knowledge Navigator to visualize conference proceedings in six dimensions: region, industry, event, topic, content, and people and to show how these relate. [56] One epidemiologist "combined multivariate categorical analyses and interactive statistical graphics to provide a novel interface to a multimedia data set (text, images, audio) dealing with Vietnam War trauma [57]." SmartMoney (smartmoney.com) uses "Map of the Market" to show changing financial trends dynamically with intuitive graphic interfaces, color coding, and detailed data-mining drill-down boxes. It has sparked interest in adaptation for audiences with varying quantitative literacies, including cross disciplinary teams [58].

Simulations with haptics and other sensor technologies are incorporated into games, training and problem-solving. Pharmaceutical companies such as Entelos, are borrowing from aircraft engineering. Simulations for Boeing's 777, which has 3 million parts, ran computer flights and crashes under all weather conditions before building any physical models. Entelos is testing drugs for diseases like asthma, by distilling scientific article data into parameters and equations for "in silico" biology. These simulations mimic the body's complex interactions between genes and molecular events [59]. Avatars and semi-immersive virtual environments are conveying a sense of personal connection for patients and teens [60]. Commercial simulations for individuals are popular, such as Microsoft's "Flight Simulator", which sold 21million copies by 1999 [61], and SimHealth, a variant of SimCity, which challenged players during the 1990's: "Tame the beast that brought Capitol Hill to a screeching halt. No, not Socks the cat – the health care crisis. You make the tough political choices to reform the system – and you live with the consequences." [62]

4. Wealth and Health Decisions: Very Personal, Very Critical to Our Quality of Life

In health and wealth, as in aviation and law, the decisions we make are some of the most difficult in our lives. They share characteristics which can illuminate how we choose. Some of these are inherent and some are "bound" to current resources and systems. Others carry seeds of the technology symbiosis which is evolving.

Table 1
Characteristics of Decisions in Health and Bellwether Industries

---

INHERENT

Decisions have great consequences
- Poor decisions can have irrevocable consequences for the quality of our life (i.e., loss of liberty, of life).

Decisions are time-bound
- Decisions made during our youth may have great consequences for our future (i.e., not smoking, exercise, diet;, saving habits).
- They are dependent upon the state-of-the-science at the time the decision is made (i.e., physicians endorsed smoking in the 1940's).

Decisions are resource-bound
- Our level of education and access to information resources determine the quality of the data upon which we base our decisions.

Decisions are based on incomplete and dynamic data which:
- Change constantly
- Reside in different places (peer-reviewed literature, professional and consumer anecdotes, gray literature)
- Blur in info smog overload

Decisions are made in the ineffable realm of values, emotions, and intuition, which are factors often not included in risk calculators
- There is an emotional charge to these decisions – a valence, if you will.
- We don't often understand our own decision-processes.
- We need to factor in our individual styles of making decisions, weights for rationale and intuitive processes, and involving others' experiences.

RESOURCE-BOUND

Decisions are subject to the limitations of current tools and often are made without understanding:
- Consequences (i.e., without the perspectives of robust simulations, or of personalized data, or of examples of choices made by people who most resemble us)
- Risks and our tolerance for them
- Knowledge domains of the context (i.e., having literacies in health, science, statistics and probability, finance, economics, environment, and public/private institutional interactions, technology)

SYSTEM-BOUND

Decisions still reflect stakeholder power imbalances and incentive structures of social and economic systems.
- They are based on the underestimation of the consumer's capacity for information.

Decisions are still often made without a consumer-centric menu of professional services and roles
- There is a "bundling" of professional services that doesn't encourage consumers to select the content, level of technical discourse, or the role and level of professional help they need.
- The professionals, as the only authorized door into wealth and health information, have until recently, chosen the content, the level, and set the professional/consumer roles.
- Although financial planners are pioneering changes, most doctors and lawyers still don't advertise access by roles (from expert to coach to partner). In the last twenty years, the right to second, third, and more medical opinions has become accepted, but is jeopardized during economic downturns.

Decisions are made with the help of professionals who don't always form opinions uniformly or objectively
- Especially in medicine, geographic practice variations reflect striking differences in how care is delivered and how more or less unrelated it is to evidence.

With all these tools, consumers need assurance of privacy, quality, evaluation, protection, and evidence-based criteria. Various government and private groups are addressing standards (e.g., Health on the Net, the Internet Healthcare Coalition, the American Medical

Association, the World Wide Web) with various laws and reports, (e.g., The Health Insurance Portability and Accountability Act of 1996, and the 1999 report "Wired for Health and Well-Being: the Emergence of Interactive Health Communication").

A Wall Street Journal article noted that a March 2001 report on healthcare quality from the U.S. Institute of Medicine, a governmental advisory agency, declares, "Between the health care we have and the care we could have lies not just a gap, but a chasm." Even when there is strong scientific evidence, it can take 15 to 20 years for new drugs and devices to be used in general practice by doctors and hospitals [63]. Despite pitfalls and perils, these decision tools hold promise for bringing the latest evidence into practice much earlier. Evidence-based medicine and meetings on risk communication, such as the 1999 conference at the National Cancer Institute, note the extraordinary opportunity afforded through the new technologies for communicating and evolving evidence-based libraries of best practices [64].

4.1 Decision Tools: Examples From Wealth

In 2000, Fidelity's website had a scenario for a surviving spouse who needed to deal with estate planning. "Karen found herself alone for the first time at age 62, when her husband died suddenly of a massive heart attack at the age of 67. All of her life, Karen had focused her energies on caring for her family and household. She had neither the training nor the experience to prepare her for the weighty financial decisions that now befell her. What is her financial status and how can she best make decisions to preserve her quality of life?"

The scenario works through various assets, a monthly pension income, a 401(k), and IRA, and an annuity contract from a life insurance company. What should Karen do with these assets? Should she opt for the monthly income or choose the lump sum pension distribution? Should she consolidate assets, or keep them where they are?"

In the commercial sector we find places like Fidelity coming forward with many decision tools for people like Karen, and a commitment to multi-modal education, (phone, e-mail, voice, and in person). Industry-wide we can expect to see increasingly sophisticated online financial planning tools with updated capabilities, which will integrate customer data and spending habits to highly personalize action plans. Business strategists envision web interactions like the following in the near future, using the web's ability to dynamically customize content similar to the following: "Hello, Peter. When you last visited and completed your learning profile and long-term plans, you said you financed your home at 8%. We wanted you to know that rates have dropped to 7% and we've run some calculations. By refinancing now, you would save $400 a month after fees. Attached are forms which are mostly completed, in case you decide to refinance with Sue Barlett from Eagle Mortgage, one of our valued partners." [65]

4.2 Decision Tools: Examples From Health

Understanding and evaluating medical information is a difficult task for laypeople. Even individuals who are highly skilled in risk assessment and analyzing quantitative data can be frustrated when it comes to their own illness.

Intel's Co-Founder and Chair, Andy Grove, Ph.D., addressed this dilemma in Fortune's May 1996 cover story "Taking on Prostate Cancer". With no clear consensus on treatment and few tools to predict risks of side effect, prostate cancer has left those affected without good decision-support data. Dr. Grove, concluded that: "There is no good gatekeeper in this business. Your general internist is not; the field of prostate cancer is a complex and changing specialty. Neither is your urologist; urologists have a natural preference toward surgery, perhaps because urologists are surgeons and surgery is what they know best. Any other treatment is deemed experimental even if it has just as much data associated with it. My review of the data led me to conclude that there are viable alternatives.....

The whole thing reminds me of the uncomfortable feeling I experienced when I first sought our investment advice. After a while, it dawned on me that financial advisers, well-intentioned and competent as they might have been, were all favoring their own financial instruments. I concluded that I had to undertake the generalist's job myself; I had to take the high –level management of my investments into my own hands. Similarly, given the structure of the medical practice associated with prostate cancer, that's the only viable choice any patient has. If you look after your investments, I think you should look after your life as well. Investigate things, come to your own conclusions, don't take any one recommendation as gospel."[66]

Fortunately, in the years since Dr. Grove drew this conclusion, technology developers began work on new decision-support tools, although the scientific evaluation of these tools is still in early stages. One firm is NexCura (operator of cancerfacts.com), a developer of an online data-driven tool called The Cancer Profiler™ [67]. This tool was created by a medical device inventor who had recently developed a new method to stage prostate cancer. While lecturing to patients around the country, he discovered that men were confused about how to use the vast quantities of data from the Internet for their individual situation. When the developer's own father was diagnosed with prostate cancer, he researched this dilemma further. He was stunned to find that there were no good resources for helping patients weigh scientific data, treatment options, and side effects against significant quality of life issues, such as the risk of impotence and incontinence.

The Prostate Cancer Profiler was his answer to this problem and people have responded. From the fall of 2000 to the spring of 2001, cancerfacts.com grew from 10,000 to over 21,000 users, employing all 16 cancer Profilers online to help frame discussions with themselves, their families, and their doctors. The Profiler provides extensive personalized information based on 128 data points that patients enter online. These entries relate to medical history, test results, and personal preferences for quality of life, which the Profiler then matches with scientific data from cancer studies in the literature and prepares an interactive bibliography with links to research studies.

Surprisingly, NexCura found people running simulations with their online files, sometimes several times a month, to try different lab data and personal quality of life preferences. They tried scenarios such as "What if the tumor grew? What if I changed my ratings of this side effect? Would my treatment choices change?"

This new tool has hit a critical nerve for providing online, interactive quantitative data analysis and simulations and informing stakeholder discussions between patients, families and health care providers, as well as peers.

We can expect ahead, that, just as retirement tools in the personal finance arena are moving to more complex simulations, and more critical evidence-based evaluation, so will these health decision tools

4.3 Decision Tools: Examples From Aviation

As technology moves through industries and flattens the information asymmetries, power shifts. In health care, power is shifting between physicians and patients. In general aviation, between air traffic controllers and private pilots. One physician who understands this power shift and embraces the value of aviation as a bellwether industry is Richard Rockefeller, M.D.

Dr. Rockefeller practices primary care in Maine. He is the founder and President of Health Commons Institute, an instructor in family medicine in the Maine Medical Center-

Mercy Hospital Family Practice Residency Program, and Chair of the U.S. Advisory Board of Doctors Without Borders. He is also a private pilot.

Dr. Rockefeller uses the concept of "onboard medical guidance" to draw parallels between the PKC Knowledge Coupler, a "point-of-care" software program which links patient data to scientific literature, which he uses in his medical practice, and onboard navigation guidance systems for small planes. His institute champions "information technologies that support better medical decisions and free up health care participants for the human work of wellness and healing." [68]

As a physician, Dr. Rockefeller feels that it is unrealistic to expect the professional to keep abreast of the 20,000 new articles in the biomedical literature each year. He believes that using computers in discussions with his patients leverages his skills and medical art. As a pilot, he observes that even small planes can now afford sophisticated aviation onboard graphical systems which keep pilots abreast of critical information such as weather, land features, other aircraft, etc., giving pilots more independence from controllers. He notes that "...given patients' growing desire to understand and control their care, and given the extent to which online tools and services are already empowering them to do so, the default relationship between doctor and patient is bound to change...This relationship will more likely come to resemble that of pilot and copilot rather than pilot and passenger. And even the question of who gets to play which role may alternate depending on circumstances." [69]

4.4 Decision Tools: Examples From Law

The legal field traditionally has had great imbalances of information among stakeholders. But Internet technologies are accelerating the shift of power from lawyers to the non-professionals. Like healthcare, law is moving from professional- to consumer-centrism.

Thirty-five years ago, the legal self-help movement began with one book, How to Avoid Probate. Now, a leading publisher, Nolo Press, has more than 100 titles, and projects over $13 million in sales for 2001. Its online consumers access an encyclopedia, a dictionary, legal updates, and "Auntie Nolo's" commonsense advice [70]. Academics are publishing curricula online, with 47 cyberlaw course websites free at a University of Pittsburgh site. And, state governments are joining: Arizona set up a self-service center in 1995 with access by phone, Web or in-person. Without using a lawyer, a battered spouse can obtain a domestic violence protection order on the same day of application.

Ralph Warner, Executive Publisher at Nolo found that in just five years, consumers online could: find the law, get legal questions answered, prepare and file documents, resolve disputes (online mediation is just emerging), find a lawyer, and buy unbundled, tailored services from lawyers. These tailored services are a striking departure from the past: "Lawyers have traditionally dictated fees, conditions of representation and legal strategy to their clients. For most problems, this meant the attorney would quote a hefty hourly fee, insist on handling the entire job, and assert whatever professional gravitas was necessary to call the shots. People who wanted to save some money by doing some of the legal work themselves, making key decisions, or consulting a lawyer only for coaching on particularly difficult aspects of a case, were usually scolded that a 'person who represents himself has a fool for a client.' In just a very few years, the Internet has transformed the way legal services are bought and sold. ... For example, lawyers might offer, separately, information only, document review, legal opinions, dispute resolution and coaching." [71] Imagine parallel unbundling for healthcare services.

5. Bellwether Cockpit Scans

A pilot's bodily senses may not always relay trustworthy perceptions; when flying in clouds, you can't tell if the plane is flying level by how you feel. So, when flying under instrument flight rules, pilots perform routine visual cockpit scans to check data from the plane's instruments and adjust their piloting. Hopefully, we'll be able to do that for our bodies in the future, but for right now, this is a helpful metaphor for healthcare strategic planners. And for people committed to building bridges for sharing knowledge between societal sectors.

Four levels of scanning are useful: the bellwether industries, the business horizons within them, edited sources, and the sources for earliest market intelligence. Each level brings its own opportunity for strategic intelligence and potential partners to ensure that the interests of the healthcare consumer and the behavioral scientific community are adding value to the product development cycle. This is crucial for the evaluation and diffusion/dissemination areas, where there long has been a disconnect between the "feast of research and the famine of diffusion and dissemination". [72]

Scanning bellwether industries, like finance, aviation, and law, reveals new technology tools and consumer patterns linked to those industries' decision characteristics. Within those bellwether industries, we can be watching for trends and product development across the business horizons (short-range of 12-24 months, mid-range of 2-5 years, and long-range of 5-15 years). At these points, it is easiest to determine, with appropriate partners (i.e., research and development groups in technology companies and industry-partnered academic centers) how the consumer and scientific communities bring value to the table.

There are many "edited" sources of information and strategic partners. These include research firms such as Forrester, digest subscription services such as COR Healthcare Resources, newsletters such as SNS Newsletter, and Release 1.0, conferences such as TED (Technology, Entertainment and Design), RoundTable, Agenda, and Pop!Tech, high-tech industry online and hardcopy magazines, such as Industry Standard (R.I.P.), Red Herring, and Upside, e-mail 'zines such as the Kaiser Daily Health Policy Report and email lists such as venturewire.com. For earliest market intelligence, outside corporate and government research and development labs, hints can be gathered from:

- technology convergence (when two or more technologies reach a mass for broad acceptance of an application; usually discussed at engineering conferences),
- people flows (recruiters helping to place high-profile executives or serial entrepreneurs into new sectors, bringing validation and money),
- fund flows (revealed by early-stage venture capital investments and strategic alliances, best seen in the top 20 U.S. "blue chip" VC firms with substantial early-stage investments, such as Kleiner Perkins and Crosspoint, as listed in the National Venture Capital Association Yearbook.) [73]

Hopefully, these public and private sector dialogues will become more accepted practice as the benefits are examined and publicized by new groups researching and supporting inter- and trans-disciplinary work in health and environmental sciences, such as the Hybrid Vigor Institute [74,75], and as government agencies require cross-sector partnering in research.

6. The Far Horizon

Technology, ethics, and global thinking are shaping our approaching future. Researchers at the Oxygen Project, at MIT, and the Endeavor Project, at the University of California at Berkeley, are working on what the early ubiquitous computing environments might look like. Many think that the supercomputers, desktop PCs, handhelds, smartphones, and

MEMs (microelectromechanical systems) of the current networks will simply disappear and become pervasive, like today's electrical power grid or like a future "smart dust" [76].

As we develop these technologies, we must simultaneously develop programs for examining their ethical implications. The rapid development of these networks and other converging technologies hold great promise and great peril [77]. Ubiquitous networks, genetic engineering, nanotechnology, and robotics, all tax our social dialogue and our wisdom. Profound ethical questions arise for us as individuals and as members of our global community.

After visiting a wired senior-care facility that provides health monitoring, Bill Donahue in the Atlantic Monthly asked: Will we equate surveillance with freedom? Oatfield Estates in Portland, Oregon, e-monitors every move of elderly residents via an infrared badge and sensors in ceilings and walls. Beds transmit weights and record restless sleep to attending staff, and if an Alzheimer patient wanders into the kitchen, the burners lose power [78].

Bill Joy, Co-Founder of Sun Microsystems, noted in his provocative WIRED article, "Why the Future Doesn't Need Us", that we need to have planetary level safeguards on how we use new technologies that are converging: "The 21st-century technologies - genetics, nanotechnology, and robotics (GNR) - are so powerful that they can spawn whole new classes of accidents and abuses. Most dangerously, for the first time, these accidents and abuses are widely within the reach of individuals or small groups. They will not require large facilities or rare raw materials. Knowledge alone will enable the use of them. Thus we have the possibility not just of weapons of mass destruction but of knowledge-enabled mass destruction (KMD), this destructiveness hugely amplified by the power of self-replication." [79]

An example of wise foresight was the establishment of the Ethical, Legal, and Social Implications Program, (ELSI) as an integral part of the U.S. National Human Genome Research Institute (NHGRI). NHGRI has committed 5 percent of its annual research budget to study ELSI issues at the same time the basic science is being studies so that ELSI solutions can be developed before the science is integrated into healthcare practice [80].

Global and systems thinking are increasingly informing the strategies of private corporations and public institutions as they seek to understand individuals, communities, nations, and the world. The World Resources Institute's Digital Dividends online database captures case studies for public/private partnerships to bring "the benefits of connectivity and participation in the e-economy to all of the world's people" [81]. Diverse partners, including the Rockefeller Foundation, BBC World Service, the European Union, and WHO fund another global venture, the Communication Initiative, which tracks and shares the use of electronic communications in international development [82]. The use of complexity theory for understanding how the nonlinear dimensions of social, cultural, economic, technical, and ethics meet in the "crucible" of telehealth is increasingly acknowledged [83]. Multidisciplinary research in health, prevention, and chronic disease management is also moving to a larger playing field as it reviews how individual choices, the physical and social environments, and the economy play into disease or health.

UNESCO's Observatory on the Global Information Society, the U.S. Central Intelligence Agency, and Sandia Labs, are all factoring health into their agendas in new ways, citing public health or aging populations, as security threats due to potential destabilization of national infrastructures. The World Health Organization and the United Nations have put the interrelatedness of public and private health, economies, and social justice on high agendas, particularly with the increased scale of terrorist attacks in September 2001.

Health as a broad concept for our bodies, our communities, and our world will become firmly anchored by the myriad of datapoints woven into understandable interfaces by the metamanaging technologies. As these transparent interfaces evolve, it will become increasingly clear how our personal health is tied to that of our neighbors, our nations and our world and how our ethical decision processes will affect everyone.

6.1 The Far Horizon: Our Bodies

For our bodies, imagine using an electronic scanner to find real time data on pathogens coupled with a functional MRI reading. Overlay this with pertinent genetic information, complete with timetables spanning our lifecycles, as well as any exposure factors (data from our home, clothes, and swallowables) that might be relevant at the onset of an illness. Correlate these data with symptoms or subclinical signs. Just as Smart Money's Market-Map gives a slice snapshot of how the stock market is doing, this graphically interfaced metamanager could quickly picture for us the state of our bodies and put it into a context for prevention or disease management. For example, it could reveal novel patterns from biological, behavioral, and environmental data that could correlate chronic vague symptoms with mold colonies in residential crawlspaces, a common but often missed health factor, in areas of the U.S. like the Northwest and Texas.

6.2 The Far Horizon: Our Communities

For our communities, imagine if everyone from the pre-school parent to the utilities chair to the manufacturing plant owner could program personalized interfaces for viewing overlays of data from the environment (air and water quality), health (school and hospital records), and compare their local data with the efforts of other communities and national agendas like the U.S. Department of Health and Human Services' Healthy People 2010 health indicators. Mike McDonald, envisions, a "middleware/service" layer to the national health information infrastructure, which would consist of networking software providing bridges to information resources for everyone from the schoolchild to the government policymaker: "Where datasets are available and understood, decision-makers – now including the engaged public – are beginning to utilize community health assessment algorithms within interdisciplinary community knowledge bases…that draw upon powerful simulation (models) and heuristic (rules for judgment) capabilities in order to participate and guide the evolution of their community." He continues, "This new aspect of community governance through citizen participation, based upon an intimate knowledge of the socio-ecological factors, provides much greater understanding and participation by the people most affected by the problems at hand. There are a multiplicity of tools that aid the public in participating more fully in the process of governance, starting with their ability to visualize the nature and functioning of their community as well as mechanisms for identifying problems."[84]

6.3 The Far Horizon: Our Planet

For our planet, imagine these metamanagers, with their layered collaboratories and personalized visual, haptic, and auditory interfaces, giving us hope for a shared stewardship of our planet. We could analyze social and environmental factors such as pollution levels, green house emissions, population densities and dynamically inventory and track speciation [85]. Data visualization tools [86] and the sciences of complexity could unmask the relationships between our decisions and their social and environmental consequences. Very-long term scientific studies would reveal the power in long-term trends, and counter the commercial pace of research, which can be confused by tracking "noisy" signals too closely [87]. Even now, NASA technologies that allow for GIS mapping of various biological events enable interfaces with health events so that we can see the connections between ocean temperatures, algae blooms off the coast of Peru, and cholera outbreaks inland [88].

7. Symmetries, Transparencies And Symbiotic Stewardship

These new ways of addressing asymmetries in information and of transparent seeing, accurate mirrors, and deep understanding will do several things, if we choose. They will address imbalances of power by expanding the partners at the decision-making table from policy makers and trained specialists to include all stakeholders, including laypersons [89]. They will release the harvests of research, too often trapped in isolated silos of academia, to enrich our daily lives and long-term social and environmental decisions. They will unmask the relationships between our decisions and their consequences, even across generations. They will mirror how foolish or wise we have been in creating our virtual progeny - the global mind of technology – who will be our partners in extending our intelligence. And they will infuse a sense of responsibility toward ourselves, our families and communities, our nation, and our fellow nations, because we will be able to see, and virtually experience, how our decisions will affect our collective future.

Which brings us back to the quotes at the beginning. Our wealth and our health are both important resources for ensuring happiness and our ability to contribute during our lifetimes. How we handle these resources and how we develop our intelligent technology partners is a reflection of our stewardship values. It has been suggested, "In the end, a symbiotic culture composed of human and digital individuals may be a more effective steward of the earth's resources than humans would be by themselves."[90]

"Symbiotic stewards" - intelligences for personal, community, and world wealth and world health. How fascinating it will be to witness how we, as humans, mature in collaboration with the intelligences we are now shaping – and which, in turn, are shaping us.

Note: The above article reflects personal opinions, not institutional affiliations, nor acknowledged persons, unless specifically stated.

Acknowledgements

Mary Akers (Poppy Lane Enterprises); Rita Altamore and Fran Lewis (University of Washington); Dean Anderson (CORHealth); Mark Anderson (SNS Newsletter); Stewart Brand (The Long Now Foundation); Renata Bushko (Future of Health Technology Institute); Maggi Cary (Vox Medica) and Adam Darkins (U.S. Veterans Administration); Denise Caruso (Hybrid Vigor Institute); Mary Jo Deering, (U.S. Office of Disease Prevention and Health Promotion, DHHS); Tom Eng (EvaluMetrix and eHealth Institute); Philippe Fauchet, Cecelia Horowitz, and Alice Pentland (University of Rochester's Center for Future Health); Warren Feek (Communications Initiative); Tom Ferguson (Harvard Institute of CyberMedicine and Online Health, Pew Internet & American Life Project); Scott Griffen, Deb Cablao, Virginia Meade, Roger Finger, Stephen McGeady (Intel); Bob Croyle, Bernard Glassman, James W. Hansen, Jon Kerner, Gary Kreps, Janice Nall, Barbara Rimer, Chris Thomsen, Stacy Vandor, Paula Zeller, (National Cancer Institute, Division of Cancer Control and Population Sciences, and Cancer Information Service); Edward E. Harbour (IBM WebSphere Foundation); Deborah J. Bowen, Nigel Bush, Ann-Marie Clark, Robert W. Day, Lee Hartwell, Peggy Means, Robert Robbins, and Heidi Unruh (Fred Hutchinson Cancer Research Center); Joseph V. Henderson, (Dartmouth College, Interactive Media Lab); Will Homes (Porivo), Pattie Maes, Sandy Pentland, Roz Picard (MIT Media Lab); Michael D. McDonald (Global Health Initiatives); Molly Mettler (HealthWise); Kathleen Miller (Miller & Associates); Laura Landro and Walt Mossberg (Wall Street Journal); Kent Murphy (Center for Excellence in Medical Multimedia, USAF); Darin Murphy (Computech Information Services); Cyndi Ohmann (Ohmann Productions); Roy Pea (SRI Center for Technology in Learning), Ryan Phelan (Medical Advanced Research Applications and All-Species Foundation); Richard Rockefeller (Health Commons Institute); Beth Short and Joanna Schade (St. Cloud Communications); Tad Simon (IDEO); Kathy Stanley (eAdvisor, joint venture with Ernst & Young and E*Trade); Karla Steele (Steele and Associates); Eve Stern, Catherine Hennings, and Michael O'Leary (NexCura/cancerfacts.com); Linda Stone (Microsoft); Chris Stout (Stout Ventures); Ted Stout (ROI), Jeff Sutherland (PatientKeeper), and Christine Thompson (Informing Arts).

References

[1] Andy Grove, "Taking on Prostate Cancer" *Fortune*, May 13, 1996, pp. 54-72.

[2] Donald Chamberlin, "Sharing Our Planet", *Beyond Calculation: the Next Fifty Years of Computing*, Peter Denning and Robert Metcalfe, Eds. Copernicus, Springer-Verlag, New York, 1997, p.242, Association for Computing Machinery

[3] Renata G. Bushko, "Knowledge-Rich Analogy: Adaptive Estimation with Common Sense", thesis, Massachusetts Institute of Technology, Cambridge, MA USA, 1991

[4] Eric Roston, "In Brief: Cyber-CFP", Time, January 15, 2001

[5] Mark R. Anderson, Strategic News Service (SNS) Newsletter, "Who's the Customer?" June 12, 2001, P.3

[6] Roy Pea, Director, Stanford Research Institute's Center for Technology in Learning (CTL) and NSF Center for Innovative Learning Technologies (CILT) http://www.sri.com/policy/ctl and http://cilt.org (October 24, 2000) (personal communication, October 24, 2000)

[7] Isabella Fonseca and S. Lee, "Ranking the Online Financial Planning Services," Celent Communication, Cambridge, MA, August 2000.

[8] Tom Ferguson, "Online Patient-helpers and Physicians Working Together: A New Partnership for High Quality Health Care," *British Medical* Journal, Vol. 321, pp. 1129-1132.

[9] Tom Ferguson, "From Industrial-Age Medicine to Information-Age Health Care", The Millennium Whole Earth Catalogue, A Point Foundation Book, Harper, San Francisco, CA, 1994, p. 170

[10] "Putting People at the Center of HealthCare", WellMed (http://www.wellmed.com/wellmed/c/c0000.htm), April 12, 2001

[11] U.S. Department of Health and Human Services, Office of Disease Prevention and Health Promotion, "Partnerships for Networked Consumer Health Information", http://odphp.osophs.dhhs.gov/confrnce/ (May 30, 2001)

[12] National Institute of Standards and Technology's Advance Technology Program Focused Program on Information Infrastructure for Healthcare, http://www.atp.nist.gov/atp/focus/iifhc.htm (June 3, 2001)

[13] Consumer Union of U.S., Inc., "How to Research a Medical Topic Online", Consumer Reports Online, http://www.consumerreports.org/Special/Samples/Reports/0009med0.htm. (January 29, 2001)

[14] William A. Herman, Donald E. Marlowe, and Harvey Rudolph, "Future Trends in Medical Device Technology: Results of an Expert Survey", Center for Devices and Radiological Health, FDA, April 8, 1998 http://www.fda.gov/cdrh/ost/trends/toc.html (May 30, 2001)

[15] Richard D. Klausner, Foreword, in Barbara Rimer, J. Paul Van Nevel, Eds. "Cancer Risk Communication: What We Know and What We Need to Learn", *Journal of the National Cancer Institute Monograph*, 1999, Number 25, Oxford University Press, Bethesda, MD, p. 1

[16] Stacy Vandor, National Cancer Institute, "Extraordinary Opportunities in Cancer Communications" http://www.cancer.gov/initiatives/grp-communicate.html (May 28, 2001)

[17] "Informing the Future: Critical Issues in Health", Institute of Medicine, Washington, D.C., (http://www.iom.edu/IOM/IOMHome.nsf/Pages/Recently+Released+Reports), January 10, 2001

[18] "Crossing the Quality Chasm: A New Health System for the 21st Century", Institute of Medicine, Washington, D.C., (http://www.iom.edu/IOM/IOMHome.nsf/Pages/Recently+Released+Reports), March 1, 2001

[19] Thomas R. Eng. et al, "The eHealth Landscape: A Terrain Map of Emerging Information and Communication Technologies in Health and HealthCare", Evalumetrix for The Robert Wood Johnson Foundation, Princeton, NJ, June 2001.

[20] Alex Pentland, "Prospectus", MIT Media Lab Special Interest Group on Health, Cambridge, MA (http://www.media.mit.edu/health/html/prospectus/prospectus.html), April 10, 2001

[21] David Talbot, "The Digital Sky," *MIT Technology Review*, Cambridge, MA, March 2001, pp. 51-67

[22] Ralph Warner, "Online Law: Why the Legal System Will Never Be the Same Again", Nolo Publishers, (http://www.nolo.com/democracy_corner/online-law.html), March 31, 2001

[23] Ray Kurzweil, The Age of Spiritual Machines: When Computers Exceed Human Intelligence, Penguin Books, New York, NY, 1999

[24] Michael D. McDonald, "Future Focus: Transforming HealthCare through Information" in Hospitals & Health Networks Profiles in Leadership, American Hospital Publishing, Chicago, IL, 1997

[25] Michael D. McDonald, dissertation for doctorate in public health, "The Public Health Communications Toolbox: The role of the intelligent network and the sciences of complexity in advancing health and human prosperity", University of California at Berkeley, CA, 1995

[26] Bill Joy, "Why the Future Doesn't Need Us", *WIRED*, April 2000 archive http://www.wired.com/wired/archive/8.04/joy.html (February 3, 2001)

[27] Howard Bloom, Global Brain: The Evolution of Mass Mind from the Big Bang to the 21st Century, John Wiley & Sons, Inc., New York, NY, 2000

[28] George Johnson, "Only Connect: From swarms of smart dust to secure collaborative zones, the Omninet comes to you", Wired, January 2001, http://www.wired.com/wired/archive/8.01/nets.html. (May 31, 2001)

[29] Wendy Everett et al, "Health and HealthCare 2010: The Forecast, The Challenge", Institute for the Future for the Robert Wood Johnson Foundation, Princeton, NJ , February 2000

[30] Carol Lewis, "Home is Where the Heart Monitor Is", *FDA Consumer*, May-June 2001, pp. 11-15

[31] Larry Armstrong, "The Skinny on Diet Dot-Coms", Business Week, October 16, 2000, pp. 200E8-E12.

[32] Greg Dalton, "A Shirt That Thinks – Imagine an outfit that takes your pulse, changes color and radiates heat. Interactive textiles aren't in stores yet, but they're on the way", *The Industry Standard*, June 18, 2001, pp. 52-53.

[33] William A. Herman, "The Last Word: Health Technology is Coming Home (And How!), *FDA Consumer*, May-June 2001, p. 36

[34] William A. Herman, Donald E. Marlowe, and Harvey Rudolph, "Future Trends in Medical Device Technology: Results of an Expert Survey", Center for Devices and Radiological Health, FDA, April 8, 1998 http://www.fda.gov/cdrh/ost/trends/toc.html (May 30, 2001)

[35] P. Weiss, "Chair Becomes Personalized Posture Coach", *Science News*, Vol. 158, Nov. 18, 2000, p. 327

[36] Joseph Henderson, "Comprehensive, Technology-Based Clinical Education: The 'Virtual Practicum'", *International Journal of Psychiatry in Medicine*, Vol. 28, 1998, pp.41-79.

[37] Isabella Fonseca and S. Lee, "Ranking Online Financial Planning Services," Celent Communications, Cambridge, MA, August 2000

[38] Jeff D. Opdyke, "Tools to Trade By – Technology is giving investors the ability to do all kinds of new things", *The Wall Street Journal*, June 11, 2001, p. R-8

[39] Russell Coile and Jeffrey Bauer, "What's Up Cyberdoc?" *Advance for Health Information Executives*, March 2001, p.63-66

[40] Larry Armstrong, "Who Says Safety isn't Sexy?" *Business Week*, February 5, 2001, p.16-117.

[41] U.S. Department of Health and Human Services' Office of Minority Health, "Assuring Cultural Competence in Health Care: Recommendations for National Standards and an Outcomes-Focused Research Agenda, http://www.omhrc.gov/clas/. (May 30, 2001)

[42] "Coffee Break", National Center for Biotechnology Information at the National Library of Medicine, http://www.ncbi.nlm.nih.gov/Coffeebreak/ (April 30, 2001)

[43] Healthfinder (http://www.healthfinder.gov) and CancerNet (http://www.cancernet.nci.nih.gov) (April 12, 2001)

[44] Consumer Union of U.S., Inc., "How to Research a Medical Topic Online", Consumer Reports Online, http://www.consumerreports.org/Special/Samples/Reports/0009med0.htm. (January 29, 2001)

[45] Molly Mettler, "The Patient is Not Diabetes Case #1155491", an editorial review of the disease management section of Health and Health Care 2010, Healthwise, Inc., February 2000. http://www.healthwise.org/as_disease.mgmt.html. (January 29, 2001).

[46] Russell Coile, "Ten Blockbuster Impacts of the Human Genome", Healthcare Leadership Review, January 2001, p. 6

[47] Richard Saul Wurman, *Information Architects*, Zurich, Switzerland; Graphis Publications; 1996

[48] Edward R. Tufte. *Envisioning Information*. Graphics Press, Cheshire, CT, 1990.

[49] Danny Hakim, "Essay: The New 'Bots' Tell Us How to Invest – Online", The New York Times on the Web, April 8, 2001, http://www.nytimes.com/2001/04/08/technology/08ESSA.html. And http://www.pioneerfunds.com (May 31, 2001)

[50] Linda Stone, "Microsoft's Linda Stone to Present Her Virtual World to the National Cancer Institute This Week", http://www.microsoft.com/PressPass/features/1998/9-14stone.asp , September 14, 1998 (May 30, 2001), and Ann-Marie Clark, Director, Arnold Digital Library, Fred Hutchinson Cancer Research Center, Seattle, WA (personal communications, 1997-1999)

[51] Software Agents Lab, MIT Media Lab, Cambridge, MA http://agents.www.media.mit.edu/groups/agents/projects/ (June 3, 2001)

[52] IBM, Geographic Information Systems, Collaborative GIS, http://giswww.pok.ibm.com/gis.html. (January 30, 2001)

[53] David Lipschultz, "Letting the World Plug into Your PC – For a profit", New York Times, June 3, 2001 http://www.nytimes.com/2001/06/03/technology/03HARN.html (June 3, 2001)

[54] Affective Computing Research Group, MIT Media Lab, Cambridge, MA http://www.media.mit.edu/affect/AC_about.html (June 3, 2001)

[55] Blue Eyes Project, IBM Almaden Research Lab, CA   http://www.almaden.ibm.com/cs/blueeyes/ (June 3, 2001)

[56] World Economic Forum, Knowledge Navigator using The Brain technology http://www.weforum.org/whatwedo.nsf/Documents/What+We+Do+-+Knowledge+Navigator (October 2, 2001)

[57] Joseph V. Henderson, Interactive Media Lab, Dartmouth College Medical http://iml.dartmouth.edu/about/staff/fulltime/joe.html (June 3, 2001)

[58] SmartMoney, Map of the Market, http://www.smartmoney.com/marketmap/. (November 4, 2000)

[59] Zina Moukheiber, "Technology – The Virtual Patient – If software can simulate something as complex as a plane crash, why not an asthma attack?" *Forbes*, January 8, 2001, pp. 234-236

[60] Kent Murphy, Founder and Director, Center for Excellence in Medical Multimedia, U.S. Air Force Academy, Colorado Springs, CO (personal communications, 1997-2000) (http://www.cemm.org) (June 3, 2001)

[61] James Fallows, "Around the World in Eighty Megabytes", The Atlantic Monthly, March 2001, pp. 72-74.

[62] SimHealth, http://gamezone.com/gamesell/p1793.htm. (April 7, 2001)

[63] Laura Landro, "Health Advocates Seek Guidelines That Stick to Proven Treatments", *Wall Street Journal*, May 11, 2001, p. B1

[64] Barbara Rimer, J. Paul Van Nevel, Eds, "Monograph:Cancer Risk Communication: What We Know and What We Need to Learn", *Journal of the National Cancer Institute*, 1999, Number 25, Oxford University Press, Bethesda, MD, p. 1

[65] Kathy Stanley, eAdvisor (joint venture between Ernst & Young and E*Trade) (personal communication, January 28, 2001)

[66] Andy Grove, "Taking on Prostate Cancer", *Fortune*, May 13, 1996, p. 72

[67] Eve Stern, Executive Vice President, Business Development, NexCura, http://www.nexcura.com and Catherine Hennings, Director of Business Development, Michael O'Leary, Managing Editor, Robert W. Day, Medical Advisor, cancerfacts.com http://www.cancerfacts.com (personal communications, 2000-2001)

[68] Richard G. Rockefeller, "Onboard Medical Guidance", *Partnerships*, Vol. 11, Summer 2000, Health Commons Institute, http://www.healthcommons.org/vision/onboard_medical_guidance.html. (May 30, 2001)

[69] Richard G. Rockefeller, "Onboard Medical Guidance", Health Commons Institute, http://www.healthcommons.org/vision/onboard_medical_guidance.html. (May 30, 2001)

[70] Matthew Benjamin, "Legal Self-Help: Cheap Counsel for Simple Cases", *U.S. News and World Report*, February 12, 2001, pp. 54-55.

[71] Ralph Warner, "Online Law: Why the Legal System Will Never Be the Same Again", Nolo, http://www.nolo.com/democracy_corner/online_law.html. (May 30, 2001)

[72] Jon Kerner, Ph.D., Assistant Deputy Director for Research Dissemination and Diffusion, Office of the Director, Division of Cancer Control and Population Sciences, National Cancer Institute, Bethesda, MD (presentation May 16, 2001, COLT – Committee on Leading Technologies, DCCPS, NCI)

[73] John Hershey and Jamie Earle, "Catching the Next Wave", *Upside*, Nov. 2000,p.179-185

[74] Denise Caruso, The Hybrid Vigor Institute, http://www.hybridvigor.org (personal communication, April 11, 2001)

[75] Mark Anderson, Strategic News Services, *SNS Newsletter*, April 4, 200, http://www.stratnews.com/ (April 4, 2001)

[76] George Johnson, "Only Connect: From swarms of smart dust to secure collaborative zones, the Omninet comes to you", *WIRED*, January 2001, http://www.wired.com/wired/archive/8.01/nets.html. (May 31, 2001)

[77] E. Tenner, *Why things bite back—technology and the revenge of unintended consequences*. New York (NY): Alfred a. Knopf, 1996

[78] Bill Donahue, "Byte, Byte, Against the Dying of the Light", *The Atlantic Monthly*, May 2001, pp.28-30

[79] Bill Joy, "Why the Future Doesn't Need Us", *WIRED*, April 2000 archive http://www.wired.com/wired/archive/8.04/joy.html (February 3, 2001)

[80] ELSI (Ethical, Legal and Social Implications of Human Genetics Research), National Human Genome Research Institute, http://www.nhgri.nih.gov/ELSI/ (April 7, 2001)

[81] Allen L. Hammond, World Resources Institute, http://www.digitaldividends.org (August 11, 2001)

[82] Warren Feek, The Communication Initiative, http://www.comminit.com (200-2001)

[83] Adam William Darkins, Margaret Ann Cary, *Telemedicine and Telehealth: Principles, Policies, Performance, and Pitfalls*, Springer Publishing Company, NY, NY, 21000, p. viii

[84] Michael D. McDonald, "The Public Health Communications Toolbox: The role of the intelligent network and the sciences of complexity in advancing health and human prosperity", dissertation for doctorate in public health, University of California at Berkeley, CA, 1995

[85] Planetary inventory of all life, All-Species Foundation, http://www.all-species.org (June 3, 2001) and (personal communication Stewart Brand and Rylan Phelan, TED12, February 2001)

[86] "The Wired World Atlas", *Wired*, November 1998 http://www.wired.com/wired/archive/6.11/mediamap.html (June 1, 2001)

[87] Stewart Brand, *The Clock of the Long Now*, Basic Books, Perseus Books Group, NY, NY 1999

[88] National Science Foundation, "Tracking a Killer: Following Cholera with Every Available Means", *Frontiers: The Electronic Newsletter of the National Science Foundation*, October 1996, http://www.health.gov/healthypeople/. (May 30, 2001)
[89] Jean A. Wooldridge, "Technology Features of a Public Health Internet Collaboratory: Acknowledging Stakeholder Diversity and Public/Private Roles in Complex Global Systems", thesis for masters, University of Washington, School of Public Health and Community Medicine, June, 2000.
[90] Donald Chamberlin, "Sharing Our Planet", *Beyond Calculation: the Next Fifty Years of Computing*, Peter Denning and Robert Metcalfe, Eds. Copernicus, Springer-Verlag, New York, 1997, p.242

Future of Health Technology
R.G. Bushko (Ed.)
IOS Press, 2002

Impact of Voice- and Knowledge-Enabled Clinical Reporting – US Example

Renata G. Bushko, M.S.

Chair, Future of Health Technology Institute, Hopkinton, MA, US

Penny L. Havlicek, Ph.D.

American Medical Association, Chicago, IL, US

Edward Deppert

Compaq Corporation, Phoenix, AZ, US

Stephen Epner, M.D.

Primary Care Physician, Chicago, IL, US

Abstract

This study shows qualitative and quantitative estimates of the national and the clinic level impact of utilizing voice and knowledge enabled clinical reporting systems. Using common sense estimation methodology, we show that the delivery of health care can experience a dramatic improvement in four areas as a result of the broad use of voice and knowledge enabled clinical reporting: (1) Process Quality as measured by cost savings, (2) Organizational Quality as measured by compliance, (3) Clinical Quality as measured by clinical outcomes and (4) Service Quality as measured by patient satisfaction [1]. If only 15 percent of US physicians replaced transcription with modern clinical reporting voice-based methodology, about one half billion dollars could be saved. $6.7 Billion could be saved annually if all medical reporting currently transcribed was handled with voice-and knowledge-enabled dictation and reporting systems.[1]

1. Introduction

According to Dr. J. Michael Fitzmaurice, Senior Science Advisor for Information Technology Immediate Office of the Director, Agency for Healthcare Research and Quality: "Speech to data conversion and wireless technologies are keys to improving health care

---

[1] Approximately 67 billion lines of medical transcription annually in US

quality by enabling health professionals to capture vital clinical data in a non-intrusive and intuitive way at the point of care. Complete, accurate and structured clinical data is a necessary base for outcomes studies leading to quality improvement."

Despite the 15 years of research and development invested in voice-enabled intuitive clinical reporting systems, their prevalence in US medicine is very low. One reason for this situation is the generally low computerization level of American physicians in the clinical area (about 5%-10% according to some estimates [2]). Another reason is the lack of awareness of the potential savings and quality improvements that can result from the use of voice-enabled clinical reporting systems.

Taking an example from the national impact study initiated by the former Secretary Louis Sullivan, we estimated the national impact and clinic level impact of utilizing voice-enabled clinical reporting in terms of cost, compliance, clinical outcomes and patient satisfaction. Results imply that the introduction of voice-enabled clinical reporting to physicians' practices is of national importance.

2. Voice-enabled and Guidelines-based Clinical Reporting

Guidelines-based and voice-enabled clinical reporting is a versatile, intelligent and easy-to-use reporting methodology that will reduce medical transcription costs, increase reimbursement revenues and reduce the liability risk resulting from incomplete documentation. With such products, twenty to sixty spoken words can generate a comprehensive multiple-page report that meets practice guidelines.

Voice-enabled, clinical reporting should integrate a medical knowledge base utilizing the standard SOAP[2] or problem oriented-note format. The voice interface should be used to assure intuitive collection of patient data and creation of medical reports. The clinician could be presented with an appropriate set of questions to answer and guided through the entire process of producing a comprehensive patient report. This methodology ensures the complete and consistent recording of patient encounter information.

Designated information can then be extracted for use in clinical databases and clinical data repositories. In addition to voice, input from touch-screen, pen, mouse, bar code and the keyboard can also be supported. This versatility ensures maximum efficiency - the clinician can use whatever approach is easiest and quickest. It should also provide the user the ability to move seamlessly to and from structured reporting and free-text dictation that is extremely easy with emerging medical continuous speech dictation.

3. Learning Process: Unstructured Digital Dictation as a Starting Point

Physicians currently use free-text unstructured dictation with transcription service. They can easily adapt to newly available, inexpensive digital medical dictation systems since they do not introduce any change into their work pattern. Over time healthcare professionals will also discover and use intelligent natural language technology that allows fast and intuitive editing of medical information. This will eliminate the need for the back end correction. Eventually physicians and nurses will develop a need for system with medical knowledge bases guiding them through the dictation and data capture process.

---

[2] Subjective, Objective, Assessment, and Plan

This three-step approach: (1) first unstructured dictation with voice-enabled systems with back-end correctionist then (2) unstructured dictation with voice-enabled systems with Natural Language Technology (no correctionist) and eventually (3) structured dictation with voice and knowledge-enabled system, should assure progress in actual acceptance and massive use by the medical community.

4. Process Quality - Cost Savings

Voice-enabled, knowledge-based clinical reporting simplifies the care management process by eliminating transcription and clerical work of filing the reports. The following assumptions were used in order to estimate the cost savings:

1. In a large physician group, $100-$250 is spent per physician per week for transcription. In a four or five physician group, about $1800 per month is spent on transcription.

2. A physician handles on average about 3000 patient-visits a year (15 per day).

3. On average 10% are new patients, 90% are returning patients, and 5% of returning patients are worker's compensation patients.

4. It costs from 7.5 to 13 cents per line to transcribe medical reports.

5. The average length of a report for new patients is 2-3 pages (60 lines).

6. The average length of a report for returning patients is 1/2 page (15 lines).

7. The average length of a report for worker's compensation cases is 4 pages (120 lines).

8. It is a myth that primary care physicians do less transcription because they do not need it - they are among the lowest paid physicians and often the economics of health care delivery does not allow them the luxury of transcription service.

9. Younger physicians are more interested in the use of new technologies.

10. Fifty percent of physicians are involved in some worker's compensation cases.

5. Estimation Equation - National Example

Let's assume that 100,000 American physicians have moved to voice-enabled medical systems based on new continuous speech and intelligent natural language technology. This is an equivalent to 300 million[3] patient visits per year. 30 million new visits, and 270 million of returning visits out of which 13.5 million visits are worker's compensation visits.

---

[3] 3000 visits per year *100,000 physicians

Table 1. Estimation of ambulatory transcription cost for 100,000 physicians based on the workload in millions of dollars

Type of visit	Number of Visits in millions	Number of Pages in millions	Number of text lines in billions	Transcription Cost in millions 10cents per line
New[4]	30	60	1.8	$180
Repeat/ non worker's comp[5]	257.5	129	3.9	$390
Repeat/ worker's comp[6]	13.5	54	1.6	$160
Total	301	243	5.3	$730 million

Thus, if only 14 percent of all US physicians[7] adopted voice enabled clinical dictation systems, a potential of about 730 million health care dollars could be saved. Non-transcription related savings could add additional 30-50% savings.

6. Large Clinic Example

Let's assume that 100 physicians in a large clinic have moved to voice-enabled clinical reporting and data capture. This is equivalent to 300,000[8] patient visits per year. 30,000 new visits, and 270,000 returning visits out of which 13,500 visits are worker's compensation visits.

Table 2. Estimation of ambulatory transcription cost for a clinic with 100 physicians based on the workload

Type of visit	Number of Visits	Number of Pages	Transcription Cost 10cents per line
New	30,000	60,000	$180,000
Repeat/ non worker's comp	257,500	129,000	$390,000
Repeat/ worker's comp	13,500	54,000	$160,000
Total	301,000	243,000	$730,000

---

[4] The average length of a report for new patients is 2-3 pages (30 lines per page, minimum 60 lines per report).
[5] The average length of a report for returning patients is 1/2 page (15 lines).

[6] The average length of a report for worker's compensation cases is 4 pages (30 lines per page, minimum 120 lines).
[7] 720,325 physicians in US according to 1996/97 AMA update of Physician Characteristics and Distribution in the US
[8] 3000 visits per year *100 physicians

7. Structured Voice-enabled and Guidelines-based Dictation

7.1 Entry Cost

If we assume that the cost of purchasing and installing voice-enabled and guidelines-based clinical reporting software and related hardware is about $6,000 per physician, then the cost of the clinical reporting system the first year is about $600,000 per100 physicians. Break-even point is achieved in 10 months - the system pays for itself in 10 month at the rate of $60,833 per month and the funding comes from the transcription budget.

7.2 First Year Savings and ROI

With annual transcription costs estimated to be $730,000, the annual savings during the first year of using the system are about $130,000.   Thus, for each dollar invested in voice-enabled and guidelines driven software, the clinic will be getting 20 cents in operational savings the same year (Return On Investment equal to about 20%).

7.3 Five-year Scenario

Over the period of five years, for each dollar invested in voice-enabled system, the clinic will be getting about $5 in operational savings (ROI=500%) assuming a high $120,000 annual maintenance, support and training cost. This is based on the $2,450,00 savings over the 5-year period.

8. Unstructured Free-text Dictation

8. 1 Entry Cost

Currently, the cost of free-text continuous medical dictation systems with natural intelligent language technology is as low as $499 per physician. Including hardware then the cost of purchasing and installing free-text voice enabled systems can be as low as $2,500 per physician, $250,000 per100-physician practice. Break-even point is achieved after 4 months.

8.2 First Year Savings and ROI

Under this scenario first year savings amount to $460,000. Thus, for each dollar invested in a free-text voice-enabled (continuous) medical dictation software, the clinic will be getting $1.84 in operational savings the same year (Return On Investment = 184%). Further savings can be derived from introducing templates for frequently occurring reports (e.g, new patient visit template) and using macros to automate frequently repeated tasks.

8.3 Five-year Scenario

Over the period of five year, for each dollar invested in voice-enabled system, the clinic will be getting about $11.20 in operational savings (ROI=1120%) assuming a high $100,000 annual maintenance, support and training cost.

9. Unstructured Free-text Dictation with Back-end Correctionist

9.1 Entry Cost

If we assume that an entry cost per physician for the system that captures physician's dictation in both acoustic and electronic (typed) formats is comparable with the free-text system[9] (no workflow management included) then savings are approximately 50% smaller due to the cost of correctionist. Break-even point can be achieved after 6 months.

9.2 First Year Savings and ROI

Under this scenario first year savings amount to $230,000. Thus, for each dollar invested in a free-text voice-enabled (continuous) medical dictation software with correctionist at the back end, the clinic will be getting $0.92 in operational savings the same year (Return On Investment = 92%).

9.3 Five-year Scenario

Over the period of five years, for each dollar invested in free-text voice-enabled system with back-end correctionist, the clinic will be getting about $5.60 in operational savings (ROI=560%).

Table 3. Break even point and ROI comparison of free text dictation,
free-text with correctionist, and structured knowledge-based voice-enabled systems

Type of Voice-recognition System	Break-even Point System is Paid off	Return on Investment 1-year	Return on Investment 5-year	Level of Additional Qualitative Benefits
Free-text Dictation	4 months	184%	1120%	Medium
Free-text Dictation with a Correctionist	6 months	92%	560%	Medium
Structured Knowledge-based Clinical Reporting	10 months	20%	500%	Very High

---

[9] Most voice recognition systems allow to capture voice via digital recording devices. Then correctionist can compare a draft automatically generated by the system with a recorded voice of the physician (50% less work for the correctionist).

10. Organizational Quality - Compliance (Accreditation & Audits)

10.1 Outcomes Analysis Requirements

With managed care forcing the proliferation of capitated contracts, the ability to capture data for use in outcomes management is rapidly becoming crucial to long term survival and profitability. (1) Low-end, voice-enabled dictation systems can have macros that allow for tagging pieces of clinical data needed for outcomes studies. (2) High-end systems supported by knowledge bases can have that information requirement embedded in the software. It appears to the clinician reading the report that the report has been transcribed while the report is actually generated with hidden character fields. These fields allow for flagging and then capturing pertinent information. This information in turn can be used to populate fields within an outcomes database (HL-7 data transmission standards). For example, a HEDIS requirement to provide statistics on the number of children under two receiving immunization, as compared with the total number of children under two in the plan, can be easily satisfied.

10.2 Audits

Accurate & complete documentation complying with government and industry rules and regulations decreases liability risk and problems during audits. It has been stated by a leading practitioner that: "Periodical audits by insurance companies would be a piece of cake with a system that could provide automatic ICD9 codes and compliance with HCFA regulations."

10.3 Liability

More accurate medical records that result from the use of voice-enabled systems reduce liability exposure. With a medical knowledge base designed for a specific medical specialty and its reporting needs, the users should be prompted to enter all pertinent information, providing a detailed and accurate report. With an editor which allows a physician to easily modify the structure of the knowledge base or templates, he/she can be certain of ensuring that his/her entire staff consistently provides the same high level of patient care. Improved quality control will lead to reduced liability exposure for a hospital or a clinic and might lower insurance costs.

Use of voice and knowledge-enabled clinical reporting systems may permit physicians to negotiate lower premiums for their malpractice insurance (e.g., 15% reduction in insurance premiums that accounted to $37,500 for a 4-physician group – about $10,000 per physician annually). Typically, in exchange for the reduction in premiums, physicians must agree to attend a risk management program and employ structured reporting system.

11. Clinical Quality - Clinical Outcomes

11.1 Data Quality Increased - Fewer Errors

With voice-enabled clinical data acquisition systems, speaking generates all the reports. The doctor can immediately verify the report by listening to it and edit any changes he/she wants using natural language technology. Thus proof reading stacks of transcribed reports can be eliminated. There are no delays caused by transcriptionist mistakes which need to be retyped, proof read again and possibly changed again.

It seems that continuity of the review process enabled by the immediate and automatic transcription should improve accuracy of the information in the report. Reporting involving: (1) initial dictation (2) transcription (3) verification and signing by the very nature of being distributed in time seems to be more error-prone than a one-time reporting event immediately after the encounter. If we compare it to a hand-written documentation, readability is another factor that has a great impact on the quality of the clinical data. While not all physicians can afford transcription service, the cost of modern voice technology is not prohibitive.

11.2 Diagnostic Quality - Sociotechnological Learning Loop

According a physician who has been using voice-enabled and knowledge-based system for three years now: "Structured reports and dictation allows you to invoke all sorts of useful templates that make diagnosis more effective. For example, the headache template includes all necessary objective findings." What he refers to can be characterized as a "sociotechnological[10] learning loop."

(1) Clinical guidelines, best practice knowledge and reporting requirements are embedded in templates and knowledge-base driven prompting system.

(2) Physicians internalize guidelines and new medical knowledge while doing medical reporting with the knowledge-based system on daily bases. Repetition encodes knowledge in memory[11]. It can be done with ease because of the intuitive, voice-enabled interface.

(3) Physicians are more prone to follow guidelines and collect pieces of clinical information needed for future outcomes studies, so there is more quality clinical data for analysis.

(4) This leads to the improved pool of information available for creation of physician guidelines, eliminating a potential false learning phenomenon that occurs when we base research on poor quality of data or incomplete data sets.

(5) New guidelines get embedded in knowledge-based systems and the "sociotechnological medical learning loop" closes and repeats itself continuously improving diagnostic quality.

---

[10] Based on sociotechnological process as described in [Bushko 95]
[11] Based on Ulric Neisser, Memory Observed, Remembering in Natural Contexts, 1982

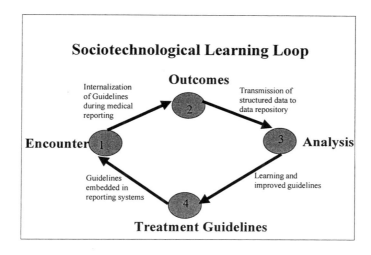

Figure 1. Sociotechnological Medical Learning Loop showing practice guidelines
internalization process supported by voice and knowledge-enabled system

12. Service Quality - Patients' Satisfaction

Reporting time is reduced down to instantaneous generation. The reports are generated on
the system monitor "as doctor dictates". They can be instantly transmitted, also with voice
command, to the information system thus being made available to other specialists and the
patient. This assures continuity of care and puts less administrative burden on the patient.
As one physician who uses voice-enabled and guidelines-based clinical dictation systems
says: "When my patients need some notes for another doctor, they are pleased with clear,
structured, and detailed report that I can give them." Voice-enabled and knowledge-based
systems also enable physicians to generate real-time, patient-specific instructions in any
language (automatic translation). This increases patients' compliance with the treatment
plan which is a big problem in achieving good clinical outcomes that are the base for
overall patient satisfaction.

13. Conclusions and Recommendations

We have demonstrated, with common sense estimation methodology and the personal
testimonials of users, that voice-enabled clinical reporting systems can significantly and
positively impact health care costs, compliance, clinical outcomes and patient satisfaction.
Some of these aspects of quality are touched upon by the following quote from a committed
user of voice-enabled and knowledge-based methodology: "My voice-generated notes are
immediately available for the chart or to be sent to a colleague. And of course once the

system is in place, there are no ongoing transcription fees. In my own office, despite vigorous efforts at cost control, conventional transcription was costing $0.075 per line. With implementation of voice-enabled medical dictation systems we were able to save more than $6,000.00 per physician per year."

Our opinion is that the introduction of voice-enabled clinical reporting to American physicians' practices is of national importance. We recommend a national initiative aimed at the accelerated computerization of American physicians and nurses through the use of intuitive, voice-enabled clinical reporting systems, similar in design to the EDI movement initiated by the former Secretary Louis Sullivan. The first important step is to increase awareness of the savings and quality improvements that can result from the use of voice-enabled clinical reporting systems. The goal is to define an action plan for changing the current situation and achieving 75% computerization of American physicians by the year 2005. Our vision is to provide physicians and nurses with intuitive, voice & knowledge enabled access to the Health Information Infrastructure, enabling health professionals to capture vital clinical data in a non-intrusive and intuitive way at the point of care. This will allow them to manage, monitor and coordinate patients' healthcare and wellness in a uniform, risk-free, and cost-effective way while capturing quality clinical data and providing patient satisfaction.

References

[1] Bushko R., Leadership Challenges in the 21st Century: 7 Strategies to Leadership, Workshop P-6, Healthcare Executive's Challenges in the 21st Century: Leadership, Quality, Technology, and Innovation-driven Process Management, IMIA'95, Vancouver Canada, 1995.

[2] Presentation at the National Managed Care Congress, Information Systems Role in Developing and Implementing Outcomes Monitoring Strategies, Bushko R., McCormick K.A., Alexander, C., Washington D.C., April, 16, 1997.

[3] Neisser, U. Memory Observed, Remembering in Natural Contexts, W.H. Freeman and Company, 1982.

[4] Minsky, M., Why People Think Computers Can't, Technology Review, November 1983

[5] E.H. Shortliffe and L.E. Perreault (eds.), *Medical Informatics: Computer Applications in Healthcare,* Reading, MA, Addison Wesley, 1990.

[6] Bushko, R. *Knowledge-Rich Analogy: Adaptive Estimation with Common Sense*, Massachusetts Institute of Technology, Department of Electrical Engineering and Computer Science, 1991

[7] Jesse W., Health Outcomes Data Workshop presentation, Federation of American Systems', Las Vegas, 1992

[8] R. Kurzweil, *When Will HAL Understand What We Are Saying? Computer Speech Recognition and Understanding?* in HAL'S Legacy: 2001's Computer as Dream and Reality, p 131-169, Edited by David G. Stork, MIT Press, 1996.

[9] Fitzmaurice, J.M., The American Perspective for the Future, in Health in the New Communications Age, M. Ladeira, J. Christensen, eds. ISO Press, 646-650.

[10]] Renata G. Bushko, Poland: Socio-technological Transformation – its Impact on Organizational, Process, Clinical and Service Quality of Health Care. In: W. Wieners (ed.), Global Healthcare Markets. Jossey-Bass Publishers, John Wiley & Sons, Inc. 2000, pp. 194-201.

[11] J. Bos, R.G. Bushko, Towards Outcomes Analysis and Shareable Medical Records: Voice and Knowledge-enabled Clinical Reporting for Primary Care, Proceedings of Towards Electronic Patient Record 1997.

Contributors' Professional Backgrounds

Editor

Renata G. Bushko, M.S.

Renata G. Bushko, M.S. is Chair of the **Future of Health Technology Institute**, www.fhti.org, a health technology think-tank dedicated to defining the health technology agenda for the 21st century. Ms. Bushko founded Future of Health Technology Institute in 1996 and has since chaired six Future of Health Technology Summits. These summits engage leading minds from the technology and healthcare fields in envisioning the future of technology for global healthcare. Under her leadership, the Future of Health Technology Institute has been recognized as the premiere health technology research and training organization. Previously Ms. Bushko served on national healthcare programs organized by Vice President Albert Gore, Dr. C. Everett Koop, and former secretary of Health and Human Services, Dr. L. Sullivan. She was an advisor on health technology investment issues in the US, UK, Puerto Rico, Australia, New Zealand, & Poland. She holds a Master of Science degree in Electrical Engineering and Computer Science with specialization in intelligent systems from the Massachusetts Institute of Technology (MIT) and a BA in Computer Science and Economics from Smith College and University of Warsaw. She has been selected by Professor Marvin Minsky – one of the founders of the field of Artificial Intelligence (AI) – to develop intelligent agents and study machine intelligence at the MIT AI Lab.

Chapter Authors

Marina U. Bers, Ph.D.

Marina Umaschi Bers is assistant professor at the Eliot-Pearson Department of Child Development at Tufts University. She received her Ph.D. from the MIT Media Laboratory. Her research involves the design and study of technological learning environments to support children's exploration of issues of personal identity and moral values. Marina has applied her research in the areas of educational technology and mental health care and has designed and implemented diverse prototypes ranging from virtual worlds to robotics that have been used in schools, museums and hospitals. She has worked on projects in the US, Argentina, Costa Rica, Colombia and Thailand. Marina is originally from Buenos Aires, Argentina.

Maria I. Busquets, M.A.

Maria I. Busquets, MA, is Chief of the Communication, Management and Training Division in the Population, Health and Nutrition Center at the U.S. Agency for International

Development. She is an expert in the area of international development with particular focus on sustainability and capacity building issues. Most recently she has focused on how applications of IT can improve the impact and reach of donor technical assistance in the developing world context and how to improve south-to-south and south-to-north information flows.

Mary Jo Deering, Ph.D.

Mary Jo Deering, Ph.D. is Director of Health Communication and eHealth in the Office of Disease Prevention and Health Promotion (ODPHP), U.S. Department of Health and Human Services (HHS). She had co-lead responsibility in ODPHP for overseeing the development of Healthy People 2010, the third decade-long national prevention initiative. She oversees www.healthfinder.gov, the official Federal consumer health information gateway on the Internet which won the prestigious Hammer Award. She is the lead HHS staff for the National Health Information Infrastructure Work Group of the National Committee on Vital and Health Statistics, which is preparing recommendations for the HHS Secretary and Congress. She created the Science Panel on Interactive Communication and Health, which produced Wired for health and well being: the emergence of interactive health communication (HHS 1999) and now oversees the follow up work. She chairs the steering committee of Partnerships for Networked Consumer Health Information, which presents national conferences and the innovative Technology Games. Dr. Deering served on the Federal Communication Commission's Advisory Committee on Telecommunications and Health Care.

David R. DeMaso, M.D.

David R. DeMaso, M.D., is an Associate Professor of Psychiatry at Harvard Medical School and the Associate Psychiatrist-in-Chief at Children's Hospital Boston. His clinical work and research has centered on the interface of psychiatry and pediatrics examining adaptation and coping in children with medical illnesses. Increasingly he has explored the risk and protector factors that determine clinical outcome in children facing adversity.

Ed Deppert

Ed brings 28 years of healthcare industry expertise to his position of Director of Healthcare for North America. Ed is responsible for setting strategy and implementing market programs that drive incremental revenue. He provides industry expertise to the field sales force and internal product groups. Ed has a platinum track record of providing executive level consulting to Healthcare CIOs and other executives. Having been a CIO for a 500-bed hospital he can interact with customers on their own level, bringing a true understanding of their requirements to the table. Ed's past history includes Director of New Health Ventures for Wang Healthcare; Senior Healthcare Executive for Data General Corporation and diverse healthcare positions with Digital Equipment Corporation and Honeywell.

Stephen Epner, M.D.

Dr. Epner practices medicine in Chicago at the UROMED Ltd. Clinic. He is a graduate of Brandeis University in Waltham Massachusetts and he received his Medical Degree from the Boston University School of Medicine in 1984. He completed his internship and residency in 1987 at the University of Illinois in Chicago. He is board certified in Internal Medicine since then. Dr. Epner uses modern technologies in his daily practice to improve quality and efficiency of care.

Robert A. Freitas Jr.

Robert A. Freitas Jr. is the author of Nanomedicine, the first book-length technical discussion of the potential medical applications of molecular nanotechnology and medical nanorobotics. Volume I was published in October 1999 by Landes Bioscience while Freitas was a Research Fellow at the Institute for Molecular Manufacturing in Palo Alto, California. Freitas is completing Volumes II and III as a Research Scientist at Zyvex Corp., a nanotechnology R&D startup company headquartered in Richardson, Texas.

Barbara B. Friedman, M.A., M.P.A. FAHRMM

Ms. Barbara B. Friedman has over twenty years of expertise as a health care administrator in both the public and private sectors. She is an Assistant Vice President, Support Services Saint Peter's University Hospital. Previously she was a Regional Consultant for the Joint Purchasing Corporation and as an instructor at Baruch College, City University of New York. Ms. Friedman serves currently on the Board of Directors for the Association for Healthcare Resource and Material Management, of the American Hospital Association. She served as President and President-elect for the New York Chapter of AHRMM, and won "Chapter-of-the-Year" for 1997 and 1998. Her educational credentials are a M.P.A, Health Care Administration from New York University, M.A. Sociology from the State University of New York at Stony Brook, and B.A, Sociology from the State University of New York at Buffalo. Ms. Friedman has lectured extensively on a national basis and has published numerous articles on a variety of topics in journals such as Hospital Materiel Management Quarterly, HAPM Insights, American Health, and Medical Focus.

Jean Garnier, Ph.D.

Jean Garnier received his first degree in Agronomy Sciences at the National Institute of Agronomy in Paris in 1952 then was graduated from the Sorbonne University in Paris where he obtained a Ph.D. degree in Physical Sciences in 1962. He also received a degree in Microbiology and Immunology from the Pasteur Institute. He held a Post doc position at the Massachusetts Institute of Technology. He has been a visiting Professor at the University of Manchester, UK, at Boston University, MA and Scholar-in-Residence at the National Institutes of Health. Besides a two year Professorship in Biophysics in Bordeaux, he did all his research work at the University of Paris-Sud at Orsay. He is presently a Visiting Professor at the National Institutes of Health, USA, and charge de mission for Bioinformatics at the National Institute for Research in Agronomy in France. He is Vice-President of the International Union of Pure and Applied Biophysics (IUPAB) and Chairman of the Inter-Union on Bioinformatics Group.

G. Scott Gazelle, M.D.

G. Scott Gazelle, MD, is an associate professor of radiology at Harvard University and an associate radiologist at Massachusetts General Hospital. Dr. Gazelle also serves as director of the Decision Analysis and Technology Assessment Group for the Department of

Radiology at MGH, and co-director of the Brigham and Women's Hospital–MGH Center for Clinical Trials in Radiology. Dr. Gazelle's research interests include development and evaluation of contrast agents for computerized tomography and ultrasound, development and optimization of techniques for in situ tumor ablation, and analytic methods for technology assessment. He also concentrates on experimental study design and data analysis, decision modeling and analysis, and technology assessment and its policy applications.

Joseph Gonzalez-Heydrich, M.D.

Joseph Gonzalez-Heydrich, M.D. is Assistant Professor of Psychiatry at the Harvard Medical School and Medical Director for the Outpatient Psychiatry Programs at Children's Hospital in Boston. In addition to work on traditional clinical trials, his research has focused on the application of computer science to important needs in psychiatry and neuroscience. His work has ranged from using simulations to study personality development to building an electronic medical record system for the outpatient psychopharmacology clinic. He and his colleagues at Children's Hospital, the MIT Media Lab, and MERL have also successfully piloted several computer applications to help children and families facing serious medical illness. The results have been published in the proceedings of CHI, Med Info, in the Journal of the Academy of Child and Adolescent Psychiatry and in the International Journal of Medical Informatics among others.

Robert A. Greenes, M.D., Ph.D.

Robert A. Greenes has an M.D. degree and Ph.D. in applied mathematics/computer science, both from Harvard, and is Board Certified in Diagnostic Radiology. Radiology Residency was at Massachusetts General Hospital. He is Professor of Radiology at Harvard Medical School, and Radiologist, Brigham and Women's Hospital. He is also Professor of Health Policy and Management, Harvard School of Public Health; and Professor of Health Informatics, in the Health Science and Technology Division (HST), a joint division of Harvard Medical School and Massachusetts Institute of Technology. In 1978 Dr. Greenes established the Decision Systems Group (DSG) a Harvard-based medical informatics research and development laboratory at Brigham and Women's Hospital which he directs, to pursue methodologies for health care education and decision support. He is the Program Director of the Harvard–MIT–NEMSC Research Training Program in Medical Informatics, with support by the National Library of Medicine. He is a Fellow of the American College of Medical Informatics as well as its past President, a Fellow of the American College of Radiology, a member of the Institute of Medicine of the National Academy of Sciences, and serves on a number of editorial boards.

Penny Havlicek, Ph.D.

Penny Havlicek, Ph.D., holds doctorate in Sociology from the University of Illinois at Chicago. Dr. Havlicek has worked in the health care industry for nearly 17 years collecting, maintaining, and disseminating data on physicians and their practices. Her research interests include the changing nature of the health care delivery system. While at the American Medical Association, she has been responsible for producing a key set of publications describing the population of medical group practices and the trends in this increasingly important practice mode.

James Kaput, Ph.D.

James Kaput is a Chancellor Professor in the Department of Mathematics at the University of Massachusetts, Dartmouth specializing in elementary students' development of algebraic reasoning, and the development of affordable technologies for mathematics education. Dr. Kaput has recently turned his attention to the massive implementation of technology-based innovations to democratize access to powerful mathematics, especially among disadvantaged populations. He is on the editorial board of six mathematics education journals and is a founding co-editor of a series of volumes sponsored by the Conference Board of the Mathematical Sciences on Research in Collegiate Mathematics Education.

Colleen Kigin, M.P.A.

Colleen Kigin facilitates and integrates targeted research projects to programs, and assists with translation of research to practice. A physical therapist by background, Ms. Kigin was formerly the director of physical therapy services at Massachusetts General Hospital (MGH). Today, she also serves as an assistant professor at the MGH Institute of Health Professions in the physical therapy program. At Partners HealthCare System, Ms. Kigin directed the system's cost reduction efforts. Ms. Kigin received her Masters in Public Administration from the Kennedy School of Government, Harvard.

Gary L. Kreps, Ph.D.

Gary L. Kreps (Ph.D. in Communication, 1979, University of Southern California) is Chief of the Health Communication and Informatics Research Branch of the National Cancer Institute's Behavioral Research Program, Division of Cancer Control and Population Sciences. In this position he plans, develops, and coordinates major new national research and outreach initiatives concerning risk communication, health promotion, behavior change, technology development, and information dissemination to promote cancer prevention and control. Dr. Kreps has published more than 20 books and 130 scholarly articles and chapters examining the important roles performed by communication in society.

Jo Lernout, M.S.

Jo Lernout is an expert in voice technologies. He holds a degree in physics, a diploma from the Vlerick Management School in Ghent, Belgium, and training in Computer Science and office automation. He started working as a biology teacher. After two years of teaching he worked at the sales department of Merk Sharp & Dome and Bull. Later on he became Sales Manager for Wang, Commercial Director of Wang Belgium and General Manager of Barco Industries, Graphic Division, in Boston, USA. In 1987 he founded Lernout & Hauspie Speech Products. Jo Lernout was a guest lecturer at the University Sint Ignatius Antwerpen (UFSIA), Belgium, the Vlerick Management School in Ghent, Belgium, the University Sint Aloysius (EHSAL), Brussels, Belgium, the Catholic University Leuven (KUL), Belgium, and the University Ghent (RUG), Belgium.

Henry Lieberman, Ph.D.

Henry Lieberman has been a Research Scientist at the MIT Media Laboratory since 1987. A member of the Software Agents group, his work tries to bring learning, proactive agents, and other ideas from artificial intelligence to make user interfaces more intelligent, personalized and responsive. Among his major research interests is Programming by Example, a technique for teaching new behavior to a machine by demonstrating examples in an interactive interface. Before that, he worked at the MIT Artificial Intelligence Laboratory, from 1972–87. He holds a doctoral-equivalent degree from the University of Paris VI and was a Visiting Professor there in 1989-90. His book, "Your Wish is My Command: Programming by Example" was published by Morgan Kaufmann in 2001.

Cindy Mason, Ph.D.

Cindy Mason is an Assistant Research Engineer at the University of California, Berkeley. Cindy's research interests include intelligent agents, distributed systems, and speech interfaces. She received her Ph.D in 1992 and was awarded Outstanding Student Contribution to the field of Distributed Artificial Intelligence for her work on collaborative belief revision. She was recipient of the National Research Council Research Associateship at NASA Ames Research Center from 1992 to 1995 and a Research Fellow in the Stanford School of Medicine in 1996. She joined the Berkeley Initiative on Soft Computing in 1995. She teaches courses on intelligent agents and is active in the area of multi-agent systems, and the development of human centered computing technologies, including speech interfaces and affective computing.

Blackford Middleton, M.D., MSc, M.P.H.

Dr. Blackford Middleton is Associate Director of Clinical & Quality Analysis for the Partners Healthcare System, and Assistant Professor of Medicine at Harvard Medical School. He received an MD from SUNY-Buffalo, an MPH in Epidemiology from Yale, and an MSc in Health Services Research, focusing on medical informatics, from Stanford University, and he is a Board Certified practicing academic internist. Dr. Middleton has held both academic and corporate executive positions. He was Medical Director of Information Management and Technology at Stanford Health Services, 1992–1995, and Senior Vice President for Clinical Informatics and Chief Medical Officer for MedicaLogic/Medscape 1995–2001 before moving to Partners. Dr. Middleton is frequently invited to speak and consult nationally and internationally on computer-based patient records, and the Internet in healthcare. Dr. Middleton is a Fellow of the American College of Medical Informatics, a Fellow of the American College of Physicians-American Society for Internal Medicine, an active member of the Healthcare Information Management and Systems Society, and is past chair of the Computer-based Patient Record Institute (CPRI).

Alex P. Pentland, Ph.D.

Alex (Sandy) Pentland is the Academic Head of the MIT Media Laboratory, Founder and Director of the Center for Future Health and the LINCOS Foundation. Newsweek magazine has recently named him one of the 100 Americans most likely to shape the next century, and he has won awards from several academic societies, including the AAAI, IEEE, and Ars Electronica. He is one of the 50 most-cited authors in Computer Science. His work has received extensive coverage by organizations such as the NY and LA Times, Newsweek and Vogue, ABC and NBC TV, and named 'idea of the year' by Parade Magazine. His overall focus is on using digital technology for the worldwide reinvention of health, education and community. Towards this end he has done research in wearable computing, human–machine interface, computer graphics, artificial intelligence, machine and human vision, and has published more than 200 scientific articles in these areas. Popular summaries of this research can be found in the April 1996 and November 1998 issues of Scientific American.

Alice P. Pentland, M.D.

Alice P. Pentland M.D. is the Medical Director of the Center for Future Health. She has twenty years of experience in scientific and clinical research in photobiology and skin cancer. Her research at the Center focuses on skin mapping and clinical applications in dermatology, and on the cellular and molecular aspects of the research effort on biomedical sensors. She received her M.D. degree and B.S. in biology in 1978 from the University of Michigan. She taught at Washington University School of Medicine until 1996 when she became the James H. Sterner Professor and Chair of Dermatology in the School of Medicine and Dentistry at the University of Rochester. She is also the Director of Telemedicine for the Strong Health System. Dr. Pentland spent a sabbatical at the MIT Media Laboratory in 1996. She has published extensively in scientific and clinical journals, and served as principal investigator on numerous NIH research grants, clinical trials, and as a member of various boards, including the Society for Investigative Dermatology

Rosalind W. Picard, Ph.D.

Professor Rosalind W. Picard is founder and director of the Affective Computing Research Group at the Massachusetts Institute of Technology (MIT) Media Laboratory. She holds Bachelors in Electrical Engineering from the Georgia Institute of Technology and Masters and Doctorate degrees, each in Electrical Engineering and Computer Science, from MIT. The author of over 80 peer-reviewed scientific articles in pattern recognition, multidimensional signal modeling, computer vision, and human–computer interaction, Picard is known internationally for pioneering research on content-based video retrieval and on giving computers the ability to recognize and respond to human emotional information. She is co-recipient with Tom Minka of a "best paper" prize (1998) from the Pattern Recognition Society for their work on interactive machine learning with a society of models. Her award-winning book, Affective Computing, (MIT Press, 1997) lays the groundwork for giving machines the skills of emotional intelligence. Her group's research on affective and wearable technologies has been featured in national and international public forums such as The New York Times, The London Independent, Scientific American Frontiers, Time, New Scientist, Vogue, as well as PBS and BBC specials. Picard is married and lives in Newton, Massachusetts with her husband, two sons, and seven non-affective computers.

Scott C. Ratzan, M.D., M.P.A., M.A.

Scott C. Ratzan, MD, MPA, MA is Senior Technical Advisor in the Global Bureau at the U.S. Agency for International Development. He also is Editor-In-Chief, for the Journal of Health Communication: International Perspectives and holds faculty appointments in the Department of Epidemiology and Public Health at Yale University School of Medicine,

Department of Family Medicine and Community Health at Tufts University School of Medicine and international public health at George Washington University. Dr. Ratzan recently was principal author of Attaining Global Health: Challenges and Opportunities. Other publications include the Mad Cow Crisis: Health and the Public Good (NYU Press/UCL Press) and AIDS: Effective Health Communication for the 90s (Taylor & Francis).

Barry Robson, Ph.D., D.Sc.

Barry Robson is an IBM executive and Strategic Advisor, Professorial Lecturer at Mount Sinai School of Medicine, NY, and CEO & Chair of the Dirac Foundation, a learned body promoting theoretical chemistry and biology in medicine and veterinary science at the Royal Veterinary college, U. London. According to an article in Nature (389,418–420,1997) he was a pioneer in bioinformatics, protein modeling, and computer-aided drug design. He was awarded a Ph.D. (University of Newcastle Upon Tyne) for experimental studies in protein folding in 1972, a D.Sc. (University of Manchester) for international recognition in computational chemistry and biochemistry in 1984, and Distinguished Engineer for contributions to bioinformatics by IBM in 1998. He is a recipient of Future of Health Technology Award 2001.

David Williamson Shaffer, Ph.D.

David Williamson Shaffer is currently an Assistant Professor of Cognitive Science in Education at the University of Wisconsin at Madison. A former teacher, curriculum developer, teacher-trainer, and school technology specialist, Dr. Shaffer has taught grades 4–12 in the United States and abroad, including two years working with the Asian Development Bank and US Peace Corps in Nepal. Dr. Shaffer's M.S. and Ph.D. are from the Media Laboratory at the Massachusetts Institute of Technology, where his work focused on the development and evaluation of technology-supported learning environments. After completing his doctoral studies, Dr. Shaffer taught and conducted research at the Technology and Education Program at the Harvard Graduate School of Education. He developed curricula and online tools the help students understand the impact of technology on society, and created technology-based learning systems for new medical devices and procedures. Dr. Shaffer's research interests are in how computational media change the way people think and learn.

Richard Spivack, Ph.D.

Richard Spivack is an economist in Advanced Technology Program's (ATP) Economic Assessment Office focusing on the long-term results of the ATP. ATP's mission of generating "broad-based economic impacts" occupies most of his time as it is his responsibility to oversee the development of the economic modeling necessary to evaluate the success(es) of the program. Richard's background includes over 18 years of college level teaching at both the undergraduate and graduate levels. Richard received his M.A. degree from the University of Rhode Island and his Ph.D. degree from the University of Connecticut. His areas of expertise include Healthcare economics as well as Urban/Regional economics in which he has published several scholarly articles.

Albert J. Sunseri, Ph.D.

Albert J. Sunseri, Ph.D. has worked in associations for over twenty years. Dr. Sunseri is currently an Executive Director, American Society of Healthcare Engineers, of American Hospital Association. He began his association career at the American Heart Association-Metropolitan Chicago. While in Chicago he wrote and managed a Phase 4 grant from the National Heart, Lung and Blood Institute of the National Institutes of Health. Dr. Sunseri served as the CEO of the American Dental Hygienists' Association and the Association for Healthcare Resource and Materials Management. He was the Director of Education for the Joint Commission on Accreditation of Healthcare Organization and the Heart Attack Prevention Program. In addition, He served as Vice President of the Healthcare Financial Management Association. Dr. Sunseri has been involved in numerous international and national meeting as an organizer and presenter. In addition, Dr. Sunseri served on the Board of the American Hospital Association Insurance Resource Institute. Prior to entering the association management, he was an Associate Profession and Faculty President at Point Park College, and Associate Professor, Teacher Corps, University of Pittsburgh.

Graziella Tonfoni, Ph.D.

Dr. Graziella Tonfoni teaches Computational Linguistics at the University of Bologna, Italy. She is currently Visiting Research Professor in Documentation Management at the School of Engineering and Applied Science at the George Washington University, in Washington D.C. A former Visiting Scholar at the Massachusetts Institute of Technology, Harvard University and University of California at Berkeley, she has also been Visiting Professor in Information Design at the University of Maryland College Park. She is the author of more than 100 publications and the author of the CPP-TRS methodology and of CTML. Her book on "Writing as a visual art" was published with Prof. Marvin Minsky's foreword.

Kevin Warwick, Ph.D.

Dr. Kevin Warwick is Professor of Cybernetics at the University of Reading, UK where he carries out research in artificial intelligence, control and robotics. His favourite topic is pushing back the frontiers of machine intelligence. Kevin began his career by joining British Telecom with whom he spent the next 6 years. At 22 he took his first degree at Aston University followed by a Ph.D. and research post at Imperial College, London. He subsequently held positions at Oxford, Newcastle and Warwick Universities before being offered the Chair at Reading, at the age of 32. Kevin has published over 350 research papers and his paperback "In the Mind of the Machine" gives a warning of a future in which machines are more intelligent than humans. He has been awarded higher doctorates both by Imperial College and the Czech Academy of Sciences, Prague and has been described (by Gillian Anderson of the X-Files) as Britain's leading prophet of the robot age. He appears in the 1999 Guinness Book of Records for an Internet robot learning experiment. In 1998 he shocked the international scientific community by having a silicon chip transponder surgically implanted in his left arm. A series of further implant experiments is now planned in which Kevin's nervous system will be linked to a computer. This research led to him being featured in February 2000, as the cover story on the US magazine "Wired". He received the Future Health Technology 2000 Award from Future of Health Technology Institute, USA. Kevin had the honour of presenting the Year 2000 Royal Institution Christmas Lectures.

Gio Wiederhold, Ph.D.

Gio Wiederhold is a professor of Computer Science at Stanford University, with courtesy appointments in Medicine and Electrical Engineering. Since 1976 he has supervised 30 Ph.D. theses in these departments. His research focuses on the application and development of knowledge-based techniques for large-scale information systems, and their transitioning to software construction in general. Recent subtopics have been in image processing and the protection of privacy. Wiederhold has authored more than 350 published papers and reports, on computing and medicine. He has been editor-in-chief of ACM's Transactions on Database Systems, and is an associate editor of Springer Verlag's M.D.Computing. He has been on ACM's publication board, encouraging their move to electronic publications. During a three-year assignment to DARPA (1991–1994) he focused on Intelligent Integration of Information and Digital Libraries to deal with the flood of data that is becoming available over our computing networks. He on the advisory board of several institutions and consults for international as well as Silicon Valley companies. Wiederhold received a degree in Aeronautical Engineering in Holland in 1957 and a Ph.D. in Medical Information Science from the University of California at San Francisco in 1976. He has been elected fellow of the ACMI, the IEEE and the ACM.

Meg Wilson, M.S.

Meg Wilson is currently teaching in IC^2's Science and Technology Commercialization Executive M.S. program at the University of Texas at Austin, and has since its inception in 1996. Wilson was Vice President for Business Development at MCC, the Austin-based research consortia, and while there, helped MCC create a companion consortium, the Healthcare Open Systems and Trials consortium (HOST) and served on its board on behalf of MCC, to accelerate the implementation of computer based patent record and related healthcare information systems. Wilson coordinated the Center for Technology Development and Transfer at UT Austin, commercializing research from Texas universities and worked in the Texas Governor's Office for 6 years, most notably as Governor White's Science and Technology Coordinator. She is currently president-elect of the Technology Transfer Society and also has served on the board of Project Bluebonnet, a Texas telecommunications research and education organization for 10 years and has been its president since 1995.

Jean Wooldridge, M.P.H.

Jean A. Wooldridge, M.P.H., is Strategic Advisor for Cancer Communication Technologies, Office of the Director, Division of Cancer Control and Population Sciences, National Cancer Institute, Bethesda, MD. She is on loan from the Cancer Prevention Research Program of the Fred Hutchinson Cancer Research Center, Seattle. She is Principal, St. Cloud Communications, whose mission is to link communities of shared imagination and practice for ensuring cross-sector dialogue supporting consumer e-health.

Author Index

572 020000 048572